DATE DUE

MAR 2 3 2006	
JUL 0 5 2006	
MAR 2 4 2011	

Revision Total
Knee Arthroplasty

Revision Total Knee Arthroplasty

James V. Bono, MD

*Associate Clinical Professor, Department of Orthopaedic Surgery,
Tufts University School of Medicine; Attending Orthopaedic Surgeon,
New England Baptist Hospital, Boston, Massachusetts*

Richard D. Scott, MD

*Professor of Orthopaedic Surgery, Harvard Medical School;
Chief, Joint Arthroplasty Service, New England Baptist and Brigham
and Women's Hospitals, Boston, Massachusetts*

Editors

Forewords by Chitranjan S. Ranawat, MD,
and Roderick H. Turner, MD

With 275 Illustrations in 365 Parts, 82 in Full Color

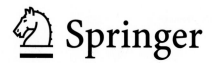

James V. Bono, MD
Associate Clinical Professor
Department of Orthopaedic Surgery
Tufts University School of Medicine
and
Attending Orthopaedic Surgeon
New England Baptist Hospital
Boston, MA 02120
USA

Richard D. Scott, MD
Professor of Orthopaedic Surgery
Harvard Medical School
and
Chief
Joint Arthroplasty Service
New England Baptist and Brigham and
  Women's Hospitals
Boston, MA 02120
USA

Library of Congress Cataloging-in-Publication Data
Revision total knee arthroplasty / James V. Bono, Richard D. Scott, editors ; forewords by
  Chitranjan S. Ranawat and Roderick H. Turner.
       p. ; cm.
    Includes bibliographical references and index.
    ISBN 0-387-22352-5 (alk. paper)
     1. Total knee replacement—Reoperation. I. Bono, James V. II. Scott, Richard D.
(Richard David), 1943–
    [DNLM: 1. Arthroplasty, Replacement, Knee. 2. Knee–surgery. 3. Reoperation. WE
870 R45481 2005]
    RD561.R4923 2005
    617.5′820592—dc22   2004058912

ISBN 0-387-22352-5   Printed on acid-free paper.

Printed in China.   (BS/EVB)

9 8 7 6 5 4 3 2 1   SPIN 10938447

springeronline.com

To my wife, Meg
To my children, Andrew, Olivia, Caroline, and Thomas
To my father for his guidance and inspiration
To Rod Turner for his pioneering work in revision
surgery
JVB

To my wife, Mary
To my sons, Jordan and Andrew
To our residents and fellows through the years
RDS

FOREWORD I

Revision Total Knee Arthroplasty, edited by Drs. James V. Bono and Richard D. Scott, is a comprehensive review of revision arthroplasty. The book includes discussions on all aspects of this technically challenging surgery, including detailed surgical techniques, exposure issues, allographs, custom implants, alignment, and TKA after other failed procedures. Invaluable pointers on technique, the authors' personal experience, useful illustrations, and an in-depth review of published literature further enhance the value of this wide-ranging text. This volume is indispensible to any surgeon who performs knee arthroplasty, including surgeons in practice, fellows, and senior residents.

This book is especially useful as a compendium of the editors' personal philosophy, which has been tested and forged by many years of concentrated practice. I hope all total knee surgeons will partake of the wisdom that these surgeons have so willingly and capably dispensed in this book.

Chitranjan S. Ranawat, MD
Chairman, Department of Orthopedics
Lenox Hill Hospital

FOREWORD II

As senior editor of this excellent treatise on complicated knee surgery, Dr. Richard D. Scott brings three decades of experience in arthroplasty surgery to focus sharply on the title subject. Dr. Scott serves as Chief of the Implant Service at the two of the busiest orthopedic implant services in the nation: New England Baptist Hospital and Brigham and Women's Hospital. He is a proven educator at all levels: medical student, resident, fellow, and postgraduate.

In addition to lectures and surgical demonstrations in over a dozen different countries, Dr. Scott has authored more than 200 scientific publications. These publications include 35 book chapters in well-established orthopedic texts.

Working primarily with Dr. Thomas Thornhill, Dick Scott has designed entire implant systems for primary and revision knee arthroplasty. These designers have made many innovations, such as the use of modular tibial wedges for bone deficiency. They also have designed a total hip replacement system.

Working with Drs. Insall, Dorr, and W.N. Scott, Dick Scott designed and published the Knee Society Clinical Rating System, which is universally accepted as the gold standard knee rating system.

To enumerate Dr. Scott's lectureships and professional presentations for any given year would take several pages. A legion of postgraduate fellows from the United States and elsewhere have come to study with him at both the Brigham and Baptist Hospitals.

Perhaps most important of all is the high regard which Dr. Scott's peers have for his judgment and technical ability. Many physicians, including a number of orthopedic surgeons, have sought out Dr. Scott when they needed major joint replacement. He is truly a surgeon's surgeon.

Dr. James V. Bono is some 18 years younger than Dr. Scott, but his career is following a similar pattern to that of the senior author. His list of publications, chapters, and presentations would number well over 150. He was a pioneer, over a decade ago, in the use of computer graphics in medical presentations and digital templating in joint replacement surgery. These presentations by Dr. Bono are made with skill, clarity, and always come across with strong visual impact.

Jim Bono was the lead author of a text entitled *Revision Total Hip Arthroplasty* with Drs. McCarthy, Bierbaum, Thornhill, and myself.

I have read the current volume *Revision Total Knee Arthroplasty* in its entirety and have found it to be thorough, accurate, readable, and very helpful. I congratulate the skillful co-editors and all of the contributors for putting together a classical and excellent orthopedic text.

Roderick H. Turner, MD
Clinical Professor, Orthopaedic Surgery
Tufts University School of Medicine
Honorary Trustee
New England Baptist Hospital

PREFACE

Revision Total Knee Arthroplasty was proposed as a "how-to" text for the diagnosis and management of the failed total knee arthroplasty, with step-by-step descriptions of surgical techniques of revision total knee arthroplasty. The text was intended to be a practical reference for students, residents, fellows, and attending surgeons engaged in the treatment and follow-up of patients who have undergone knee replacement surgery.

In Part I, the need for reoperation after total knee arthroplasty is summarized from the prospective of one surgeon's practice and brings to light Dr. Scott's vast experience in total knee arthroplasty. This is complemented nicely by Dr. Thornhill's chapter on the painful total knee arthroplasty, where it is emphasized that the etiology of the patient's pain must be elucidated prior to embarking on revision surgery. Part I also includes the definitive treatise on ultra-high molecular weight polyethylene in knee arthroplasty as well as a compendium of the radiological evaluation of the failed total knee arthroplasty.

Part II emphasizes general principles of revision surgery, including management of skin, surgical exposure, and removal of femoral and tibial implants at the time of revision. The fundamental aspects of revision total knee arthroplasty, alignment, management of bone defects, and use of constrained implants are discussed in the ensuing chapters. Management of the extensor mechanism is included as a separate entity.

Part III draws attention to the wide dimension of complicating issues that frequently occur in revision knee surgery. These chapters address the topics of infection, periprosthetic fracture, and stiffness and discuss the complexities of total knee arthroplasty after failed high tibial osteotomy, after fractures about the knee, and after prior unicompartmental and hinged knee replacement. The topics of insert exchange, aseptic synovitis, and the economics of revision total knee arthroplasty are discussed individually. The final chapter discusses the role of arthrodesis as a salvage procedure.

We feel fortunate to have received the support of so many well-known master surgeons who have contributed to the text. We are grateful to all of them and are honored to have been able to present their combined experience in the ensuing pages.

We are especially grateful to Dr. Ranawat for writing the foreword and acknowledge the profound personal impact he has had on our understanding of joint replacement surgery through his commitment to patient care, teaching, and musculoskeletal research.

James V. Bono, MD
Richard D. Scott, MD

CONTENTS

CONTRIBUTORS

Michael E. Ayers, MD, Partner, South Shore Orthopedic Associates, South Weymouth, MA 02190, USA.

Nigel M. Azer, MD, Surgeon-in-Chief, Washington Orthopaedic Center for Orthopaedic Subspecialists, Washington, DC 20037, USA.

William P. Barrett, MD, Director, Center for Joint Replacement, Proliance Surgeons, Renton, WA 98055, USA.

Burak Beksaç, MD, Attending Surgeon, Department of Orthopaedics and Traumatology, SSK Göztepe Education Hospital, Istanbul 81070, Turkey.

Daniel J. Berry, MD, Professor, Department of Orthopedics, Mayo Clinic College of Medicine; Consultant, Department of Orthopedic Surgery, Mayo Clinic, Rochester, MN 55905, USA.

James V. Bono, MD, Associate Clinical Professor, Department of Orthopaedic Surgery, Tufts University School of Medicine; Attending Orthopaedic Surgeon, New England Baptist Hospital, Boston, MA 02120, USA.

Peter P. Chiang, MD, Fellow in Adult Reconstruction, Department of Orthopaedic Surgery, Massachusetts General Hospital, ACC 537, Boston, MA 02114, USA.

Michael J. Christie, MD, Associate Clinical Professor, Department of Orthopaedic Surgery, Vanderbilt University Medical Center; Director, Southern Joint Replacement Institute, Nashville, TN 37203, USA.

David K. DeBoer, MD, Assistant Clinical Professor, Department of Orthopaedic Surgery, Vanderbilt Medical Center; Chief, Department of Orthopaedics, Baptist Hospital; Southern Joint Replacement Institute, Nashville, TN 37203, USA.

Carl Deirmengian, MD, Orthopaedic Resident, Department of Orthopaedic Surgery, Pennsylvania Hospital, Philadelphia, PA 19107, USA.

Douglas A. Dennis, MD, Adjunct Professor, Department of Biomedical Engineering, University of Tennessee; Colorado Joint Replacement, Denver, CO 80222, USA.

Rahul V. Deshmukh, MD, Instructor in Orthopaedic Surgery, Harvard Combined Orthopaedic Surgery Program, Boston; Department of Orthopaedic Surgery, New England Baptist Hospital, Boston, MA 02114, USA.

Michael C. Dixon, MBBS, FRACS, Attending Surgeon, Department of Orthopaedics, Harvard Medical School, Boston, MA 02115, USA.

Gerard A. Engh, MD, Director, Knee Research, Anderson Orthopaedic Research Institute, Alexandria, VA 22306, USA.

Thomas K. Fehring, MD, Charlotte Hip and Knee Center, Charlotte Orthopedic Specialists, Charlotte, NC 28207, USA.

David A. Feiock, MD, Fellow, Musculoskeletal Imaging, Department of Radiology, New England Baptist Hospital, Boston, MA 02120, USA.

Wolfgang Fitz, MD, Instructor, Department of Orthopaedic Surgery, Harvard Medical School, Brigham and Women's Hospital, MA 02115, USA.

xvii

Andrew A. Freiberg, MD, Associate Professor, Department of Orthopaedics, Harvard Medical School; Department of Orthopaedic Surgery, Massachusetts General Hospital, Boston, MA 02114, USA.

Reuben Gobezie, MD, Clinical Fellow, Department of Orthopaedic Surgery, Massachusetts General Hospital and Brigham and Women's Hospital, Boston, MA 02115, USA.

A. Seth Greenwald, DPhil (Oxon), Orthopaedic Research Laboratories, Lutheran Hospital, Cleveland Clinic Health System, Cleveland, OH 44113, USA.

William L. Healy, MD, Chairman, Department of Orthopaedic Surgery, Lahey Clinic, Burlington, MA 01805, USA.

Christine S. Heim, BSc, Orthopaedic Research Laboratories, Lutheran Hospital, Cleveland Clinic Health System, Cleveland, OH 44113, USA.

Ginger E. Holt, MD, Assistant Professor, Department of Orthopaedics, Vanderbilt University Medical Center, Nashville, TN 37232-2550, USA.

James Huddleston, MD, Clinical Fellow, Department of Orthopaedic Surgery, Massachusetts General Hospital, Boston, MA 02114, USA.

Richard Iorio, MD, Assistant Professor, Boston University School of Medicine; Department of Orthopaedic Surgery, Lahey Clinic, Burlington, MA 01805, USA.

Richard S. Laskin, MD, Professor, Clinical Orthopaedic Surgery, Weill Medical College of Cornell University; Co-chief, Knee Service, Attending Orthopaedic Surgeon, Department of Orthopaedics, Hospital for Special Surgery, New York, NY 10021, USA.

Jess H. Lonner, MD, Attending Orthopaedic Surgeon, Pennsylvania Hospital; Booth Bartolozzi Balderston Orthopaedics; Director, Orthopaedic Research, Pennsylvania Hospital, Philadelphia, PA 19107, USA.

David W. Manning, MD, Assistant Professor of Surgery, Department of Surgery and Division of Orthopaedics, University of Chicago, Chicago, IL 60637, USA.

J. Bohannon Mason, MD, Chief, Department of Orthopedics, Presbyterian Orthopedic Hospital; Charlotte Hip and Knee Center, Charlotte Orthopedic Specialists, Charlotte, NC 28207, USA.

Brian McDermott, MD, Fredericksburg Orthopaedic Associates, Fredericksburg, VA 22401, USA.

Samir Mehta, MD, Orthopaedic Resident, Department of Orthopaedic Surgery, Pennsylvania Hospital, Philadelphia, PA 19107, USA.

J. Craig Morrison, MD, Attending Surgeon, Southern Joint Replacement Institute, Nashville, TN 37203, USA.

Arthur H. Newberg, MD, Professor of Radiology and Orthopaedics, Tufts University School of Medicine; Department of Radiology, New England Baptist Hospital, Boston, MA 02120, USA.

Joel S. Newman, MD, Associate Clinical Professor, Department of Radiology, Tufts University School of Medicine; Associate Chairman, Department of Radiology, New England Baptist Hospital, Boston, MA 02120, USA.

Donald T. Reilly, MD, PhD, Attending Surgeon, Department of Orthopedics, New England Baptist Hospital, Boston, MA 02215, USA.

Harry Rubash, MD, Chief of Orthopaedics and Edith M. Ashley Professor, Department of Orthopaedics, Massachusetts General Hospital, Boston, MA 02120, USA.

Richard D. Scott, MD, Professor of Orthopaedic Surgery, Harvard Medical School; Chief, Joint Arthroplasty Service, New England Baptist and Brigham and Women's Hospitals, Boston, MA 02120, USA.

Van P. Stamos, MD, Attending Orthopaedic Surgeon, Department of Orthopaedic Surgery, Illinois Bone and Joint Institute, Glenview, IL 60025, USA.

Thomas S. Thornhill, MD, Head, Department of Orthopaedic Surgery, Brigham and Women's Hospital, Boston, MA 02115, USA.

William L. Walter, MB, BS, Sidney Northside Hip and Knee Surgeons, Waverton, NSW 2060, Australia.

Steven R. Wardell, MD, Director, Joint Replacement Services, Parkview Musculoskeletal Institute, Palos Heights, IL 60463, USA.

Russell E. Windsor, MD, Professor, Department of Orthopaedic Surgery, Weill Medical College of Cornell University; Co-chief, Knee Service, Hospital for Special Surgery, New York, NY 10021, USA.

PART I

Diagnosis and Evaluation

CHAPTER 1

Reoperation After Total Knee Arthroplasty

Richard D. Scott

The specific incidence and causes for reoperation after total knee arthroplasty continue to change with time. In the early experience with hinge and condylar knees, reoperations were most frequently required for prosthetic loosening, knee instability, and sepsis. Fifteen to 20 years ago, patellofemoral complications accounted for up to 50% of reoperations.[1] With improved prosthetic designs and better surgical technique, reoperations are becoming less frequent. Polyethylene wear is now the leading cause for reoperation, while prosthetic loosening, instability, and patellofemoral problems are rare.

In this chapter, the incidence and causes of reoperation after 2000 consecutive posterior cruciate retaining primary total knee arthroplasties followed for a mean of 11 years are discussed. Some of the incidence and causes will obviously be prosthesis specific. Nevertheless, this large consecutive series by one surgeon gives an overview of the complications most likely to be seen today in any surgeon's arthroplasty practice.

FEMORAL COMPONENT LOOSENING

In the early experience with these 2000 consecutive knees, hybrid fixation was popular.[2] Seven hundred eighty-six of the femoral components were implanted without cement, while 1214 were cemented. Among the cementless components, only one had clinically loosened. This patient had a dysplastic femur with an additional 5-degree valgus bow that was not visible on her short x-rays (See Figure 1-1A, B).

Her mechanical axis, therefore, was in 5 degrees more valgus than was apparent on a short film. Over a 4-year period, the femoral component loosened and subsided into valgus. She required revision with a long-stem femoral component inserted in 5 degrees of varus to counteract her metaphyseal deformity (Figure 1-2A, B). Ironically, her opposite knee was one of the 2 loose cemented components among the series and required the same treatment with a varus long stem. While the cementless femur failed at 4 years, the cemented femur loosened at 15 years. This time difference could be coincidental, but could reflect the probability that cemented femoral fixation is more forgiving to adverse forces across the fixation interface than a cementless component.

FRACTURED FEMORAL COMPONENTS

An interesting complication seen in this early series of cementless femoral components is the occurrence of stress fracture of one metal condyle. Although this problem is somewhat prosthesis specific, it has been reported in other designs.[3] There were 7 such cases among the 786 cementless porous coated components. All but one occurred in active men weighing between 90 and 140kg, and involved the larger component sizes. All fractures occurred in otherwise well-fixed components at the junction between the distal medial condyle and the posterior medial chamfer (Figure 1-2), except the one female patient who had a fracture at the anterior medial chamfer. All presented with accelerated medial polyethylene wear due to the abrasion from the rough edge of the fracture line. The fracture was missed preoperatively in most cases and only apparent in retrospect on some lateral roentgenograms.

Examination of all 7 retrieved components showed that the stress fracture was initiated at the porous surface on the inside of the component. This would imply that the force causing the fracture was one of expansion of the posterior condyle away from the trochlear flange as the

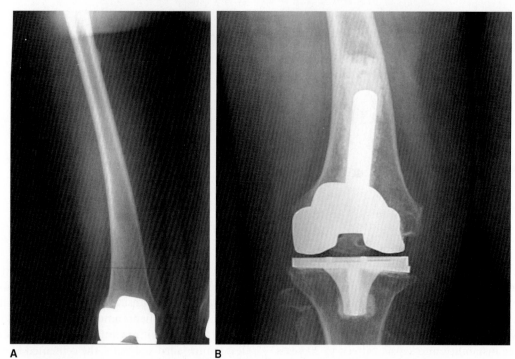

A   **B**

FIGURE 1-1. (A) A femoral shaft with a significant valgus metaphyseal bow not visible on standard short roentgenograms. The femoral component failed by subsiding into increased valgus. (B) Salvage at revision by the use of a 5-degree varus stem to offset the 10-degree valgus femoral shaft deformity.

FIGURE 1-2. (A and B) A fractured femoral component.

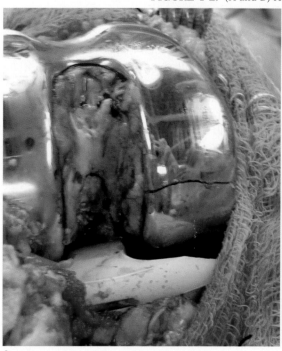
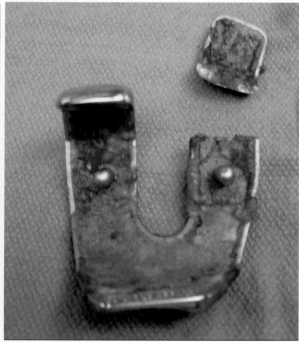

A   **B**

bone was loaded. This is in contrast to a compression force on the posterior condyle implicated in femoral component loosening that might occur as a patient ascends a stair or gets up from a chair.[4] No fractures were seen in cemented components. Subsequently, the femoral component used in this series was redesigned and reinforced at the chamfers, and no fractures have been seen since that time.

TIBIAL COMPONENT LOOSENING

Tibial component loosening (among cemented components) is also infrequent. Among the 2000 consecutive knees, cementless tibias were implanted in only 38 knees or approximately 2% of patients and never with ancillary screw fixation. Among these 38 knees, 3 loosened for an incidence of 8%. Eighty-seven knees were implanted with the so-called hybrid technique. In these knees the plateau was cemented but the tibial keel was not. One of these 87 knees loosened. Hybrid tibial fixation was initially attractive as a bone-sparing technique. There has been only one tibial loosening, however, among the 1875 fully cemented tibias, and several long-term follow-up studies have shown an increased incidence of tibial radiolucent lines or loosening with the "hybrid" technique.[5] Most surgeons now fully cement all tibial components.

Advocates of cementless tibial fixation prefer and succeed with ancillary screw fixation. There are long-term concerns with this technique, however, in regard to potential screw migration, as the tibial tray normally undergoes some long-term subsidence. This would allow well-fixed screws to begin to penetrate into the undersurface of the polyethylene, and the screw holes in the tray would allow ingress of wear debris into the bone with subsequent osteolysis. Examples of both of these complications have been described in the literature.[6]

METAL-BACKED PATELLA

When tibial components adopted metal-backing in the late 1970s and early 1980s, the same rationale was used to metal-back the patella. The metal-backing would add support to the polyethylene and decrease focal forces across the fixation interface. It would also allow for the application of a porous surface for bone ingrowth, permitting cementless fixation. In the mid-1980s, failures of metal-backed patellae were reported due to accelerated polyethylene wear with early designs.[7] In retrospect, it was appreciated that the application of a metal-backing diminished the polyethylene thickness to such an extent that accelerated wear would occur, especially if the patella

tracked asymmetrically (usually with some lateral tilt). In this series, 7 of the 87 implanted metal backed patellae failed due to wear. Most surgeons now avoid metal-backed patellae except with the mobile bearing variety, which has not reported the same high incidence of failures.[8]

ALL-POLYETHYLENE PATELLAR REPLACEMENT

Since the mid-1980s, a 3-pegged, all polyethylene patellar component has become the state of the art. Among 1723 all-polyethylene patellae in this series, none have been revised for wear or patellar instability. There have been 3 traumatic fractures, but all were treated conservatively and did not require surgery.

A small number of avulsion fractures were seen that usually involved a few millimeters of the superior pole of the patella (Figure 1-3). Most often, these were incidental findings at routine follow-up. Occasionally, they were symptomatic for approximately 6 weeks, during which time the patients were advised to avoid high forces across the patellofemoral articulation, such as ascending stairs and arising from a sitting position without arm support.

FIGURE 1-3. An asymptomatic avulsion fracture of the superior pole of the patella.

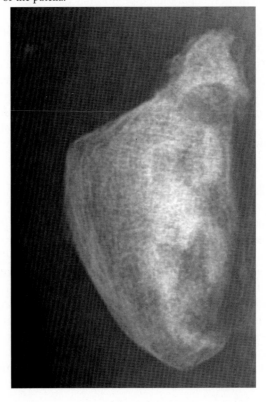

There were 4 reoperations due to patellar complications. Three of these involved shearing-off of the 3 lugs in an early design. The junction between the lug and the patellar component was reinforced, eliminating this complication. Its etiology would also involve the presence of an abnormal shearing force caused by imbalance in the quadriceps mechanism. The conformity of the articulation would tend to keep the patella located in the trochlear groove while the soft tissue imbalance would attempt to pull the patella toward the lateral side.

A third reoperation involving cemented 3-pegged, all-polyethylene patellae was a rare case of patellar loosening. This patient had undergone a lateral retinacular release, and examination of the patellar bone at reoperation showed signs of osteonecrosis, possibly contributing to the loosening.

THE UNRESURFACED PATELLA

Among the 2000 consecutive primary knee arthroplasties, 175 patellae were left unresurfaced. In this series, there were specific indications for not resurfacing the patella.[9,10] At average 15-year follow-up of these unresurfaced patients, 4 had required secondary resurfacing at 1, 5, 10, and 12 years, respectively, after initial arthroplasty. Only 2 of these 4 patients had complete relief of their pre-resurfacing pain, emphasizing the point that the unresurfaced patella invites reoperation even if it may not be the source of persistent discomfort.

Because the complications of resurfacing with a cemented 3-pegged, all-poly patella are so rare, most surgeons now consider not resurfacing only young, active, osteoarthritic male patients who fulfill specific selection criteria and only after a careful discussion with them of the pros and cons of not resurfacing. There are regional and individual exceptions to this philosophy where leaving the patella unresufaced is common.

POLYETHYLENE INSERT WEAR

Polyethylene wear has now become the most frequent cause of reoperation after total knee arthroplasty. In this series of 2000 consecutive knees at mean 11-year follow-up, wear complications have necessitated reoperation in 47 knees. This gives an incidence of 2.3% at 11 years, or slightly over 0.2% per year of follow-up. Twenty-nine of the inserts exhibited wear with synovitis and osteolysis. Eleven had insert wear with synovitis only. Seven had insert wear without symptoms. These 7 were detected at routine follow-up screening and exchanged electively within a year after their detection. In 2 cases, residual

varus alignment was corrected by the use of a custom angle bearing to modify the alignment. One bearing was angled at 3 degrees and the second at 5 degrees (Figure 1-4).

Osteolysis was extremely rare in knees implanted in the 1980s. Its incidence began to slowly climb in the early 1990s, peaked in 1995, and then subsided. The reasons for this are unclear. Multiple factors are most likely responsible, including increased top side conformity, oxidation due to gamma radiation in air, polyethylene resin changes, and other factors.

MISCELLANEOUS CAUSES FOR REOPERATION

Recurrent Hemarthrosis
Recurrent hemarthrosis is an unusual complication, with 4 cases requiring open synovectomy among these 2000 knees. An additional number of incidents of acute, late bleeding occurred that did not require surgery.[11]

Recurrent Rheumatoid Synovitis
This is also a very unusual complication, with 4 cases of documented recurrent active rheumatoid synovitis seen following a total knee arthroplasty that included resurfacing of the patella. In these cases, infection was ruled out because their presentation often simulated that of metastatic infection. Medical treatment of a rheumatoid flare can help relieve the synovitis. Occasionally, a steroid injection is appropriate. Rarely, an open synovectomy may be necessary and was curative in the 3 cases in which it was employed.

Stiffness Requiring Arthroscopic Manipulation
This specific need for reoperation comes from a desire to improve postoperative range of motion in a select group of patients who have passed the time when closed manipulation might still be effective. There were 5 such cases from among these 2000 knees. Four of the 5 patients gained and maintained sufficient flexion and/or extension following the procedure for them to consider it a success.

Laxity After Total Knee Arthroplasty
Six knees required surgical intervention due to late-onset knee instability. Three were associated with trauma and 3 developed insidiously over a period of many months. The 3 trauma cases involved falls. Two of the patients were status post patellectomy with persistent quadriceps weakness and episodes of giving way. The third patient had muscle weakness and imbalance due to a syringomyelia.

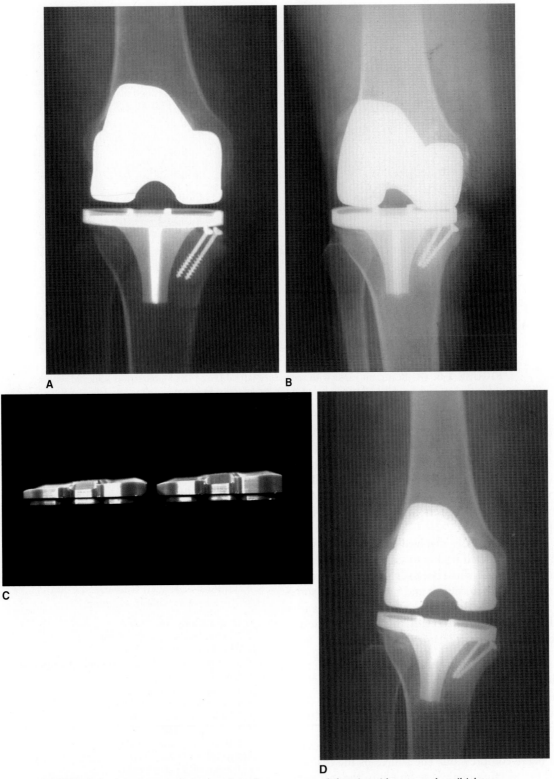

FIGURE 1-4. (A) Postoperative correction of a severe varus deformity with a cementless tibial component and bulk allograft of the deficient medial tibial plateau. (B) Asymptomatic polyethylene wear 8 years after initial surgery, with subsidence of the tibial component into varus. (C) Trial 5 degree angled bearings. (D) Postoperative correction achieved by the angled bearing insert exchange.

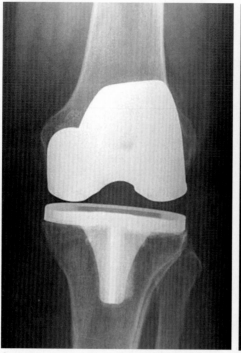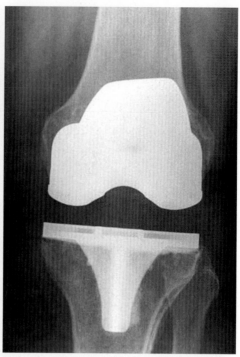

A   B

FIGURE 1-5. (A) Recurrent varus with secondary lateral laxity. (B) Stabilization achieved with a thicker insert and a medial release to balance the lax lateral side.

All 3 were treated with thicker inserts. The neurologic deficit progressed in the syringomyelia patient, and repeated falls continued until she became wheelchair bound. Thicker inserts stabilized the 2 patellectomized patients, although one required revision of the femoral component and insert to a posterior-stabilized topography.

The 3 atraumatic cases involved preoperatively varus knees that slowly drifted back into varus, associated with lateral laxity. All 3 knees had been slightly undercorrected regarding their mechanical axis and most likely had some residual lateral laxity that then progressed as the varus recurred. They were treated with thicker inserts and a medial release to improve ligament balance (Figure 1-5).

Ganglion Cysts

Two patients have required reoperation to excise a ganglion cyst that arose from the tibiofibular joint.[12] Neither cyst appeared to communicate directly with the knee joint. One of the cysts intermittently caused symptomatic peroneal nerve compression. The source of the cyst was identified by injecting methylene blue into the mass and following the dye to the tibiofibular joint. The joint was excised with a rongeur, and neither cyst had recurred at 4 and 8 years, respectively.

A third patient required excision of a popliteal cyst involving the semimembranosus bursa.

SUMMARY

In Table 1.1 are listed all the operations reported among these 2000 consecutive knees at average 11-year follow-up (range 3 to 19 years). At that point, there had been 116

TABLE 1.1. 116 Reasons for Reoperation in 2000 Knees (mean 11-year follow-up).

47 insert wear problems
    29 insert wear with lysis (most implanted in 1995)
    11 insert wear with synovitis
    7 insert wear without symptoms

- 16 metastatic infections
- 7 metal-backed patellar wear
- 7 broken femoral components
- 5 stiffness requiring arthroscopic manipulation
- 4 recurrent hemarthrosis
- 4 recurrent rheumatoid synovitis
- 4 unresurfaced patellar pain
- 3 loose cementless tibias
- 3 traumatic laxity
- 3 atraumatic lateral laxity
- 3 ganglion cysts
- 3 shear-off of patellar lugs
- 2 loose cemented femur
- 1 loose cementless femur
- 1 loose cemented tibia
- 1 loose hybrid tibia
- 1 traumatic tibial fracture
- 1 patellar loosening (associated with AVN?)

reoperations for an incidence of 5.8% at average 11 years, or approximately 0.5% per year. Insert wear was the most frequent reason, with 47 reoperations or 2.3% at 11 years. These account for 40% of the total reoperations. The next most frequent cause was a metastatic infection. Sixteen had been recorded coming from various remote sites. There were no early primary infections in this series. Other reasons for reoperation in decreasing incidence of frequency were the following: 7 cases of worn metal-backed patellae and broken femoral components; 5 cases of stiffness requiring arthroscopic manipulation; 4 cases each of recurrent hemarthrosis, recurrent rheumatoid synovitis, and unresurfaced painful patellae; and 3 cases each of loose cementless tibias, shear-off of patellar lugs, traumatic laxity, atraumatic lateral laxity, and ganglion cysts. There were 2 loose cemented femurs. There was 1 loose cementless femur, 1 loose cemented tibia, 1 loose hybrid tibia, 1 traumatic tibial fracture involving the tibial component, and 1 case of patellar loosening associated with osteonecrosis.

A review of these reasons for reoperation indicates that cemented and cementless femoral components, cemented tibial components, and cemented three-pegged, all-poly patellar components have excellent longevity. Components needing attention are metal-backed patellae, cementless tibias, and polyethylene inserts. Two of these, the metal-backed patella and the cementless tibia, are no longer used in most practices. This leaves the tibial insert polyethylene as the only significant factor needing attention. This is being addressed in a number of ways, including the increased use of mobile bearing articulations that can provide high topside conformity without constraint being imparted to the insert tray interface. Some surgeons are also making more use of nonmodular, metal-backed or all-polyethylene tibial components to eliminate the potential of backside wear. Finally, all manufacturers are pursuing improvements in the quality and fabrication of polyethylene and in modular locking mechanisms to maximize polyethylene performance.

In summary, total knee arthroplasty has a very high initial success rate. Patients can expect a successful outcome at 1 year after surgery in up to 99% of cases and the need for reoperation at a rate of approximately 1% per year over the first 15 years.

REFERENCES

1. Brick GW, Scott RD. The patellofemoral component of total knee arthroplasty. *Clin Orthop.* 1988;231:163–178.
2. Wright JR, Lima JRN, Scott RD, Thornhill TS. Two- to four-year results of posterior cruciate sparing condylar total knee arthroplasty with an uncemented femoral component. *Clin Orthop.* 1990;260:80–86.
3. Whiteside LA, Fosco DR, Brooks JG Jr. Fracture of the femoral component in cementless total knee arthroplasty. *Clin Orthop.* 1993;286:160–167.
4. King TV, Scott RD. Femoral component loosening in total knee arthroplasty. *Clin Orthop.* 1985;194:285–290.
5. Schai PA, Thornhill TS, Scott RD. Total knee arthroplasty with the PFC system. *J Bone Joint Surg.* 1998;80B:850–858.
6. Berger RA, Lyon JH, Jacobs JJ, Barden RM, Berkson EM, Shienkop MB, Rosenberg AG, Galante JO. Problems with cementless total knee arthroplasty at 11 years follow-up. *Clin Orthop.* 2001;392:196–207.
7. Bayley JC, Scott RD, Ewald FC, Holmes GB. Failure of the metal-backed patellar component after total knee replacement. *J Bone Joint Surg.* 1988;70-A:668–674.
8. Buechel FF, Rosa RA, Pappas MJ. A metal-backed rotating-bearing patella prosthesis to lower contact stress. an 11-year clinical study. *Clin Orthop.* 1989;248:34–49.
9. Levitsky KA, Harris W, McManus J, Scott RD. Total knee arthroplasty without patellar resurfacing. *Clin Orthop.* 1993;286:116–12l.
10. Kim BS, Reitman RD, Schai PA, Scott RD. Selective patellar non-resurfacing in total knee arthroplasty. *Clin Orthop.* 1999;367:81–88.
11. Kindsfater K, Scott RD. Recurrent hemarthrosis after total knee arthroplasty. *J Arthroplasty.* 1995;10(s):52–55.
12. Gibbon AJ, Wardell SR, Scott RD. Synovial cyst of the proximal tibiofibular joint with peroneal nerve compression after total knee arthroplasty. *J Arthroplasty.* 1999;14:766–768.

CHAPTER 2

Ultra-High Molecular Weight Polyethylene in Total Knee Arthroplasty

A. Seth Greenwald and Christine S. Heim

THE PROBLEM

The enduring success of the low-friction arthroplasty, advanced by Sir John Charnley as a solution for hip arthrosis, may be appreciated by the fact that in 2002 almost 700000 primary and revision hip and knee arthroplasties were performed in the United States, a number more than doubling on a global basis[1] (Table 2.1). The prevalence of aseptic loosening attributed to ultra-high molecular weight polyethylene (UHMWPE) wear debris-induced osteolysis is in the single digits in most contemporary knee series, with some reports describing prosthesis survival beyond 20 years.[2–12] Despite this obvious success, UHMWPE wear is an inescapable consequence of total joint articulation and is of contemporary concern particularly as our population grays and lifestyle demands increase.[13–22] Appreciating both the causes and remedies of *in vivo* UHMWPE failure assists the goal of avoiding total knee arthroplasty revision as an endpoint.

THE MATERIAL

The UHMWPE used in joint arthroplasty components results from polymerization of ethylene gas into a fine resin powder of submicron and micron size distribution. A number of resin mixtures exist, but GUR 1050 is the prevalent polymer used in contemporary devices. They are consolidated with the use of ram extrusion or compression-molding techniques. Structurally, UHMWPE is made up of repeating carbon-hydrogen chains that are arranged in ordered (crystalline) and disordered (amorphous) regions.[23]

Processing Shortcomings

Inadequate quality control during manufacture has resulted in fusion defects arising from incomplete polymerization, voids, and foreign body inclusions, which ultimately contribute to the *in vivo* degradation of the final part.[24–26] Previous attempts to improve UHMWPE performance have included carbon fiber reinforcement (Poly-2)[27] and polymer reprocessing by hot isostatic pressing (Hylamer).[28] The former was withdrawn from the market because of an unexpectedly high wear rate[29] (Figure 2-1), while the latter has been linked to debris-induced osteolytic response, especially when sterilized by gamma irradiation in air[30] (Figure 2-2). Heat pressing was yet another attempt to improve the finish of the articular surface, but was associated with UHMWPE fatigue and early delamination[31] (Figure 2-3). These material innovations describe checkered pasts as they moved from the laboratory to clinical application.

Sterilization Oversights

Gamma irradiation in air has, until recently, been the predominant method of UHMWPE component sterilization and, despite current concerns, represents the only gold standard against which contemporary material improvements will be measured over time. However, recent attention drawn to an increasing prevalence of tibial component failures associated with debris-induced osteolysis has raised concerns over the long-term durability of contemporary devices.[32,33] A clinical follow-up study reported by Bohl et al. suggests that this may be accounted for by the prolonged shelf storage prior to implantation of UHMWPE components gamma irradiated in air.[34] A 12% to 20% reduction in *in vivo* survival is noted for shelf storage ranging from 4 to 11 years with a mean *in vivo* time to revision of 2.5 years (Figures 2-4 and 2-5).

TABLE 2.1. Hip and Knee Arthroplasty Procedures Performed in the United States in 2002.

	Primary	Revision	Total
Knees	321 084	31 159	352 243
Hips	300 434	43 082	343 816
Total	621 518	74 241	696 059

Data from *Orthopaedic Network News.*[1]

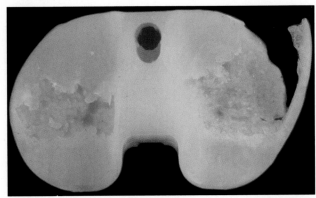

FIGURE 2-3. Six-year retrieval of a heat-pressed tibial component associated with polyethylene fatigue and early delamination.

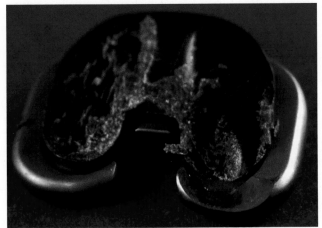

FIGURE 2-1. Five-year retrieval of a failed Poly-2 tibial insert demonstrating a high component wear rate with infiltration of carbon fibers and polyethylene debris into surrounding tissue.

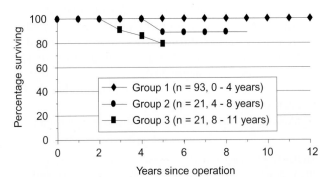

FIGURE 2-4. The influence of shelf storage on survival of a prosthetic knee plateau following gamma irradiation in air. (From Bohl, Bohl, Postak, et al.[34] by permission of *Clin Orthop.*)

FIGURE 2-5. A Group 2 plateau implanted after 7.6 years of shelf storage and retrieved 3.8 years after implantation. Gross delamination and pitting, characteristics of fatigue failure, are observed. (From Bohl, Bohl, Postak, et al.[34] by permission of *Clin Orthop.*)

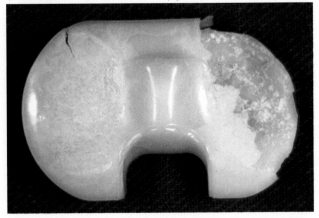

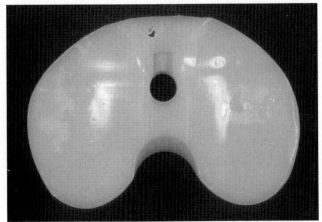

FIGURE 2-2. Three-year retrieval of a failed Hylamer-M tibial plateau demonstrating an unexpectedly high wear rate with corresponding wear and debris-induced inflammatory tissue response.

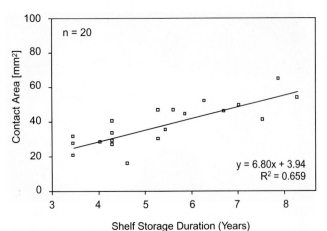

FIGURE 2-6. Tibial-femoral contact area for a 5.6-mm thick tibial plateau carrying >20 MPa stresses during articulation dramatically increases with lengthening shelf storage periods.

Further, laboratory studies indicate that as shelf storage increases, the amount of UHMWPE exposed to high surface stresses during articulation increases dramatically and is a contributing factor to early *in vivo* polymer failure[35–37] (Figure 2-6).

The explanation for these observations lies in the mechanics of the sterilization process, which facilitates breakage of polymer chains by the incoming gamma radi-

FIGURE 2-7. Depicted polymer chain breakage following irradiation in air and combination with oxygen facilitating oxidative degradation of UHMWPE.

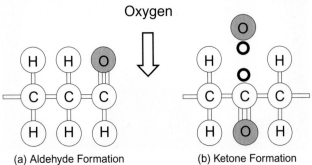

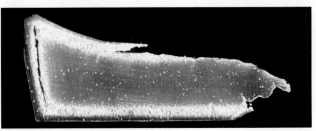

FIGURE 2-8. Three-year retrieval of a fully oxidized, gamma irradiated in air, UHMWPE tibial component demonstrating a circumferential white band indicative of polymer embrittlement after prolonged shelf life. Fusion defects from incomplete consolidation are noted.

ation, creating free radicals, which preferentially combine with available oxygen[38,39] (Figure 2-7). The onset of mass UHMWPE component production and device modularity resulted in extended component shelf storage before use. This was not a previous consideration, but ongoing shelf life oxidation offers an explanation for mechanical compromise of the polymer *in situ*[36,38,40,41] (Figure 2-8). It is also noted, in this regard, that *in vivo* component oxidation occurs, but to a lesser degree.[42]

Component Manufacturing Deficiencies

As knee designs have evolved, a growing appreciation of the avoidance of round-on-flat geometries through the ranges of knee flexion in favor of round-on-curved surfaces emerged.[32] The ability of a given design to minimize contact stresses during walking gait contributes to UHMWPE tibial component longevity. The increased tibial-femoral conformity realized in posterior cruciate ligament (PCL) sacrificing knee plateaus serves to enhance UHMWPE service life by attenuation of peak contact stresses responsible for material damage. This is appreciated in the comparison shown between PCL preserving and PCL sacrificing plateau geometries articulating against their respective, common femoral component (Figure 2-9).

The trend toward more conforming design geometries also has associated with it the expectation that femoral component tolerances be maintained during the manufacturing process. Failure to achieve this can dramatically decrease contact surfaces, elevate peak stresses, and, concurrent with articulation, is the harbinger of material damage[44] (Figure 2-10). This is of particular import with the current interest in mobile bearing knee designs, whose cited advantage is the maximization of contact surfaces during gait.[45]

Third-Body Wear

The interaction of third-body particulate between articulation surfaces in knee replacement consistently demonstrates catalysis of UHMWPE damage. Surface scratching of the metallic counterface resulting from these interactions further contributes to the wear process. Foreign

FIGURE 2-9. Contact areas by surface stress range of PCL-preserving and PCL-sacrificing tibial-femoral conformities at 0 degrees extension. The overall bar height depicts the total contact area. (From Heim, Postak, Greenwald[43] by permission of AAOS.)

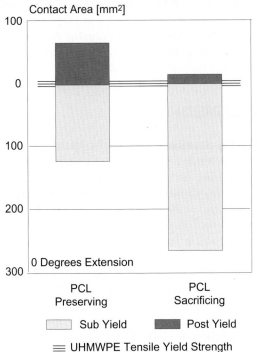

body inclusions may derive from acrylic bone cement, entrapped bone, and beads from an incomplete sintering process or hydroxyapatite (HA) particulate (Figure 2-11).

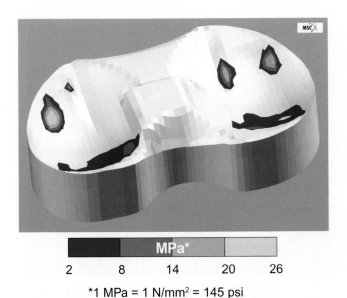

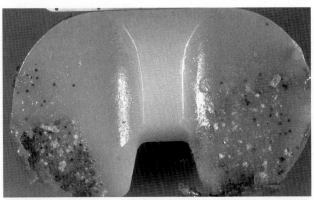

FIGURE 2-11. An early retrieval of a cementless, metal-backed tibial component demonstrating the effects of third-body entrapment. Bead embedment as well as delamination and pitting are observed in the posteromedial quadrant.

Component Design Influences

With the introduction of modularity, the interest in the all-poly tibia diminished, despite successful, long-term clinical reports.[46,47] Monoblock components were also introduced with the goal of optimizing stress transfer to the tibial bone surface.[48] Recently, attention has been drawn to the shortcomings of modular designs by the report of backside wear and an associated link to osteolysis and aseptic loosening.[49–58] Locking mechanism deficiency has been cited as a factor in allowing displacement between the insert and tibial tray to occur resulting in UHMWPE debris generation (Figure 2-12). Particulate transport to the intramedullary canal is facilitated through gaps at the locking mechanism interface as well as through screw holes when present.

Component Malalignment: A Surgical Prodrome

The forces and torques that occur during walking gait, particularly during toe-off, promote articulation in the posteromedial quadrant of tibial inserts.[59–63] Retrieved

FIGURE 2-12. Visualization of adhesive film transfer demonstrating UHMWPE insert rotatory micromotion in a modular tibial component.

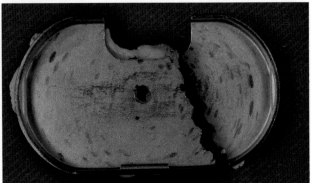

*1 MPa = 1 N/mm² = 145 psi

FIGURE 2-10. Finite element analysis of tibial-femoral contact areas and surface stresses of a contemporary mobile bearing knee design at 0 degrees extension. Poor mating of the articulating surfaces is observed resulting in peripheral contact with damaging stress levels.

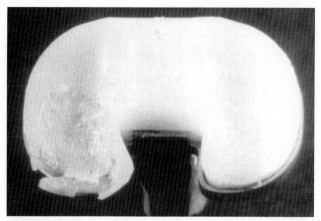

FIGURE 2-13. UHMWPE tibial component retrieval showing deformation and wear in the posteromedial portion of the insert. (From Swany, Scott,[68] by permission of *J Arthroplasty*.)

components of failed knee arthroplasties demonstrate UHMWPE damage patterns in this area[64–68] (Figure 2-13). Notwithstanding poor component design, causal factors include overloading the medial compartment, improper surgical correction or alignment of the bony structures, insufficient soft tissue balance and release, polyethylene cold flow near the edge of the tibial plateau, and surgical

malrotation of the components.[64–68] In addition, the dynamic effects of lift-off and subsequent impact loading, and unusual patient kinematics further increase the potential for posteromedial failures.[69] The influence of surgical malrotation may be appreciated in Figure 2-14A, B, which demonstrate dramatic changes in location, contact area, and peak stresses for a PCL preserving knee in laboratory investigation.[70]

THE REMEDIES

UHMWPE Sterilization Techniques

Attempts to remove oxygen from the sterilization process include the use of inert gas and vacuum environments or by avoiding gamma irradiation altogether through the use of ethylene oxide (EtO) or gas plasmas.[71–73] Acetabular components sterilized by these techniques demonstrate a reduction in UHMWPE wear in hip simulation studies (Figure 2-15).

Today, orthopedic device manufacturers avoid the use of an air environment when packaging UHMWPE components sterilized through the gamma irradiation process. Further, sterilization dates are now standard on package labeling of UHMWPE components.

FIGURE 2-14. The distribution of contact stresses at the toe-off position of walking gait for a PCL preserving design at (A) neutral rotation and (B) after the application of a 16 N-m external torque, simulating deliberate component malalignment. A dramatic increase in peak contact stresses is observed, which is contributory to component damage. (From Morra, Postak, Plaxton, et al.[70] by permission of *Clin Orthop*.)

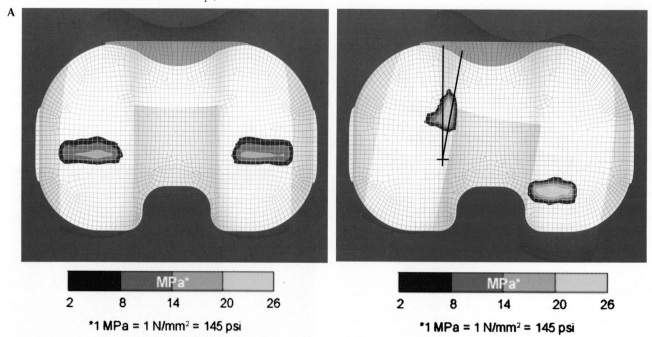

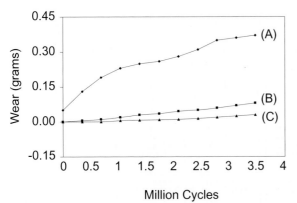

FIGURE 2-15. Hip simulator weight-loss comparison for aged (25 days at 78 degrees Celsius in O_2) compression-molded cup components: (A) gamma irradiated in air; (B) sterilized with ethylene oxide; and (C) gamma irradiated in a vacuum environment and use of barrier packaging. (From Greer, Schmidt, Hamilton,[72] by permission of *Trans Orthop Res Soc.*)

UHMWPE Processing Techniques

It is now quantitatively appreciated that increasing the gamma radiation dose above the 2.5 Mrad level used in conventional UHMWPE component sterilization, encourages free radicals to combine, creating crosslinks between the molecules of adjacent chains, which is further enhanced in an oxygen-free environment.[74–76] This graph from McKellop and coworkers is descriptive of this phenomenon in a simulator comparison of acetabular cup components (Figure 2-16). The volumetric wear per million cycles is dramatically reduced with increasing gamma radiation exposure.

There are clinical reports attributed to Oonishi and Grobbelaar, which describe *in vivo* UHMWPE wear reduction in acetabular components realized through increased crosslinking.[77–82] However, these studies employed large doses of gamma radiation (>50 Mrad), which are known to cause polymer embrittlement

FIGURE 2-16. Mean acetabular cup wear rates versus gamma dose level. (From McKellop, Shen, Lu, et al.[75] by permission of *J Orthop Res.*)

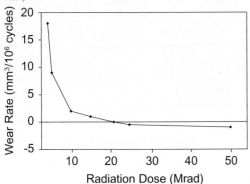

and yellowing. Wroblewski employing a chemically enhanced cross-linked polymer, achieved similar findings both *in vivo* and *in vitro*, when coupled with an Alumina articulation.[83]

In some sense these isolated studies point the way to a new class of UHMWPEs, whose common denominator is an appreciation of the importance of increased crosslinking while minimizing oxidative degradation to reduce wear. Current methods used to manufacture these moderately to highly cross-linked UHMWPEs are shown (Figure 2-17). Process differences include (1) heating above or below the melt temperature of the polyethylene, (2) the type of radiation employed, (3) the radiation dose level, and (4) the endpoint sterilization.

All have received Food and Drug Administration 510[k] clearance, allowing commercial distribution for both hip and knee components. Currently, there is a minimum of short-term clinical reports supporting the advantage of these increased cross-linked UHMWPEs for the hip[84–90] and knee.[91,92] However, impressive laboratory data have been produced, predominantly with regard to hip simulation.[93–97]

Manufacturing Optimization

The attainment of femoral component tolerances has markedly improved with the relatively recent use of computer-aided precision grinding as a standard finishing technique for metallic femoral knee components. This is particularly beneficial where small variations in surface contours have large effects on contact areas and surface stresses (Figure 2-18). The implications of this technique have potentially far-reaching consequences. As design specifications are produced with higher required tolerances, as in contemporary mobile bearing knee designs, the need for precision manufacturing is imperative (Figure 2-19).

Tibial Tray Design Improvement

Improving the capture mechanisms of UHMWPE tibial inserts is an ongoing design challenge. Minimizing insert microdisplacement over time will contribute to reduced UHMWPE debris generation. This notwithstanding, careful attention must also be paid to the tibial tray material and its surface finish. Just as polished, titanium femoral heads fell from clinical popularity as their surfaces easily scratched and wore during articulation,[98–100] modular tibial tray components should be manufactured using cobalt-chrome alloys. If, because of modular mismatch, microdisplacement is inevitable, the articulation surfaces should be optimized to reduce the potential for wear debris generation. From a design perspective, circumferential capture and the capping or avoidance of screw holes should be considered, so as to avoid potential

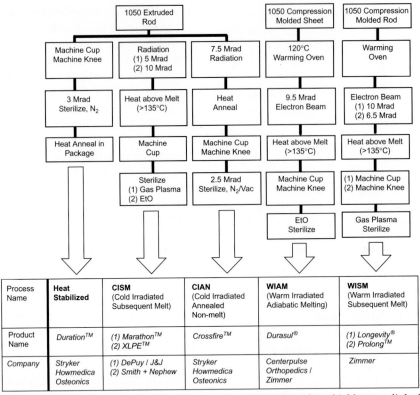

FIGURE 2-17. Current methods used to manufacture moderately to highly cross-linked UHWMPE.

FIGURE 2-19. Finite element analysis demonstrating the optimization of tibial-femoral contact areas and surface stresses resulting from quality controlled finishing of the component demonstrated earlier in Figure 2-10. It is apparent that use of the conforming geometries has been achieved with the resulting diminishment of peak contact stresses.

FIGURE 2-18. A comparison of tibial-femoral contact areas by surface stress range for belt finishing and computer-aided precision grinding techniques of a single femoral component design at 0 degrees extension. The overall bar height depicts the total contact area. (From Helm, Postak, Greenwald[43] by permission of AAOS.)

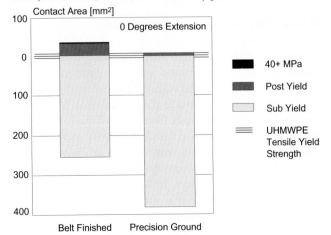

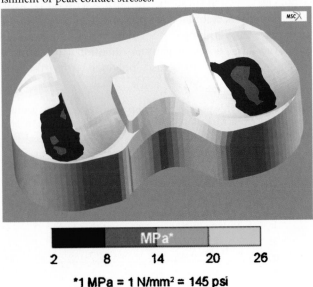

pathways for debris transport.[101–105] A further consequence of modularity is the employment of highly cross-linked UHMWPE inserts whose fracture toughness is reduced. Locking points in tray design represent foci for stress concentrators, increasing the potential for crack initiation, the propagation of which occurs more rapidly in these materials than conventional polyethylene.[106]

Surgical Optimization

The increasing emphasis on templating and the relatively recent introduction of computer-assisted navigation techniques offer the promise that component malalignment may ultimately be minimized.[107–109] Eliminating the outliers in component placement will contribute to diminishing UHMWPE material damage in knee arthroplasty. Continued improvements in instrument design go hand-in-hand with the achievement of this goal.

Patient Factors: Do They Really Matter?

Overenthusiastic patient use following total knee arthroplasty has been cited as a factor influencing failure.[110–112] Its occurrence, however, has generally been described in singular case reports in much the same way as failure attributed to obesity. Series reports do not support a relationship between increased body mass index and device failure following arthroplasty.[113–118] Surgical preference, however, weighs in favor of the lightweight patient as the ideal arthroplasty candidate.[119] However, it is known from both physical laboratory testing and finite element analysis that load magnitude in combination with displacement are factors influencing UHMWPE damage.[120–127] While a recommendation for patient weight loss before surgery may be justified from these laboratory investigations, the clinical reality of achieving this does not lie in the patient's or surgeon's favor.[128]

THE CONCERNS

Highly Cross-Linked UHMWPE Use in TKA

The proclaimed advantage of highly cross-linked UHMWPEs lies in the reduction of wear debris generation through enhanced crosslinking of the polymer chains coincident with the elimination of oxidation. However, changes in the mechanical properties of these materials, particularly in their reduced resistance to fatigue crack propagation (fracture toughness) raises concerns about their long-term suitability in hip and knee components where locking mechanisms offer foci for stress risers[106] (Figures 2-20, 2-21, and 2-22). An appreciation of the differing modes of hip (abrasion and adhesion) and knee (pitting and delamination) failure, confirmed through conventional UHMWPE component retrieval,[132–134] sug-

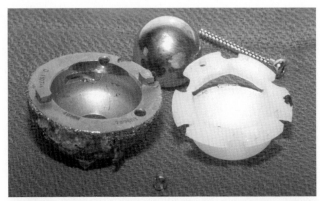

FIGURE 2-20. A 1-year conventional UHMWPE, primary acetabular liner demonstrating crack initiation and propagation. Failure initiated at a sharp edge of a locking point. (From Tradonsky, Postak, Froimson[129] by permission of *Clin Orthop.*)

gests that a universal, highly cross-linked polymer may not be appropriate.

Investigation into the means by which fracture toughness and ultimate tensile strength of these new polymers may be increased is and should be an ongoing quest, particularly if their rapid employment will lead to obsolescence of conventional UHMWPE. Its furthest hope in knee replacement application would be a reduction in the capacity for these materials to pit and delaminate or, in other words, when the knee behaves like a hip in terms of its wear process. This reality may be appreciated with designs of increasing conformity such as those found in mobile bearing knees.

FIGURE 2-21. A 10-month highly cross-linked UHMWPE, revision acetabular liner demonstrating crack initiation and propagation. The decision to retain the acetabular shell in an almost vertical and anteverted position contributed to this early failure, which was compounded by the decision to use a 40-mm femoral head and a correspondingly thin liner. (From Halley, Glassman, Crowninshield[130] by permission of *J Bone Joint Surg.*)

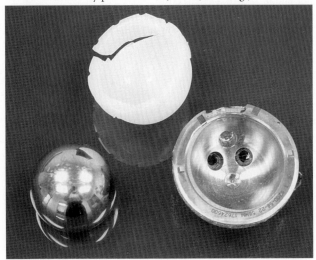

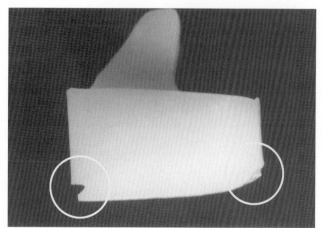

FIGURE 2-22. A 3-year failure of a constrained condylar conventional UHMWPE tibial insert. Failure of the posterior locking mechanism resulted in posterior component lift-off. (From Ries[131] by permission of *J Bone Joint Surg.*)

Particle Bioreactivity

Conventional wisdom and our experience particular to hip arthroplasty suggest that osteolytic response is associated with both particle size and debris volume. Laboratory hip simulator experiments have shown that UHMWPE particle volumes in various size ranges are dependent on radiation dose[135] (Figures 2-23 and 2-24). The greatest potential for cytokine release, the first step in the sequelae leading to osteolysis, following macrophage debris encapsulation is at the <1 micron level. Ingram et al. have suggested that highly cross-linked UHMWPE debris obtained from scratched surface articulation is bioreactive when placed in culture medium and appears to be volume dependent.[136]

The influence of surface roughness has been further investigated by Scott et al. in a hip simulator comparison

FIGURE 2-23. Comparative volumes of acetabular particle generation for different size ranges per million cycles for conventional and highly cross-linked UHMWPEs at 5 and 10 Mrads resulting from hip simulation. ECD, equivalent circular diameter. (From Ries, Scott, Jani,[135] by permission of *J Bone Joint Surg.*)

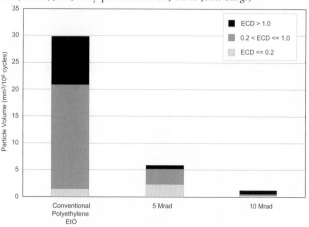

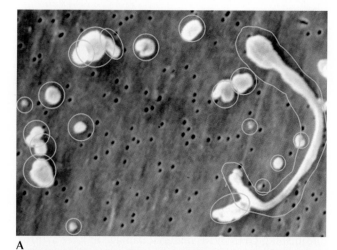

A

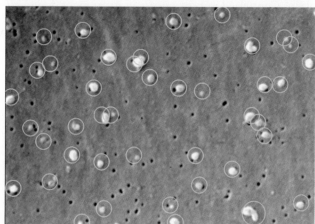

B

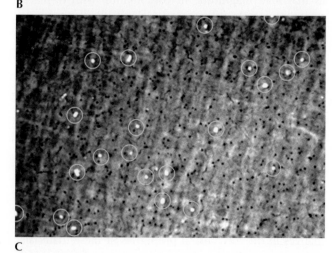

C

FIGURE 2-24. Corresponding SEM visualization (10000×) of particle distribution for (A) conventional and (B and C) highly cross-linked UHMWPEs at 5 and 10 Mrads, respectively, employing a 0.05-micron filter. The particles are highlighted for appreciation. (From Ries, Scott, Jani,[135] by permission of *J Bone Joint Surg.*)

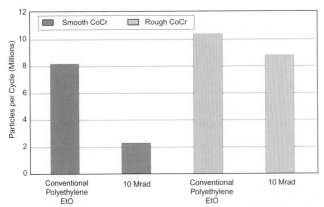

FIGURE 2-25. The influence of smooth and roughened femoral head surfaces on particle generation for conventional and highly cross-linked UHMWPE acetabular components resulting from hip simulation. (From Good, Ries, Barrack, et al.[139] by permission of *J Bone Joint Surg Am.*)

between conventional, EtO, and 10 Mrad polyethylene components.[137] As one appreciates from Figure 2-25, roughened surfaces have a negative influence on particle production where highly cross-linked polyethylenes are employed. This has been challenged most recently by Muratoglu et al. in a study in which retrieved femoral components were articulated in knee simulation against a highly cross-linked polyethylene.[138]

Alternatives to reduce the influence of surface roughness on femoral component design have recently been reported using fully oxidized zirconium surfaces. This has relevance on the long-term viability of knee articulations with conventional UHMWPE tibial inserts, but its performance is unknown with highly cross-linked materials.[139,140]

Direct-to-Consumer Marketing

Further, it is no small coincidence that almost 62% of all polyethylene acetabular components sold in the United

States today are constituted of highly cross-linked polyethylenes in their various formulations[1] (Figure 2-26). Cost as well as patient selection and the unknown clinical realities of long-term series reporting are concerns with these materials that only *in vivo* time will elucidate. The march of progress toward increasing use of these materials—in the relative absence of mid- and long-term clinical reports—portrays a rapid direct-to-consumer marketing philosophy employed by orthopedic manufacturers for both the orthopedic surgeon and the patients they serve.

THE PROMISE

The previous remarks have attempted to define problems, solutions, and unknown performance factors of both conventional and emerging highly cross-linked UHMWPE materials currently used in knee arthroplasty. What is important for the reader to appreciate is that the description of employment of highly cross-linked polymers in knee arthroplasty is an evolving experience, which will find advocacy or limitation in what is now a tandem laboratory and clinical approach. The passage of *in vivo* time, as has always been, will be the defining factor in their use.

REFERENCES

1. *Orthopaedic Network News.* 14:3, Ann Arbor, MI: Mendenhall Associates, Inc.; 2003.
2. Aglietti P, Buzzi R, De Felice R, et al. The Insall-Burstein total knee replacement in osteoarthritis: a 10-year minimum follow-up. *J Arthroplasty.* 1999;14(5):560–565.
3. Berger RA, Rosenberg AG, Barden RM, et al. Long-term followup of the Miller-Galante total knee replacement. *Clin Orthop.* 2001;388:58–67.
4. Buechel FF. Long-term followup after mobile-bearing total knee replacement. *Clin Orthop.* 2002;404:40–50.
5. Ewald FC, Wright RJ, Poss R, et al. Kinematic total knee arthroplasty: a 10- to 14-year prospective follow-up review. *J Arthroplasty.* 1999;14(4):473–480.
6. Gill GS, Joshi AB. Long-term results of cemented, posterior cruciate ligament-retaining total knee arthroplasty in osteoarthritis. *Am J Knee Surg.* 2001;14(4):209–214.
7. Gill GS, Joshi AB, Mills DM. Total condylar knee arthroplasty. 16- to 21-year results. *Clin Orthop.* 1999;367:210–215.
8. Keating EM, Meding JB, Faris PM, et al. Long-term followup of nonmodular total knee replacements. *Clin Orthop.* 2002;404:34–39.

FIGURE 2-26. Histogram illustrating the growth of highly cross-linked UHMWPE acetabular component sales in the United States. (Data from *Orthopaedic Network News.*[1])

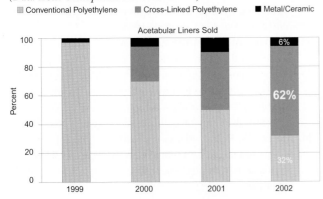

9. Kelly MA, Clarke HD. Long-term results of posterior cruciate-substituting total knee arthroplasty. *Clin Orthop.* 2002;404:51–57.

10. Pavone V, Boettner F, Fickert S, et al. Total condylar knee arthroplasty: a long-term followup. *Clin Orthop.* 2001;388:18–25.

11. Rodriguez JA, Bhende H, Ranawat CS. Total condylar knee replacement: a 20-year followup study. *Clin Orthop.* 2001;388:10–17.

12. Whiteside LA. Long-term followup of the bone-ingrowth Ortholoc knee system without a metal-backed patella. *Clin Orthop.* 2001;388:77–84.

13. Brander VA, Malhotra S, Jet J, et al. Outcome of hip and knee arthroplasty in persons aged 80 years and older. *Clin Orthop.* 1997;345:67–78.

14. Diduch DR, Insall JN, Scott WN, et al. Total knee replacement in young, active patients. *J Bone Joint Surg Am.* 1997;79(4):575–582.

15. Duffy GP, Trousdale RT, Stuart MJ. Total knee arthroplasty in patients 55 years old or younger. 10- to 17-year results. *Clin Orthop.* 1998;356:22–27.

16. Gill GS, Joshi AB. Total knee arthroplasty in the young. *J Arthroplasty.* 2004;19(2):255.

17. Hilton AI, Back DL, Espag MP, et al. The octogenarian total knee arthroplasty. *Orthopedics.* 2004;27(1):37–39.

18. Hofmann AA, Heithoff SM, Camargo M. Cementless total knee arthroplasty in patients 50 years or younger. *Clin Orthop.* 2002;404:102–107.

19. Joshi AB, Markovic L, Gill GS. Knee arthroplasty in octogenarians: results at 10 years. *J Arthroplasty.* 2003;18(3):295–298.

20. Laskin RS. Total knee replacement in patients older than 85 years. *Clin Orthop.* 1999;367:43–49.

21. Pagnano MW, Levy BA, Berry DJ. Cemented all polyethylene tibial components in patients age 75 years and older. *Clin Orthop.* 1999;367:73–80.

22. Tankersley WS, Hungerford DS. Total knee arthroplasty in the very aged. *Clin Orthop.* 1995;316:45–49.

23. Li S, Burstein AH. Ultra-high molecular weight polyethylene. the material and its use in total joint implants. *J Bone Joint Surg Am.* 1994;76(7):1080–1090.

24. Tanner MG, Whiteside LA, White SE. Effect of polyethylene quality on wear in total knee arthroplasty. *Clin Orthop.* 1995;317:83–88.

25. Won CH, Rohatgi S, Kraay MJ, et al. Effect of resin type and manufacturing method on wear of polyethylene tibial components. *Clin Orthop.* 2000;376:161–171.

26. Wrona M, Mayor MB, Collier JP, et al. The correlation between fusion defects and damage in tibial polyethylene bearings. *Clin Orthop.* 1994;299:92–103.

27. Sclippa E, Piekarski K. Carbon fiber reinforced polyethylene for possible orthopedic uses. *J Biomed Mater Res.* 1973;7:59–70.

28. Champion AR, Li S, Saum K, et al. The effect of crystallinity on the physical properties of UHMWPE. *Trans Orthop Res Soc.* 1994;19:585.

29. Busanelli L, Squarzoni S, Brizio L, et al. Wear in carbon fiber-reinforced polyethylene (poly-two) knee prostheses. *Chir Organi Mov.* 1996;81(3):263–267.

30. Collier JP, Bargmann LS, Currier BH, et al. An analysis of hylamer and polyethylene bearings from retrieved acetabular components. *Orthopedics.* 1998;21(8):865–871.

31. Wright TM, Rimnac CM, Stulberg SD, et al. Wear of polyethylene in total joint replacements. Observations from retrieved PCA knee implants. *Clin Orthop.* 1992;276:126–134.

32. Collier JP, Mayor MB, McNamara JL, et al. Analysis of the failure of 122 polyethylene inserts from uncemented tibial knee components. *Clin Orthop.* 1991;273:232–242.

33. Peters PC, Engh GA, Dwyer KA, et al. Osteolysis after total knee arthroplasty without cement. *J Bone Joint Surg Am.* 1992;74:864–876.

34. Bohl JR, Bohl WR, Postak PD, et al. The effects of shelf life on clinical outcome for gamma sterilized polyethylene tibial components. *Clin Orthop.* 1999;267:28–38.

35. Collier JP, Sperling DK, Currier JH, et al. Impact of gamma sterilization on clinical performance of polyethylene in the knee. *J Arthroplasty.* 1996;11:377–389.

36. Currier BH, Currier JH, Collier JP, et al. Shelf life and in vivo duration: impacts on performance of tibial bearings. *Clin Orthop.* 1997;342:111–122.

37. Heim CS, Postak PD, Greenwald AS. The influence of shelf storage duration on gamma irradiated UHMWPE tibial components. *Orthop Trans.* 1998–9;22:149–150.

38. Collier JP, Sutula LC, Currier BH, et al. Overview of polyethylene as a bearing material: Comparison of sterilization methods. *Clin Orthop.* 1996;333:76–86.

39. Nusbaum HJ, Rose RM. The effects of radiation sterilization on the properties of ultrahigh molecular weight polyethylene. *J Biomed Mater Res.* 1979;13:557–576.

40. Ries MD, Weaver K, Rose RM, et al. Fatigue strength of polyethylene after sterilization by gamma irradiation or ethylene oxide. *Clin Orthop.* 1996;333:87–95.

41. Rimnac CM, Klein RW, Betts F, et al. Post-irradiation ageing of ultra-high molecular weight polyethylene. *J Bone Joint Surg Am.* 1994;76:1052–1056.

42. Leibovitz BE, Siegel BV: Aspects of free radical reactions in biological systems: aging. *J Gerontol.* 1980;35: 45–56.

43. Helm CS, Postak PD, Greenwald AS. Factors Influencing the longevity of UHMWPE tibial components. In: Pritchard D, ed. *Instructional Course Lectures*, Vol. 45. Chicago, IL; American Academy of Orthopaedic Surgeons, 1996.

44. Morra EA, Postak PD, Greenwald AS. The influence of mobile bearing knee geometry on the wear of UHMWPE tibial inserts: a finite element study. *Orthop Trans.* 1998–9;22(1):148.

45. Buechel FF, Pappas MJ. The New Jersey low-contact-stress knee replacement system: a biomechanical rationale and review of the first 123 cemented cases. *Arch Orthop Trauma Surg.* 1986;105(4):197–204.

46. Brassard MF, Insall JN, Scuderi GR, et al. Does modularity affect clinical success? a comparison with a minimum 10-year follow-up. *Clin Orthop.* 2001;388:26–32.

47. Rodriguez JA, Baez N, Rasquinha V, et al. Metal-backed and all-polyethylene tibial components in total knee replacement. *Clin Orthop.* 2001;392:174–183.

48. Ritter MA, Worland R, Saliski J, et al. Flat-on-flat, non-constrained, compression molded polyethylene total knee replacement. *Clin Orthop.* 1995;321:79–85.

49. Chapman-Sheath P, Cain S, Bruce WJ, et al. Surface roughness of the proximal and distal bearing surface of mobile bearing total knee prostheses. *J Arthroplasty.* 2002;17(6):713–717.

50. Conditt MA, Stein JA, Noble PC. Factors affecting the severity of backside wear of modular tibial inserts. *J Bone Joint Surg Am.* 2004;86(2):305–311.

51. Cuckler JM, Lemons J, Tamarapalli JR, et al. Polyethylene damage on the nonarticular surface of modular total knee prostheses. *Clin Orthop.* 2003;410:248–253.

52. Engh GA, Lounici S, Rao AR, et al. In vivo deterioration of tibial baseplate locking mechanisms in contemporary modular total knee components. *J Bone Joint Surg Am.* 2001;83(11):1660–1665.

53. Li S, Scuderi G, Furman BD, et al. Assessment of backside wear from the analysis of 55 retrieved tibial inserts. *Clin Orthop.* 2002;404:75–82.

54. Parks NL, Engh GA, Topoleski T, et al. Modular tibial insert micromotion: a concern with contemporary knee implants. *Clin Orthop.* 1998;356:10–15.

55. Rao AR, Engh GA, Collier MB, et al. Tibial interface wear in retrieved total knee components and correlations with modular insert motion. *J Bone Joint Surg Am.* 2002; 84(10):1849–1855.

56. Surace MF, Berzins A, Urban RM, et al. Backsurface wear and deformation in polyethylene tibial inserts retrieved postmortem. *Clin Orthop.* 2002;404:14–23.

57. Wasielewski RC, Parks N, Williams I, et al. Tibial insert undersurface as a contributing source of polyethylene wear debris. *Clin Orthop.* 1997;345:53–59.

58. Wasielewski RC. The causes of insert backside wear in total knee arthroplasty. *Clin Orthop.* 2002;404:232–246.

59. Apkarian J, Naumann S, Cairns B. A three-dimensional kinematic and dynamic model of the lower limb. *J Biomech.* 1989;22:143–155.

60. LaFortune MA, Cavanaugh PR, Sommer HJ, et al. Three-dimensional kinematics of the human knee during walking. *J Biomech.* 1992;25:347–357.

61. Morrison JB. Function of the knee joint in various activities. *Biomed Eng.* 1969;4:573–580.

62. Murray MP, Drought AB, Kory RC. Walking patterns in normal men. *J Bone Joint Surg Am.* 1964;46:335–360.

63. Paul JP. Forces transmitted by joints in the human body. *Proc Inst Mech Eng.* 1967;181:358.

64. Cameron HU. Tibial component wear in total knee replacement. *Clin Orthop.* 1994;309:29–32.

65. Eckhoff DG, Metzger RG, Vedewalle MV. Malrotation associated with implant alignment technique in total knee arthroplasty. *Clin Orthop.* 1995;321:28–31.

66. Fehring TK. Rotational malalignment of the femoral component in total knee arthroplasty. *Clin Orthop.* 2000;380:72–79.

67. Lewis P, Rorabeck CH, Bourne RB, et al. Posteromedial tibial polyethylene failure in total knee replacements. *Clin Orthop.* 1994;299:11–17.

68. Swany MR, Scott RD. Posterior polyethylene wear in posterior cruciate ligament-retaining total knee arthroplasty: a case study. *J Arthroplasty.* 1993;8:439–846.

69. Dennis DA, Komistek RD, Cheal EJ, et al. In vivo femoral condylar lift-off in total knee arthroplasty. *Orthop Trans.* 1997;21:1112.

70. Morra EA, Postak PD, Plaxton NA, et al. The effects of external torque on polyethylene tibial insert damage patterns. *Clin Orthop.* 2003;410:90–100.

71. Fisher J, Reeves EA, Isaac GH, et al. Comparison of aged and non-aged ultrahigh molecular weight polyethylene sterilized by gamma irradiation and by gas plasma. *J Mater Sci Mater Med.* 1997;8:375–378.

72. Greer KW, Schmidt MB, Hamilton JV. The hip simulator wear of gamma-vacuum, gamma-air, and ethylene oxide sterilized UHMWPE following a severe oxidative challenge. *Trans Orthop Res Soc.* 1998;23:52.

73. McGloughlin TM, Kavanagh AG. Wear of ultra-high molecular weight polyethylene (UHMWPE) in total knee prostheses: a review of key influences. *Proc Inst Mech Eng.* 2000;214:349–359.

74. Kurtz SM, Muratoglu OK, Evans M, et al. Advances in the processing, sterilization, and crosslinking of ultra-high molecular weight polyethylene for total joint arthroplasty. *Biomaterials.* 1999;20(18):1659–1688.

75. McKellop H, Shen FW, Lu B, et al. Development of an extremely wear-resistant ultra high molecular weight polyethylene for total hip replacements. *J Orthop Res.* 1999;17(2):157–167.

76. Muratoglu OK, Bragdon CR, O'Connor DO, et al. A novel method of cross-linking ultra-high-molecular-weight polyethylene to improve wear, reduce oxidation, and retain mechanical properties. *J Arthroplasty.* 2001; 16(2):149–160.

77. Oonishi H, Kadoya Y, Masuda S. Gamma-irradiated cross-linked polyethylene in total hip replacements—analysis of retrieved sockets after long-term implantation. *J Biomed Mater Res.* 2001;58(2):167–171.

78. Oonishi H, Kadoya Y. Wear of high-dose gamma-irradiated polyethylene in total hip replacements. *J Orthop Sci.* 2000;5(3):223–228.

79. Oonishi H, Clarke IC, Masuda S, et al. Study of retrieved acetabular sockets made from high-dose, cross-linked polyethylene. *J Arthroplasty.* 2001;16(8)(Suppl): 129–133.

80. Oonishi H, Clarke IC, Yamamoto K, et al. Assessment of wear in extensively irradiated UHMWPE cups in simulator studies. *J Biomed Mater Res.* 2004;68(1):52–60.

81. Grobbelaar CJ, de Plessis TA, Marais F. The radiation improvement of polyethylene prostheses. a preliminary study. *J Bone Joint Surg Br.* 1978;60(3):370–374.

82. Yamamoto K, Masaoka T, Manaka M, et al. Micro-wear features on unique 100-Mrad cups: two retrieved cups compared to hip simulator wear study. *Acta Orthop Scand.* 2004;75(2):134–141.

83. Wroblewski BM, Siney PD, Dowson D, et al. Prospective clinical and joint simulator studies of a new total hip arthroplasty using alumina ceramic heads and cross-linked polyethylene cups. *J Bone Joint Surg Br.* 1996; 78(2):280–285.

84. Bradford L, Baker DA, Graham J, et al. Wear and surface cracking in early retrieved highly cross-linked polyethylene acetabular liners. *J Bone Joint Surg Am.* 2004;86(6): 1271–1282.

85. Bradford L, Kurland R, Sankaran M, et al. Early failure due to osteolysis associated with contemporary highly cross-linked ultra-high molecular weight polyethylene. A case report. *J Bone Joint Surg Am.* 2004;86(5):1051–1056.

86. Heisel C, Silva M, dela Rosa MA, et al. Short-term in vivo wear of cross-linked polyethylene. *J Bone Joint Surg Am.* 2004;86(4):748–751.

87. Hopper RH Jr, Young AM, Orishimo KF, et al. Correlation between early and late wear rates in total hip arthroplasty with application to the performance of Marathon cross-linked polyethylene liners. *J Arthroplasty.* 2003;18(7 Suppl 1):60–67.

88. Sychterz CJ, Orishimo KF, Engh CA. Sterilization and polyethylene wear: clinical studies to support laboratory data. *J Bone Joint Surg Am.* 2004;86(5):1017–1022.

89. Muratoglu OK, Greenbaum ES, Bragdon CR, et al. Surface analysis of early retrieved acetabular polyethylene liners. A comparison of conventional and highly crosslinked polyethylenes. *J Arthroplasty.* 2004;19(1):68–77.

90. Digas G, Karrholm J, Thanner J, et al. Highly cross-linked polyethylene in cemented THA: randomized study of 61 hips. *Clin Orthop.* 2003;417:126–138.

91. Fisher J, McEwen HM, Barnett PI, et al. Influences of sterilizing techniques on polyethylene wear. *Knee.* 2004; 11(3):173–176.

92. Muratoglu OK, Ruberti J, Melotti S, et al. Optical analysis of surface changes on early retrieval of highly cross-linked and conventional polyethylene tibial inserts. *J Arthroplasty.* 2003;18(7)(Suppl):42–47.

93. Bragdon CR, Jasty M, Muratoglu OK, et al. Third-body wear of highly cross-linked polyethylene in a hip simulator. *J Arthroplasty.* 2003;18(5):553–561.

94. McEwen HMJ, Farrar R, Auger DD, et al. Reduction of wear in fixed bearing total knee replacement using crosslinked UHMWPE. *Trans Orthop Res Soc.* 2003;28(2): 1428.

95. Kurtz SM, Pruitt LA, Jewett CW, et al. Radiation and chemical crosslinking promote strain hardening behavior and molecular alignment in ultra high molecular weight polyethylene during multi-axial loading conditions. *Biomaterials.* 1999;20(16):1449–1462.

96. Muratoglu OK, Bragdon CR, O'Connor DO, et al. Aggressive wear testing of a cross-linked polyethylene in total knee arthroplasty. *Clin Orthop.* 2002;404:89–95.

97. Muratoglu OK, Merrill EW, Bragdon CR, et al. Effects of radiation, heat and aging on in vitro wear resistance of polyethylene. *Clin Orthop.* 2003;417:253–262.

98. Bankston AB, Faris PM, Keating EM, et al. Polyethylene wear in total hip arthroplasty in patient-matched groups. A comparison of stainless steel, cobalt chrome, and titanium-bearing surfaces. *J Arthroplasty.* 1993;8(3):315–322.

99. Lombardi AV Jr, Mallory TH, Vaughn BK, et al. Aseptic loosening in total hip arthroplasty secondary to osteolysis induced by wear debris from titanium-alloy modular femoral heads. *J Bone Joint Surg Am.* 1989;71(9): 1337–1342.

100. McGovern TE, Black J, Jacobs JJ, et al. In vivo wear of Ti6Al4V femoral heads: a retrieval study. *J Biomed Mater Res.* 1996;32(3):447–457.

101. Berger RA, Lyon JH, Jacobs JJ, et al. Problems with cementless total knee arthroplasty at 11 years followup. *Clin Orthop.* 2001;392:196–207.

102. Engh GA, Parks NL, Ammeen DJ. Tibial osteolysis in cementless total knee arthroplasty. A review of 25 cases treated with and without tibial component revision. *Clin Orthop.* 1994;309:33–43.

103. Ezzet KA, Garcia R, Barrack RL. Effect of component fixation method on osteolysis in total knee arthroplasty. *Clin Orthop.* 1995;321:86–91.

104. Lewis PL, Rorabeck CH, Bourne, RB. Screw osteolysis after cementless total knee replacement. *Clin Orthop.* 1995;321: 173–177.

105. Peters PC Jr, Engh GA, Dwyer KA, et al. Osteolysis after total knee arthroplasty without cement. *J Bone Joint Surg Am.* 1992;74(6):864–876.

106. Baker DA, Hastings RS, Pruitt L. Study of fatigue resistance of chemical and radiation crosslinked medical grade ultrahigh molecular weight polyethylene. *J Biomed Mater Res.* 1999;46(4):573–581.

107. Jenny JY, Boeri C. Computer-assisted implantation of total knee prostheses: a case control comparative study with

classical instrumentation. *Comput Aided Surg.* 2001;6(4): 217–220.

108. Krackow KA, Phillips MJ, Bayers-Thering M, et al. Computer-assisted total knee arthroplasty: navigation in TKA. Orthopedics 2003;26(10):1017–1023.

109. Stulberg SD. how accurate is current TKR instrumentation? *Clin Orthop.* 2003;416:177–184.

110. Lavernia CJ, Sierra RJ, Hungerford DS, et al. Activity level and wear in total knee arthroplasty. *J Arthroplasty.* 2001; 16(4):446–453.

111. Mont MA, Rajadhyaksha AS, Marxen JL, et al. Tennis after total knee arthroplasty. *Am J Sports Med.* 2002;30(2): 163–166.

112. Seedhom BB, Wallbridge NC. Walking activities and wear of prostheses. *Ann Rheum Dis.* 1985;44:838.

113. Benjamin J, Tucker T, Ballesteros P. Is obesity a contraindication to bilateral total knee arthroplasties under one anesthetic? *Clin Orthop.* 2001;392:190–195.

114. Deshmukh RG, Hayes JH, Pinder IM. Does body weight influence outcome after total knee arthroplasty? a 1-year analysis. *J Arthroplasty.* 2002;17(3):315–319.

115. Griffin FM, Scuderi GR, Insall JN, et al. Total knee arthroplasty in patient who were obese with 1 years followup. *Clin Orthop.* 1998;356:28–33.

116. Mont MA, Mathur SK, Krackow KA, et al. Cementless total knee arthroplasty in obese patients. A comparison with a matched control group. *J Arthroplasty.* 1996;11(2): 153–156.

117. Spicer DD, Pomeroy DL, Badenhausen WE, et al. Body mass index as a predictor of outcome in total knee replacement. *Int Orthop.* 2001;25(4):246–249.

118. Wendelboe AM, Hegmann KT, Biggs JJ, et al. Relationships between body mass indices and surgical replacement of knee and hip joints. *Am J Prev Med.* 2003;25(4):290–295.

119. Vazquez-Vela Johnson G, Worland RL, Keenan J, et al. Patient demographics as a predictor of the ten-year survival rate in primary total knee replacement. *J Bone Joint Surg Br.* 2003;85(1):52–56.

120. Blunn GW, Walker PS, Joshi A, et al. The dominance of cyclic sliding in producing wear in total knee replacements. *Clin Orthop.* 1991;273:253–260.

121. Kawanabe K, Clarke IC, Tamura J, et al. Effects of A-P translation and rotation on the wear of UHMWPE in a total knee joint simulator. *J Biomed Mater Res.* 2001;54(3): 400–406.

122. Rose RM, Goldfarb HV. On the pressure dependence of the wear of ultrahigh molecular weight polyethylene. *Wear.* 1983;92:99–111.

123. Rostoker W, Galante JO. Contact pressure dependence of wear rates of ultra high molecular weight polyethylene. *J Biomed Mater Res.* 1979;12:957–964.

124. Sathasivam S, Walker PS. A computer model with surface friction for the prediction of total knee kinematics. *J Biomechanics.* 1996;30(2):177–184.

125. Szivek JA, Anderson PL, Benjamin JB. Average and peak contact stress distribution evaluation of total knee arthroplasties. *J Arthroplasty.* 1996;11(8):952–963.

126. Wimmer MA, Andriacchi TP. Tractive forces during rolling motion of the knee: implications for wear in total knee replacement. *J Biomechanics.* 1996;30(2):131–137.

127. Wimmer MA, Andriacchi TP, Natarajan, et al. A striated pattern of wear in ultrahigh-molecular-weight polyethylene components of Miller-Galante total knee arthroplasty. *J Arthroplasty.* 1998;13(1):8–16.

128. Booth RE Jr. Total knee arthroplasty in the obese patient: tips and quips. *J Arthroplasty.* 2002:17(4)(Suppl 1):69–70.

129. Tradonsky S, Postak PD, Froimson AI, et al. A comparison of disassociation strength of modular acetabular components. *Clin Orthop.* 1993;296:154–160.

130. Halley D, Glassman A, Crowninshield RD. Recurrent dislocation after revision total hip replacement with a large prosthetic femoral head. *J Bone Joint Surg Am.* 2004; 86(4):827–830.

131. Ries MD. Dissociation of an ultra-high molecular weight polyethylene insert from the tibial baseplate after total knee arthroplasty. *J Bone Joint Surg Am.* 2004;86(7): 1522–1524.

132. Blunn GW, Joshi AB, Minns, et al. Wear in retrieved condylar knee arthroplasties. *J Arthroplasty.* 1997;12(3):281–290.

133. Jasty M, Goetz DD, Bragdon CR, et al. Wear of polyethylene acetabular components in total hip arthroplasty. an analysis of one hundred and twenty-eight components retrieved at autopsy or revision operations. *J Bone Joint Surg Am.* 1997;79(3):349–358.

134. Landy MM, Walker PS. Wear of ultra-high-molecular-weight polyethylene components of 90 retrieved knee prostheses. *J Arthroplasty.* 1988;3(Suppl):S73–85.

135. Ries MD, Scott ML, Jani S. Relationship between gravimetric wear and particle generation in hip simulator: conventional compared with cross-linked polyethylene. *J Bone Joint Surg.* 2001;83(Suppl 2, Pt 2):116–122.

136. Ingram JH, Fisher J, Stone M, et al. Effect of crosslinking on biological activity of UHMWPE wear debris. *Trans Orthop Res Soc.* 2003;28(2):1439.

137. Scott ML, Ries MD, Jani S. Abrasive wear in total hip replacement: is crosslinked UHMWPE coupled to ceramic heads the answer? *Proc Am Acad Orthop Surg.* 2002;3:732.

138. Muratoglu OK, Burroughs BR, Christensen SD. In vitro simulator wear of highly crosslinked tibias articulating against explanted rough femoral components. *Trans Orthop Res Soc.* 2004;29(1):297.

139. Good V, Ries M, Barrack RL, et al. Reduced wear with oxidized zirconium femoral heads. *J Bone Joint Surg Am.* 2003;85(Suppl 4):105–110.

140. Laskin RS. An oxidized Zr ceramic surfaced femoral component for total knee arthroplasty. *Clin Orthop.* 2003;416: 191–196.

CHAPTER 3

The Painful Total Knee Arthroplasty

Nigel M. Azer and Thomas S. Thornhill

Total knee arthroplasty is one of the most successful operations performed, with 95% to 98% good to excellent results reported at 10 to 15 years.[1–3] Given the number of arthroplasties performed annually and the fact that more than 22 000 revision operations are performed as well, there are still many patients who either develop pain in their replaced knee or fail to get relief from their index procedure.[4] A thoughtful and systematic approach to these patients can help elucidate the mechanism of failure and develop an appropriate treatment paradigm. The results of exploration for debilitating pain of unknown etiology in a total knee replacement remain poor, with only 59% fair or poor results reported after surgery.[5] Thus, it is paramount to consider all potential causes of pain about a total knee arthroplasty before considering intervention. We shall consider the diagnosis and treatment of the painful total knee replacement from an anatomical perspective, stratified into intra-articular, periarticular, and extra-articular/systemic causes (See Table 3.1).

INTRA-ARTICULAR

Infection

Infection *must* be considered in the evaluation of every patient with a painful total knee replacement. It is a most devastating and feared complication that often threatens the function of the joint, the preservation of the limb, and the health of the patient. Infections are reported to occur in 0.5% to 2% of patients undergoing primary total knee replacements and 5% to 7% of revision patients.[6] Rheumatoid arthritis, diabetes, oral steroid use, obesity, concurrent infections, malnutrition, and higher degrees of prosthetic constraint all increase the relative risk of infection.[7,8] The most common organisms are

Staphylococcus aureus and *Staphylococcus epidermis.* Methicillin- and vancomycin-resistant organisms are becoming increasingly prevalent and difficult to treat. The diagnosis of infection can usually be made by a thorough history and physical examination. Persistent pain is the only consistent finding with infection, although a draining wound or history of wound problems or any erythema must also raise the suspicion for infection (Figure 3-1).[9] Serum studies including white blood cell count, erythrocyte sedimentation rate, and C-reactive protein are useful, particularly in following the course of treatment. The erythrocyte sedimentation rate is only 60% sensitive and 65% specific for infection.[10] Bone scans are also helpful, with sensitivities and specificities of approximately 84%.[10] Combining a technetium-99m-sulfur colloid scan with an indium-111 leukocyte scan improves sensitivity to 100%, specificity to 97%, and accuracy to 98% in diagnosing infected cemented total hip arthroplasties.[11] Aspiration of the knee should be performed and the fluid should be analyzed for culture, glucose, and cell count. Although recent studies quote 100% sensitivity for aspiration,[12] other studies demonstrate only a 75% positive predictive value and a 94% negative predictive value.[10] Polymerase chain reaction testing has been advocated but has such high sensitivity that it may increase the degree of false-positive results.[13] Finally, tissue taken intraoperatively may be sent for frozen section pathological examination. Greater than 10 polymorphonuclear leukocytes per high-power field is implicated in infection with a sensitivity of 84% and a specificity of 99%.[14] Hence, the diagnosis of infection must be made based on careful history and physical examination using all available data, rather than basing the diagnosis on one particular test.

Treatment of a total knee infection is often based on the timing and duration of the infection as well as the implicated organism and the status of patient's overall

TABLE 3.1. Differential Diagnosis for Painful Total Knee Arthroplasty.

Intra-articular
  Infection
  Patellofemoral
    Resurfaced vs. unresurfaced patella
    Maltracking
    Fracture
    Avascular necrosis
    Loosening
    Patellar fibrosis
    Overstuffing joint
  Wear
  Osteolysis
  Instability
    Valgus-varus
    Axial including midflexion
  Malalignment
  Arthrofibrosis
  Recurrent hemarthrosis
  Popliteus impingement
  Loose bodies
  Persistent synovitis
  Overhanging component
  Gout/CPPD
Periarticular
  Neuroma
  Fracture
  Heterotopic ossification
  Bursitis
Extra-articular
  Complex regional pain syndrome
  Hip/spine pathology
  Vascular etiology
  Unrealistic expectations
  Psychological profile

a relatively low virulence gram-positive infection is encountered in a competent host. Results with this approach are variable, with most studies reporting 50% to 75% success.[16] A recent study showed 89.2% success with single-stage exchange in which there was a gram-positive infection, absence of sinus tract, antibiotic-impregnated cement in the new prosthesis, and 12 weeks of adjuvant antibiotic treatment.[17] The most widely accepted approach is the two-stage exchange in which aggressive irrigation, debridement, synovectomy, and prosthesis removal are performed, followed by reimplantation after a period of intravenous antibiotics. During the interim, a spacer of antibiotic-impregnated methylmethacrylate is often used. Up to 97% eradication rates are reported with this technique.[12] The use of a PROSTA-LAC functional spacer made of antibiotic-laden cement with a small metal-on-polyethylene articulation is of interest because of its potential for enhanced function and maintenance of good alignment and stability of the knee. This facilitates second-stage procedures. Using this technique in a two-stage exchange with a mean 4 years' follow-up, cure rates of 91% have been demonstrated.[18] Although this is promising, further outcomes-based studies are necessary.

It is critical to always maintain a high index of suspicion for infection and to treat infections aggressively. All

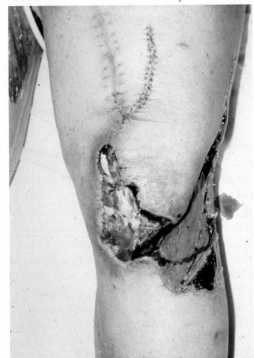

FIGURE 3-1. Infection must always be excluded.

health. Decisions must then be made whether to attempt prosthesis retention, one-stage exchange, or two-stage exchange. A glycocalyx layer formed around the prosthesis may prevent antibiotic penetration to the prosthesis, rendering antibiotic treatment alone ineffective. Success rates as low as 6% to 10% have been reported for the treatment of acute infections with antibiotics alone.[15] Surgical treatment remains the mainstay. Aggressive treatment for *superficial* wound infections is recommended, as many of these infections actually involve deeper tissues. Open surgical debridement, radical synovectomy, and antibiotic treatment are successful in only 20% to 30% of acute infections.[16] Even lower rates of success are reported for using this approach for chronic infections. Arthroscopic debridement has only seen moderate success in the eradication of acute (within 4 weeks of surgery) infections, providing eradication in 52% of patients.[17]

Prosthetic exchange is the primary mode of treatment when eradication of the infection is the goal. Single-stage exchange may be considered when an acute infection with painful total knee replacements must be evaluated for the possibility of an indolent infection.

Patellofemoral Problems

Anterior knee pain is a relatively common complication after total knee arthroplasty and is often attributed to the patellofemoral articulation. It is, however, important to exclude other causes of anterior knee pain, such as peripatellar tendinitis, bursitis, Sinding-Larsen-Johansson disease, residual from Osgood-Schlatter disease, neuromas, and complex regional pain syndrome. The prevalence of anterior knee pain after total knee replacement has been reported as high as 25.1% in knees with unresurfaced patellae and 5.3% in resurfaced patellae.[19] Overall, approximately 10% of patients with total knee replacement may be expected to have anterior knee pain.[20] Complication rates ranging from 5% to 50% in resurfaced patellae are reported and account for up to 50% of revision total knee replacements.[21] Problems with the patellofemoral articulation in a total knee may be referable to malalignment and maltracking of the patella, osteonecrosis, fracture, loosening, component failure, tendon rupture, and peripatellar fibrosis. Evaluation of this pain must first identify whether the patella has been resurfaced, as unresurfaced patellae have been shown to have a significantly higher incidence of pain. The patella should be resurfaced in obese patients, patients with inflammatory arthritis, preoperative maltracking, significant loss of cartilage and exposed subchondral bone on the patella, gross surface irregularities, and those with significant anterior knee pain preoperatively.[22] When anterior knee pain is diagnosed in a patient with an unresurfaced patella, consideration to revision to a resurfaced patella must be given after other etiologies have been excluded. With newer three-lugged, cemented, all-polyethylene components available and careful attention to technical detail, the authors advocate patellar resurfacing in all total knee arthroplasties.

Patella maltracking is evident when the patella fails to maintain a congruent articulation with the trochlear groove of the femoral component (Figure 3-2). Failure to achieve adequate tracking may cause pain and crepitance as well as wear, failure of the patellar component, loosening, and fracture. Maltracking is most commonly caused by an imbalance of the extensor mechanism, especially with tightness of the lateral retinaculum and weakness of the vastus medialis. It may also be attributed to malposition of the femoral, tibial, or patellar components themselves. Placing the femoral component into excessive valgus increases the Q-angle and elicits an increase in the lateral force vector, tending to displace the patella laterally. Likewise, internal rotation or medial shift of the femoral component also displaces the patella laterally.

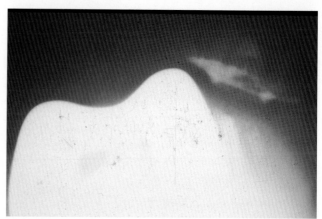

FIGURE 3-2. Mechant radiographs permit diagnosis of patellofemoral dislocation.

Internal rotation of the tibia causes lateralization of the tibial tubercle, also detrimentally increasing the Q-angle. Lateral placement of the patellar component also contributes to maltracking. It is essential to perform diligent intraoperative assessment of patellar tracking to avoid patellofemoral instability. Alteration of the joint line itself may result in patella alta or infera, which could exacerbate abnormal tracking, impingement, or recurrent dislocation. An asymmetrical patellar resection may also contribute to patellar maltracking. The medial facet is thicker than the lateral facet. Thus, it is essential to resect the same amounts of bone from the medial and lateral facets to maintain this orientation. An oblique resection, taking too much bone off laterally, results in maltracking. The diagnosis of patellar instability can usually be made by physical examination, but may be evident on Merchant radiographic views. Computed tomography may provide essential information in determining the rotational alignment of the femoral and tibial components. Treatment of patellar subluxation begins with aggressive quadriceps rehabilitation, patellofemoral bracing, and avoidance of deep squatting exercises. Malrotated components should be revised as necessary. Additional soft tissue procedures, such as lateral release and medial advance as well as tibial tubercle osteotomy, may be added as indicated.

Fractures of the patella are generally rare, reported as 0.12%, although one small study in the literature quotes a 21% incidence.[23,24] Fractures include occult stress fractures as well as intraoperative and postoperative fractures (Figure 3-3). They may be associated with trauma, patellar subluxation, inadequate resection, excessive resection, thinning the patella to less than 15 mm, and operative disruption of the patellar blood supply, particularly when median parapatellar exposure is accompanied by lateral release.[25] Treatment typically depends on the competence

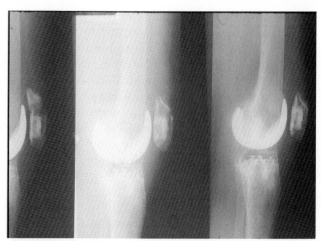

FIGURE 3-3. Fractures of the patella are generally rare and include occult stress fractures as well as intraoperative and postoperative fractures.

of the extensor mechanism, the degree of displacement, and the integrity of prosthetic fixation. Nonoperative treatment has been successful in nondisplaced fractures with a well-fixed component and a competent extensor mechanism. Surgical fixation with tension band and/or revision of the component is indicated in the more severe injuries. Patellectomy should be avoided whenever possible.

Loosening of the patellar component is exceedingly rare and has been reported in fewer than 2% of total knees.[26] It is associated more with metal-backed designs, which have largely fallen out of favor. Risk factors for failure of the patellar component include excessive body weight, recalling that the patellofemoral articulation can bear up to 7 times body weight during squatting, increased knee flexion, and a high level of activity. The diagnosis is usually apparent with symptoms of effusion and crepitance, which are more pronounced with activities that load the patellofemoral joint. Plain radiographs confirm the diagnosis, and treatment involves revision.

Patellar fibrosis or *patellar clunk syndrome* occurs when a fibrous nodule forms at the junction of the posterior aspect of the quadriceps tendon and the proximal pole of the patella (Figure 3-4). With flexion, this nodule enters the intercondylar notch. Then, as the knee is extended from 30 to 60 degrees, the fibrotic lesion *clunks* out of the notch. This syndrome is classically associated with posterior stabilized components, but has been reported in cruciate retaining designs, as well as in cases in which the patella remains unresurfaced.[27,28] Extensive excision of the synovium in the suprapatellar region may prevent this. Treatment involves debridement of the fibrotic nodule, either by arthroscopy or arthrotomy. If

the clunk involves a malpositioned patella or inappropriately sized femoral component, revision is recommended. Arthroscopic debridement has yielded 41% good results, 19% fair results, and 40% poor results. Thus, such treatment should be approached with trepidation.[29] A similar entity, synovial entrapment, is described in which hypertrophic synovium causes pain during extension from 90 degrees of flexion. Patients typically had pain when arising from a chair or climbing stairs, but had no symptoms with level walking. Treatment with synovectomy resulted in relief of symptoms in all patients studied.[30]

A number of entities may cause anterior knee pain in patients with total knee replacements. A systematic approach and inclusive differential diagnosis can yield the appropriate diagnosis and guide treatment.

Osteolysis

Polyethylene wear in total knee arthroplasty continues to affect the longevity of modern total knee replacements. Wear and aseptic loosening have been shown to be the most common modes of failure requiring surgery, collectively accounting for up to 49% of revision operations.[31] From a basic science standpoint, osteolysis is the granulomatous response to polyethylene, polymethylmethacrylate, and metal debris, which are formed by both the articulating and nonarticulating (undersurface) surfaces of the prosthetic knee. Delamination, adhesion, and abrasion cause the liberation of loose particles that contribute to osteolysis. Sixteen percent of total knees are reported to have osteolysis.[32] Risk factors include incongruent articulations, poor tibial locking mechanisms, thin polyethylene, sterilization of polyethylene with gamma irradiation in air, fixation screws in the tibial base plate, and an

FIGURE 3-4. Patellar fibrosis occurs when a fibrous nodule forms at the junction of the posterior aspect of the quadriceps tendon and proximal pole of the patella.

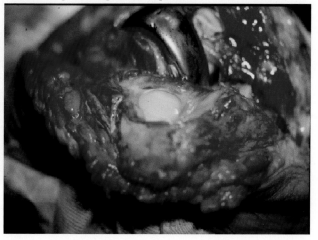

extended shelf life of the polyethylene implants. Most patients remain asymptomatic. However, some patients have a boggy synovitis and mild to moderate pain with activity. A triad of effusion, pain, and change in coronal alignment, usually into varus, is strongly suggestive of accelerated polyethylene wear. Identification of a lytic osseous defect, absence of bone trabeculae, and geographic demarcation makes the diagnosis radiographically (Figure 3-5). The presence of the components may obscure the lesions on radiography, particularly as they are most commonly found within 2 mm of the tibial component and in the posterior femoral condyles. Dynamic fluoroscopy has been advocated to overcome this.[33] Nuclear medicine studies may also demonstrate increased uptake around loose components. Osteolysis must be distinguished from radiolucent lines that are a common finding in radiographic surveillance of total knees. Lysis requires a complete radiolucent line of greater than 2 mm in length. Smaller lines are of unknown significance and may be followed clinically. Ranawat et al. noted radiolucent lines in 72% of the tibiae, 54% of the femurs, and 33% of patellae.[3] Not all of these represented osteolysis. Treatment of these lesions primarily depends on whether the osteolysis is associated with loose prosthetic components. It is essential to review serial radiographs to determine if radiolucent lines are progressive. Well-fixed components with lytic lesions may be treated with exchange of the polyethylene insert and bone grafting of the lesions. Engh et al. studied the results of isolated polyethylene exchange and discovered a 17% failure rate at 4 to 5 years.[34] They recommended that limited revision of the polyethylene should be avoided if severe delamination

is present, if there is significant undersurface wear of the polyethylene suggesting an inadequate locking mechanism, and if there is early failure within 10 years of the index operation. Revision of loose components with bone graft is indicated for lysis associated with loose components. It is important to have a full complement of revision instruments available with stems, wedges, and allograft when performing these revisions, as radiographs not only underestimate lesion size, but do not take into account bone loss with explanation of the loose components (Figure 3-6).

Instability

Symptomatic axial instability of a total knee arthroplasty, including valgus-varus and flexion-extension instability, is a potential cause for pain and disability following total knee replacement. It occurs in 1% to 2% of patients and may be present in either posterior stabilized or cruciate-retaining knees. Overall, instability accounts for 10% to 20% of all total knee revisions, following only infection and aseptic loosening in prevalence.[35] Instability may be caused by trauma, ligamentous stretch, inadequate balance at the time of surgery, or a systemic disorder such as Ehlers-Danlos disease.

Patients with mediolateral, valgus-varus instability often present with pain, buckling, giving way, and progressive weightbearing deformity. This instability may be the result of traumatic injury, but is often the result of failure to achieve appropriate soft tissue balance at the time of surgery. The diagnosis can usually be made by history and physical examination and may be confirmed by stress radiographs or video fluoroscopy. Using a sys-

FIGURE 3-5. Loose component. (A) Identification of a lytic osseus defect, absence of bone trabeculae, and geographic demarcation makes the diagnosis radiographically. (B) Additional tests such as magnetic resonance imaging and bone scans may also facilitate the diagnosis of loose components.

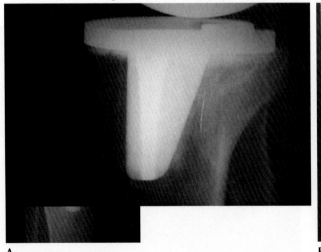
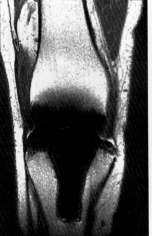
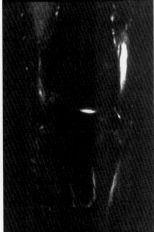

A   B

bility. Soft tissue balance and increase in prosthetic constraint were applied as indicated. Only 1% of the patients had recurrent instability.[36]

Failure to balance the flexion and extension gaps properly may lead to symptomatic instability in the sagittal plane. This entity was first recognized and reported with the obvious acute dislocation of a posterior-stabilized prosthesis. Subsequently this has been reported to occur in 1% to 2% of posterior-stabilized knees.[37] Cam-post design, large lateral soft tissue release in valgus knees, and above average range of motion have all been implicated as risk factors for the dislocation of a posterior-stabilized knee. The diagnosis is usually obvious and treatment involves reduction and revision to balance the flexion-extension gaps or increase constraint if necessary.

Flexion instability in posterior cruciate retaining knees is also evident. However, this entity is much more subtle than its counterpart in posterior-stabilized knees (Figure 3-7A). Patients typically present with anterior knee pain, a sense of instability, recurrent effusions, soft tissue tenderness of the pes tendons, and posterior instability, evidenced by a positive posterior drawer sign or sag. Symptoms may occur early in the postoperative period if there is inadequate flexion-extension or posterior cruciate ligament (PCL) balance. Late PCL rupture or attenuation may give a delayed presentation of symptoms. The diagnosis may be made by careful history and physical examination. Medial and lateral translocation of the polyethylene eminence under the medial or lateral femoral condyle performed passively with the knee flexed is a hallmark of flexion instability. Performing a posterior drawer test and examining for flexion instability should be routine in evaluating every painful total knee. A common cause for this pattern of imbalance occurs when treating patients with residual flexion contractures. Proper

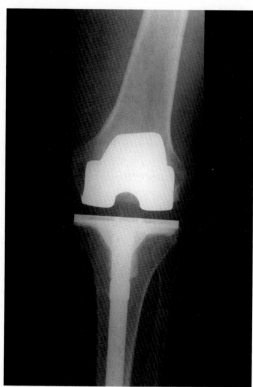

FIGURE 3-6. Revision for loose components. Radiographs often underestimate lesion size and do not take into account bone loss with explanation of the loose components.

tematic approach and meticulous technique, good results may be achieved in knees with severe varus or valgus alignment. Prevention is the best treatment. Revision to correct soft tissue imbalance or revision to a higher degree of prosthetic constraint with stems and wedges may be necessary. Haas et al. reported excellent results of revision surgery for patients with symptomatic valgus-varus insta-

FIGURE 3-7. (A) Flexion instability in posterior cruciate retaining knees. (B) The revision operation balances the flexion-extension gaps in conjunction with revision to a posterior stabilized knee.

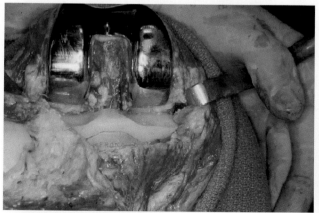

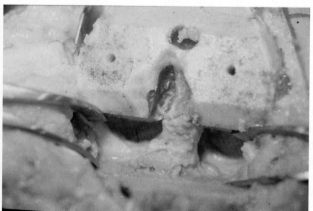

A

B

balance in flexion, but excess tightness in extension may entice the placement of a thinner polyethylene liner or further tibial resection. Although this may correct the flexion contracture, it is a setup for symptomatic flexion instability. A better remedy is to perform a posterior capsular release or resect more distal femur. The treatment of flexion instability may be difficult because it often involves considering revision of well-aligned, well-fixed components with the resultant bone loss and potential elevation of the joint line. There have been several reports on the results of treatment by isolated revision to a thicker polyethylene insert. Overall the results have been marginal. Seventy-one percent success with polyethylene liner exchange alone has been reported, with this technique being favored if the etiology was primarily soft tissue imbalance. If incompetent ligaments were identified, revision to more highly constrained components was recommended.[38] Eighty-six percent success is reported when revising to a more constrained component. A revision operation that focuses on balancing the flexion-extension gaps in conjunction with revision to a posterior stabilized knee is the most reliable treatment for symptomatic flexion instability after PCL retaining prosthesis (Figure 3-7B).[39] It is essential to always include valgus-varus and flexion-extension instability in the differential diagnosis of the painful total knee.

Arthrofibrosis

Most patients achieve a satisfactory range of motion after total knee replacement and are able to perform their activities of daily living without limitation. Typically, 63 degrees is needed for the swing phase of gait, 83 degrees for stair ascent, 84 degrees for stair descent, at least 93 degrees to rise from a chair and 106 degrees to fasten a shoelace.[40] However, postoperative stiffness occurs, and patients may not achieve these degrees of motion. This expectedly causes significant functional limitation and patient dissatisfaction. A review of total knee revisions has shown that 14.6% of revisions are for inability to achieve satisfactory range of motion.[31] Stiffness occurs in both posterior stabilized and posterior cruciate-retaining implant designs. The etiology is largely unknown, but may be biologic, related to an underlying collagen disorder characterized by rapid fibrous metaplasia of scar tissue, or mechanical, related to technical errors in operative technique, such as failure to properly balance the flexion and extension gaps or release the posterior capsule and remove posterior osteophytes when present. Actin and myosin fibrils have been identified histologically in arthrofibrotic tissue and may also be implicated. Risk factors for limited postoperative range of motion include limited preoperative range of motion, contractures, obesity in which posterior soft tissue impingement limits

flexion, excessive intra-articular scar from previous operations, and poor patient compliance with postoperative rehabilitation protocols (Figure 3-8). Excessive tension or laxity in the PCL may also result in limited motion. A lax PCL allows paradoxical anterior femoral translation with increased knee flexion, resulting in loss of flexion. It is important to recognize that arthrofibrosis may be the hallmark of other knee pathology such as infection, component loosening, periprosthetic fracture, complex regional pain syndrome, or heterotopic ossification. Thus, these must be considered in the evaluation of a stiff knee. Furthermore, it is particularly important to accurately document with a goniometer preoperative and intraoperative range of motion so that the patient, surgeon, and physical therapist appreciate realistic motion goals before embarking on an aggressive campaign to restore motion. Moreover, as shorter hospital stays mandate the majority of physical therapy as outpatient, the surgeon must convey to the therapist the patient's preoperative, intraoperative, and expected goals for postoperative motion.

Treatment of a stiff knee initially involves aggressive physiotherapy and closed manipulation under anesthesia. This is particularly advantageous in the first 3 to 6 weeks postoperatively when the scar tissue has not matured. After 8 weeks, the scar tends to mature and the risk of

FIGURE 3-8. Arthrofibrosis and patella infera limit range of motion postoperatively.

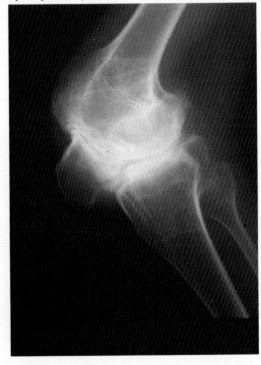

supracondylar femoral fracture increases. Although continuous passive motion (CPM) is controversial, particularly when range of motion at 1 year postoperatively is considered, it is recommended after manipulation. Barring success with this, surgical intervention with arthroscopic or open arthrolysis is considered. Arthroscopy has been shown to provide gains in range of motion in 43% of patients treated for arthrofibrosis following total knee replacement.[41] Open procedures have the benefit of allowing radical scar excision, ligament rebalancing, and exchange of the polyethylene insert if necessary. Should these fail, revision arthroplasty with definitive reestablishment of flexion-extension gaps, ligament balance, and possibly a higher degree of prosthetic constraint may be necessary. Revision has shown satisfactory results in terms of pain and range of motion in several small studies.[42,43] Finally, the off-label use of Seprafilm (Genzyme Corp., Cambridge, MA), an anti-adhesion membrane commonly used in abdominal surgery, has met anecdotal success in total knee arthroplasty in high-risk, young arthritic patients who have had multiple operations.[44]

Recurrent Hemarthrosis

Recurrent hemarthrosis is an uncommon but significantly disabling cause of pain following total knee arthroplasty. Kindsfater and Scott reviewed 30 cases of patients who experienced painful recurrent hemarthrosis after total knee replacement.[45] The patients developed their first hemarthrosis an average of 2 years after their replacements. Most experienced multiple episodes of bleeding. Approximately one-third of the patients had resolution of symptoms with aspiration, rest, ice, and elevation followed by gradual return to activities. Of the patients who underwent surgical exploration, only 43% had an identifiable etiology for their bleeding. Proliferative synovium entrapped between the prosthetic articulations or a vascular leash were both implicated and treated. Usually an associated soft tissue laxity necessitates use of a more conforming or a thicker polyethylene insert. With synovectomy, 14 of 15 no longer bled. Thus, hemarthrosis must be considered in the differential diagnosis of the painful total knee. Most resolve with aspiration, but some require open synovectomy that provides reliable relief of symptoms.

Popliteus Impingement

The popliteus tendon may subluxate anteriorly or posteriorly over a lateral femoral condylar osteophyte or an overhanging edge of the posterior femoral condylar prosthesis, causing a painful snap or even audible *popping* sensation in the posterolateral corner of the knee after total knee arthroplasty. Such symptomatic snapping is

reported in 0.2% of total knee replacements.[46] Patients with valgus deformity and female patients, who require relatively larger components in the mediolateral dimension to compensate for their larger AP dimension, appear to be at increased risk for this. The diagnosis can only be made by placing the knee through a range of motion with the capsule closed. Treatment includes releasing the popliteus or removing the offending osteophytes at the time of the total knee replacement. Barnes and Scott diagnosed and intraoperatively addressed this in 2.7% of 300 consecutive knees.[47] Successful treatment with arthroscopic release has been reported for those symptomatic cases, which present after surgery.

Miscellaneous

Other significant intra-articular causes of a painful total knee replacement include the presence of loose bodies, loose polymethylmethacrylate cement, overhanging components, or incomplete seating of modular inserts. Persistent synovitis and gout or calcium pyrophosphate deposition disease (CPPD) may also present as a painful total knee replacement. Loose bodies and cement particles may be avoided by meticulous inspection and irrigation of the joint after implantation. It is particularly important to examine the posterior aspects of the knee for the presence of loose bodies and cement particles after polymerization of the bone cement. Many loose particles in the knee are asymtomatic because the knee is self-cleansing. Most particles tend to migrate away from the prosthetic articulations. Nevertheless, some cause persistent effusion, pain, and synovitis. Patients may even report a sensation of something moving in their knees. The diagnosis is made by history and physical examination, although some loose bodies may be apparent on high-quality plain radiographs. Treatment involves their removal, either arthroscopically or by arthrotomy. Overhanging components, particularly those overhanging anteriorly or impinging the popliteus, may also be painful. Such cases present with pain, synovitis, and recurrent effusion. History, physical examination, and radiographs revealing component overhang make the diagnosis. A localized anesthetic injection may be diagnostic and therapeutic. Treatment in the most severe cases involves removal of osteophytes or revision of the component.

PERIARTICULAR CAUSES OF PAIN

Neuroma

Extensive anatomical mapping of the cutaneous innervation of the skin and soft tissues around the knee has provided significant insight into the presence of symptomatic neuromas as an etiology of pain about the knee. While the infrapatellar branch of the saphenous nerve has a distribution across the tibial tuberosity, and the medial cutaneous nerve of the thigh has a distribution across the patella, the inferior cutaneous nerve of the thigh, the proximal tibiofibular nerve, the medial retinacular nerve, the common peroneal nerve, and the lateral reticular nerve all also have specific, known cutaneous distributions about the knee.[48] This knowledge, combined with detailed mapping of the patient's pain, may provide a diagnosis for previously enigmatic complaints. When suspected, neuromas should initially be treated with physical modalities such as moist heat, massage, topical steroid-containing creams, iontophoresis, and neuropathic pain medications. Diagnosis can be confirmed by positive Tinel's sign and by selective anesthetic injections. Dellon et al. studied the results of 70 patients treated with selective surgical denervation of persistent neuroma pain about the knee. Having excluded other causes for knee pain, such as infection, they considered this procedure for patients who had persistent pain for at least 6 months and had no effusion or obvious mechanical cause for pain. Eighty-six percent of the patients were satisfied and demonstrated relief of their pain as well as significant improvement in their Knee Society scores, which increased from a mean of 51 to mean of 82.[49] Pathological confirmation of nerve resection correlated with good results.

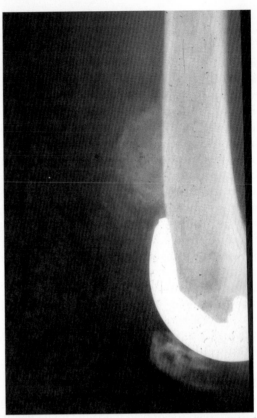

FIGURE 3-9. The formation of mature lamellar bone in the soft tissues is shown in heterotopic ossification.

Heterotopic Ossification

Heterotopic ossification (HO) is the formation of mature lamellar bone in the soft tissues (Figure 3-9). Reports suggest that the incidence of heterotopic ossification after total knee arthroplasty range from 3.8%[50] to 42%.[51] Although most cases are asymptomatic, pain and limited range of motion have been reported. Barrack et al. also demonstrated lower functional and Knee Society scores in patients with heterotopic ossification.[52] HO in the knee usually occurs in the quadriceps expansion. Predisposing factors include a previous history of heterotopic ossification, trauma, prior operations, postoperative manipulation, osteoarthritis, and immobilization, as well as intraoperative risks including excessive trauma to the muscles, periosteal exposure of the femur, notching of the femur, and hematoma formation. Infection is also a significant risk factor for HO. Prophylaxis against HO may be considered in primary or revision total knee arthroplasty if there are considerable risk factors. Treatment with a single fraction of 7-Gy radiation to the knee is effective prophylaxis with minimal documented morbidity.[53]

Bursitis

Pes anserine bursitis and patellar tendinitis may also be responsible for a painful total knee arthroplasty. Periarticular pain located approximately 5 cm below the knee joint on the anterior and medial portion of the tibia may indicate pes bursitis. The diagnosis is usually made by history and physical examination. Selective anesthetic injection including corticosteroids may also prove diagnostic and therapeutic. Patellar tendinitis presents as localized pain along the patellar tendon and tibial tubercle. Scrutiny of patella tracking and the patellofemoral articulation are necessary. Stress fractures must be excluded. Isolated patellar tendinitis responds to physical therapy, stressing hamstring stretching, bracing, and vastus medialis strengthening.

EXTRA-ARTICULAR PAIN

Complex Regional Pain Syndromes

Complex regional pain syndrome (CRPS) has been reported following total knee arthroplasty with a prevalence of 0.8%.[54] Although this syndrome is well described for the upper extremity, knowledge of its presentation in the knee and, in particular, total knee arthroplasty is evolving. Intense, prolonged pain out of proportion to physical findings, vasomotor disturbance, delayed functional recovery, and various trophic changes should raise suspicion of CRPS. Typically, arthroplasty patients have an uncomplicated postoperative course but rapidly plateau and do not achieve their expected recovery. The presence of infection or other pathological process in the knee must be excluded. The prognosis of CRPS in the knee depends on early diagnosis and treatment. Institution of treatment within 6 months is the most favorable prognostic indicator in the treatment of CRPS.[55] Initially, mobilization and physical therapy should be stressed, followed closely by a lumbar sympathetic block if rapid improvement does not ensue. A good response to the block, characterized by 75% relief of symptoms is the *sine qua non* of the diagnosis. Unfortunately, only 64% of the patients achieved some relief with sympathetic blockade. None achieved complete relief of symptoms, and most patients considered their knee replacements a failure. Patients who have had multiple operations on their knees and experience significant debilitating pain before their arthroplasties are at increased risk. Given the severity of this pathologically exaggerated physiological response, total knee arthroplasty should be approached cautiously in patients who may be at risk, and when the diagnosis is questioned, early, aggressive intervention should ensue.

Referred Pain

Pain may be referred to the knee from a number of sources including ipsilateral hip, lumbar spine, or vascular pathology. These sources of referred pain may be readily identified by complete and thoughtful history and physical examination. Ipsilateral hip pathology presents as knee pain by irritation of the continuation of the branch of the obturator nerve to the adductor magnus (Figure 3-10). Thus, the presence of arthrosis or fracture of the ipsilateral hip must be explored. Selective intra-articular injections may help distinguish the primary source of pain if both joints are arthritic. It is essential to exclude the possibility of such referred pain before performing a total knee replacement. Degeneration or spinal stenosis of the lumbar spine may also present as pain in the knee, particularly when affecting the L3/4 level. Careful history and neurological examination provide the diagnosis. CT myelography or MRI may confirm the clinical diagnosis and guide treatment accordingly. Vascular insufficiency and claudication and deep vein thrombosis may also present as pain in the knee. Once again, a careful history and physical examination make the diagnosis and permit appropriate referral. Moreover, depression,

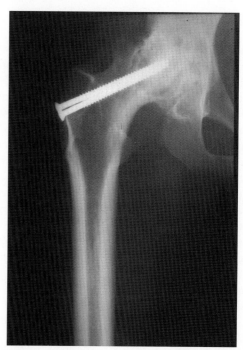

FIGURE 3-10. Ipsilateral hip pathology presents as knee pain by irritation of the continuation of the branch of the obturator nerve to the adductor magnus.

anxiety, and anger may all detrimentally affect a patient's expectations and results from a total knee replacement. Limited objective knee pathology before arthroplasty may also correlate with unsatisfactory results. Good communication between the patient and the surgeon helps clarify expectations and provide realistic goals for the patient. It is essential to take into account the patient's overall psychological and physical condition and to determine the role that the prosthetic knee plays in the patient's life. Often, counseling and pharmacological management provide important adjunctive treatment for the patient's knee pain.

SUMMARY

Although total knee arthroplasty predictably provides relief of pain and good functional results, a number of potential etiologies exist for a painful total knee replacement. It is paramount to exclude infection whenever evaluating a painful total knee. Results of treatment will not be satisfactory if the mechanism of pain or knee failure is not understood. There is no role for exploratory revision surgery. A complete history, physical examination, and thoughtful differential diagnosis help make the diagnosis and develop an effective treatment paradigm.

REFERENCES

1. Schai P, Thornhill T, Scott R. Total knee arthroplasty with the PFC system: results at a minimum of ten years and survivorship analysis. *J Bone Joint Surg.* 1998;80-B(5):850–858.

2. Ritter M, et al. Long-term survival analysis of a posterior cruciate-retaining total condylar total knee arthroplasty. *Clin Orthop.* 1994;309:136–145.

3. Ranawat C, et al. Long-term results of the total condylar knee arthroplasty: a 15-year survivorship study. *Clin Orthop.* 1993;286:94–102.

4. Anonymous. *Strategic Opportunities in Joint Replacement: The Surgeon's Perspective.* Chagrin Falls, OH: Knowledge Enterprises, Inc; 1998.

5. Mont M, et. al. Exploration of radiographically normal total knee replacements for unexplained pain. *Clin Orthop.* 1996; 331:216–220.

6. Hanssen A, et al. Instructional course lectures, AAOS: evaluation and treatment of infection at the site of a total hip or knee arthroplasty. *J Bone Joint Surg.* 1998;80(6): 910–922.

7. Wilson M, et al. Infection as a complication of total joint replacement arthroplasty. risk factors and treatment in sixty-seven cases. *J Bone Joint Surg.* 1990;72-A:878–883.

8. Poss R, Thornhill T, et al. Factors influencing the incidence and outcome of infection following total joint arthroplasty. *Clin Orthop.* 1984;182:117–126.

9. Fitzgerald RH, Jones DR. Hip implant infection. treatment with resection arthroplasty. *J Bone Joint Surg.* 1977;59-A: 847–855.

10. Levitsky KA, et al. Evaluation of the painful prosthetic joint. relative value of bone scan, sedimentation rate, and joint aspiration. *J Arthroplasty.* 1991;6:237–244.

11. Palestro CJ, et al. Total hip arthroplasty: periprosthetic Indium-111 labeled leukocyte activity and complementary technetium-99m-sulfur colloid imaging in suspected infection. *J Nucl Med.* 1990;31:1950–1955.

12. Duff GP, et al. Aspiration of the knee joint before revision arthroplasty. *Clin Orthop.* 1996;331:132–139.

13. Mariani BD, et al. Polymerase chain reaction detection of bacterial infection in total knee arthroplasty. *Clin Orthop.* 1996;331:11–22.

14. Lonner JH, et al. The reliability of analysis of intraoperative frozen sections for identifying active infection during revision hip or knee arthroplasty. *J Bone Joint Surg.* 1996;78A: 1553–1558.

15. Brien WW, Salvati E, et al. Antibiotic impregnated bone cement in total hip arthroplasty. An in vivo comparison of the elution properties of tobramycin and vancomyicin. *Clin Orthop.* 1993;296:242–248.

16. Wasielewski RC, Barden RM, Rosenberg AG. Results of different surgical procedures on total knee arthroplasty infections. *J Arthroplasty.* 1996;11:931–938.

17. Silva M, et al. Results of direct exchange or debridement of the infected total knee arthroplasty. *Clin Orthop.* 2002;404: 125–131.

18. Haddad F, Masri B, et al. The PROSTALAC functional spacer in two-stage revision for infected knee replacements. *J Bone Joint Surg.* 2000;82-B(6):807–812.

19. Waters TS, Bentley G. Patellar resurfacing in total knee arthroplasty: a prospective, randomized study. *J Bone Joint Surg.* 2003;85A:212–217.

20. Scott WN, Kim H. Resurfacing of the patella offers lower complication and revision rates. *Orthopedics.* 2001;24: 24.

21. Brick G, Scott RD. The patellofemoral component of total knee arthroplasty. *Clin Orthop.* 1998;231:163–178.

22. Boyd A, Ewald F, et al. Long-term complications after total knee arthroplasty with or without resurfacing the patella. *J Bone Joint Surg.* 1993;75(A)5:674–681.

23. Grace JN, Sim FH. Fracture of the patella after total knee arthroplasty. *Clin Orthop.* 1988;230:168–175.

24. Cameron HU, et al. The patella in total knee arthroplasty. *Clin Orthop.* 1982;165:197–199.

25. Reuben JD, et al. Effect of patella thickness on patella strain following total knee arthroplasty. *J Arthroplasty.* 1991;6: 251–258.

26. Rae PJ, et al. Patellar resurfacing in total condylar knee arthroplasty. technique and results. *J Arthroplasty.* 1990;5: 259–265.

27. Shoji H, Shimozaki E. Patellar clunk syndrome in total knee arthroplasty without patellar resurfacing. *J Arthroplasty.* 1996;11:198–201.

28. Beight JL, et al. The patellar clunk syndrome after posterior stabilized total knee arthroplasty. *Clin Orthop.* 1994;299: 139–142.

29. Markel J, et al. Arthroscopic treatment of peripatellar fibrosis after total knee arthroplasty. *J Arthroplasty.* 1996;11(3): 293–297.

30. Pollock DC, Ammeen DJ, Engh G. Synovial entrapment: a complication of posterior stabilized total knee arthroplasty. *J Bone Joint Surg.* 2002;84:2174–2178.

31. Sharkey PF, Hozack WJ, et al. Why are total knee arthroplasties failing today? *Clin Orthop.* 2002;404:7–13.

32. Peters PC, Engh GA, et al. Osteolysis after total knee arthroplasty without cement. *J Bone Joint Surg.* 1992;74-A(6): 864–876.

33. Fehring TK, McAvoy G. Flouroscopic evaluation of the painful total knee arthroplasty. *Clin Orthop.* 1996;331: 226–233.

34. Engh GA, et al. Clinical Results of Polyethylene exchange with retention of total knee arthroplasty components. *J Bone Joint Surg.* 2000;82A(4):516–523.

35. Cameron HU, Hunter GA. Failure in total knee arthroplasty: mechanisms, revisions, and results. *Clin Orthop.* 2000;170:141–146.

36. Haas SB, Insall JN, et al. Revision total knee arthroplasty with modular components with stems inserted without cement. *J Bone Joint Surg.* 1995;77A:1700–1707.

37. Diduch DR, Insall JN, Scott WN, et al. Total knee replacement in young active patients: long term follow-up and functional outcome. *J Bone Joint Surg.* 1997;79A:575–582.

38. Brooks HD, Fehring TK. Polyethylene exchange only for prosthetic knee instability. *Clin Orthop.* 2002;405:182–188.

39. Pagnano MW, Hanssen AD, et al. Flexion instability after primary posterior cruciate retaining total knee arthroplasty. *Clin Orthop.* 1998;356:39–46.

40. Laubenthal KN, et al. A quantitative analysis of knee motion during activities of daily living. *Phys Ther.* 1972; 52:34–43.

41. Bocell JR, Thorpe CD, et al. Arthroscopic treatment of symptomatic total knee arthroplasty. *Clin Orthop.* 1991; 271:125–134.

42. Ries MD, Badalamente M. Arthrofibrosis after total knee arthroplasty. *Clin Orthop.* 2000;380:177–183.

43. Christensen CP, et al. Revision of the stiff total knee arthroplasty. *J Arthroplasty.* 2002;17(4):409–415.

44. Minas T. Personal communication.

45. Kindsfater K, Scott R. Recurrent hemarthrosis after total knee arthroplasty. *J Arthroplasty.* 1995;10(suppl):S52–S55.

46. Allardyce TJ, Scuderi GR, Insall JN. Arthroscopic treatment of popliteus tendon dysfunction following total knee arthroplasty. *J Arthoplasty.* 1997;12(3) 353–355.

47. Barnes CL, Scott RD. Popliteus tendon dysfunction following total knee arthroplasty. *J Arthroplasty.* 1995;10(4): 543–545.

48. Horner G, Dellon L. Innervation of the human knee joint and implications for surgery. *Clin Orthop.* 1994;301: 221–226.

49. Dellon L, Mont M, et al. Partial denervation for persistent neuroma pain around knee. *Clin Orthop.* 1996;329: 216–222.

50. Harwin SF, et al. Heterotopic ossification following primary total knee arthroplasty. *J Arthoplasty.* 1993;8:113–116.

51. Rader CP, et al. Heterotopic ossification after total knee arthroplasty. *Acta Orthop Scand.* 1997;68:46.

52. Barrack RL, et al. Heterotopic ossification after revision total knee arthroplasty. *Clin Orthop.* 2002;404:208–213.

53. Chidel MA, et al. Radiation prophylaxis for heterotopic ossification of the knee. *J Arthroplasty.* 2001;16(1):1–6.

54. Katz MM, Hungerford DS. Reflex sympathetic dystrophy affecting the knee. *J Bone Joint Surg.* 1987;69B(5)797–803.

55. Cooper DE, DeLee JC. Reflex sympathetic dystrophy of the knee. *J Am Acad Orthop Surg.* 1994;2:79–86.

CHAPTER 4

Radiological Evaluation of Total Knee Arthroplasty

David A. Feiock, Joel S. Newman, and Arthur H. Newberg

Total knee arthroplasty (TKA) is a remarkably successful procedure. Good and excellent outcomes in greater than 90% of patients have been reported from many independent centers at long-term follow-up, and long-term prosthesis survival rates are greater than 90%.[1] Although surgical techniques and implant designs continue to improve, the potential for complications will remain. As TKAs become more common in an aging population, and as implant survival rates increase, the prevalence of patients with TKAs is rising. Due to all of these factors, the number of patients requiring imaging evaluation of their TKAs will also continue to increase.

Diagnostic imaging plays a vital role in the diagnosis and management of complications of TKA. Loosening and infection are the most troublesome complications of TKA, but several other conditions, such as component malposition, polyethylene wear, particle disease/osteolysis, periprosthetic fractures, bursitis, and tendon pathology may also result in hardware failure and/or pain. Conventional radiography can detect many of the potential complications. Arthrography remains a valuable tool, especially when paired with aspiration. Although the metal hardware of TKA presents special challenges for the more *advanced* imaging techniques of computed tomography (CT) and magnetic resonance imaging (MRI), strides that have been made in recent years in reducing artifacts have allowed both modalities to make important contributions on the evaluation of TKA. Nuclear medicine studies can also provide valuable information. Most recently, FDG PET imaging has shown promise in the evaluation of patients with orthopedic hardware.[2,3] The following discussion of the imaging of the total knee arthroplasty first gives an overview of the imaging techniques available, then covers the imaging findings of each of the potential TKA complications.

TECHNIQUES AND MODALITIES

A host of imaging techniques has been employed for the evaluation of the symptomatic TKA, including conventional radiography, fluoroscopy with or without arthrography, several types of nuclear medicine studies, ultrasound, CT, and MRI. The fact that such an array of modalities is currently used is indicative of the imaging challenges presented by TKA. There is no single ideal imaging study for the symptomatic TKA. Each of these modalities has been shown to have significant limitations, and thus they are often used in conjunction with each other to increase overall sensitivity and specificity. Significant advances have been made in recent years with several of the modalities, offering hope for improved detection of complications.

Radiography

Conventional radiography is the first-line imaging study in the evaluation of the symptomatic TKA. The American College of Radiology Appropriateness Criteria for the Evaluation of the Patient with Painful Hip or Knee Arthroplasty (1999) gives conventional radiographs (with comparison to prior studies) the highest possible appropriateness rating.[4] Radiographs offer an informative, quick, and relatively inexpensive method of evaluation of both the prosthetic components and the native bone. Radiographs are limited, however, by their 2-dimensional nature and by their inability to depict most soft tissue pathologies.

A portable AP radiograph of the knee may be obtained in the recovery room immediately after surgery. AP supine and/or standing, lateral, and tangential patellar views are obtained routinely before the patient is discharged or within 3 months of the surgery. This series serves as a baseline to which future studies can be compared. The weightbearing/standing views are necessary to assess true osseous alignment. Some authors stress the importance of using long films that include the femoral head and ankle to accurately measure the lower extremity's axial alignment. Others have found the differences in measurements between long and short films to be insignificant. The use of long films is probably most important in patients who have bowed tibias or femurs.[5]

The ability to accurately measure alignment in TKAs is compromised by variability introduced by differences in limb positioning. Limb rotation and knee flexion have been shown to have a significant effect on measured values of anatomic alignment of TKAs on radiographs. External rotation simulates decreased tibiofemoral valgus, while internal rotation simulates increased tibiofemoral valgus. Knee flexion significantly increases apparent anatomic valgus with progressive internal rotation, but does not have an effect when the knee is externally rotated. The apparent tibial axis also varies significantly with internal and external rotation, but is not affected by flexion.[5]

Fluoroscopy

Fluoroscopic assessment is a relatively quick and inexpensive means for evaluation of the TKA. Fluoroscopy allows real-time dynamic assessment of the TKA, is helpful in guiding aspiration, and is the means by which conventional arthrography is performed. Fluoroscopy can be used as a guide for obtaining radiographs. Since very small degrees of obliquity can obscure radiolucent lines adjacent to prostheses, fluoroscopy is useful as a method by which one can obtain radiographs in which each interface of the TKA is well visualized.[6] As with conventional radiography, fluoroscopy is limited in its ability to depict soft tissue pathology.

Arthrography and Aspiration

The procedure for aspiration and arthrography of the TKA is relatively straightforward. In our institution, a medial parapatellar approach is preferred. The anterior aspect of the knee is prepped and draped in the standard sterile fashion, and the skin and subcutaneous tissues over the medial aspect of the patellofemoral joint are anesthetized with a few milliliters of an 80:20 mixture of 1% lidocaine and 8.4% sodium bicarbonate. A 22-gauge, 1.5-inch needle is advanced into the superomedial aspect of the patellofemoral joint space at a roughly 45- to 60-degree angle. Fluoroscopy is of little use in the placement of the needle, as the needle tip is generally obscured by the metallic hardware. A superolateral approach is preferred by some, though the lateral facet is longer than the

medial and is oriented more parallel to the femur. In all cases, fluid is aspirated and is sent to the laboratory for aerobic and anaerobic cultures and sensitivities, Gram's stain, and cell count.

Knees with joint prostheses generally contain enough fluid that aspiration of fluid is not difficult. However, if fluid cannot be readily aspirated, contrast material may be injected into the joint and reaspirated. It is important that contrast without bacteriostatic properties (e.g. Diatrizoate Meglumine USP 60% (Reno-60), Bracco Diagnostics, Princeton, NJ) be used for this purpose, to avoid false-negative culture results.

If arthrographic assessment of the TKA is desired, scout fluoroscopic spot images in AP and lateral projections are obtained before injection of contrast to provide a baseline. Extension tubing is attached to the 22-gauge needle, and a small test injection of 1 to 2 mL of iodinated contrast material is performed under fluoroscopy to confirm intra-articular positioning. (The contrast should flow freely away from the needle, rather than pooling at the tip.) As the knee joint is voluminous compared with other joints, at least 20 mL of contrast should be injected. The knee should then be moved passively through a range of motion to ensure contrast material spreads throughout all joint recesses. During this manipulation, the operator should watch for motion of the prosthetic components within the native bone. An AP image of the knee should be obtained with the tibial tray in tangent, and a lateral image should be obtained with the prosthesis in profile. The patient is then asked to walk for several minutes to increase the likelihood of contrast extending around the prosthetic components into areas of potential loosening. AP, lateral, and patellar conventional radiographs are then performed.

Nuclear Medicine

Scintigraphic evaluation of orthopedic implants is commonly performed to investigate suspected postoperative complications, especially loosening and infection. Nuclear medicine studies reflect physiologic changes rather than anatomic changes. They are generally more sensitive than conventional radiographs, and the presence of orthopedic hardware is not a limitation. Low specificity is inherent in nuclear medicine studies, but recent innovations are showing promise for improvements in this area.

Bone scans are performed with intravenous injection of technetium (Tc) 99m-labeled diphosphonate. In the setting of orthopedic hardware such as a TKA, triple-phase bone scans are employed, as specificities are higher than single-phase. In phase 1, known as the *blood-flow* phase, images are acquired every 2 to 5 seconds for the first 60 seconds after bolus injection of the radiotracer.

This phase displays the vascular delivery of radiotracer to the area of the TKA. In phase 2, called the *blood-pool* phase, an image is obtained over a 5-minute period (or for a certain number of counts, usually 200000 to 300000), starting 1 minute after the injection. This phase depicts a combination of vascular flow and tissue extraction and distribution. In both the blood-flow and blood-pool phases, both knees should always be imaged, so that the symptomatic and asymptomatic sides can be compared. In the third (*delayed*) phase, images are acquired 2 to 4 hours after injection. This phase depicts the retention of radiotracer in bone due to chemisorption, and thus depicts osteoblastic activity. Osteoblasts assemble labeled diphosphonates into the hydration shell of hydroxyapatite crystals as they are formed and modified.[7] Thus, any cause of accelerated new bone formation may result in increased periprosthetic uptake in this phase.

One approach employed to improve specificity is to perform simultaneous bone scans and nuclear arthrograms. Immediately after the delayed-phase bone scan images are obtained, Indium (In)-111 or Tc-99m sulfur colloid (mixed with iodinated contrast) is injected into the joint. Flow of the radiotracer around the arthroplasty components is indicative of loosening.

Gallium scans may also be used in the evaluation of TKAs, most commonly sequentially with bone scans to increase specificity. Gallium localizes to sites of inflammation of all types, including infection. Localization at sites of inflammation is a function of uptake in leukocytes and possibly bacteria, transferrin and lactoferrin binding, and abnormal vascular permeability. One drawback is that scanning is usually not performed until at least 24 to 48 hours after injection.[8]

The white blood cell (WBC) scan theoretically increases specificity for infection in that white blood cells should only accumulate at sites of inflammation caused by infection. Thus, WBC scans are often performed after a positive triple-phase bone scan to rule out infection as the cause of the abnormal uptake around the TKA on bone scan. WBC scans are difficult to perform, however, in that they involve a tedious, expensive radiopharmaceutical preparation process, a long delay time before imaging if In-111 is used (18 to 24 hours), and poor count rates that result in low-resolution images. White blood cells can be labeled with either In-111 or Tc-99m HMPAO. Tc-99m HMPAO is advantageous in that it is cheaper and allows more rapid imaging (2 hours following injection).

Interpretation of WBC scans is complicated by the fact that WBCs also accumulate in reticuloendothelial cells of normal hematopoetic marrow. In adults, hematopoietic marrow is usually not present to any significant degree around the knees. However, trauma and joint replacement surgery can prompt conversion of fatty marrow to hematopoietic marrow, which results in increased "abnormal" uptake on WBC scans. In order to deal with this problem, a Tc-99m sulfur colloid marrow study may be performed immediately following the WBC scan. The Tc-99m sulfur colloid is taken up in normal hematopoetic marrow. Thus, uptake of labeled WBCs around the TKA due to infection can be distinguished from uptake in normal hematopoetic marrow. The Tc-99m sulfur colloid study adds little expense or time, with images obtained only 10 min after injection.[8]

Currently, in many institutions, the following sequence of studies for scintigraphic evaluation of the symptomatic TKA is preferred. First a triple-phase bone scan is performed. If this shows abnormal uptake, then a Tc 99m HMPAO WBC scan is performed. If this in turn shows abnormal uptake, a Tc 99m sulfur colloid marrow scan is performed. In some institutions, however, practitioners prefer to skip the bone scan and go straight to the WBC scan/sulfur colloid marrow scan combination.

Recent data show that positron emission tomography (PET) with fluorine-18 labeled fluorodeoxyglucose (FDG) is useful for the detection of musculoskeletal infections,[2] even in trauma patients with metallic implants.[3] It is unclear how effectively PET distinguishes infection from noninfectious inflammation around prosthetic joints. Patients must fast for at least 6 hours before the study, and blood glucose levels must be checked before injection. Scanning takes 15 to 60 minutes, depending on the size of the area being scanned, and is generally performed 1 hour after injection. Attenuation correction is helpful in limiting artifacts.

Ultrasound

Ultrasound (US) has the advantage over radiographs, fluoroscopy, and scintigraphy of being able to directly evaluate soft tissue structures. Additionally, artifacts caused by metallic hardware are less pronounced than on CT and MRI images and are generally limited to the area deep to the hardware producing the artifact. US is also advantageous in that it allows real-time dynamic evaluation of moving structures such as muscles, tendons, and joints. Color and power Doppler sonography allow evaluation of tissue vascularity.

The development of high-frequency transducers allows for detailed evaluation of tendons, ligaments, and muscles. In-plane resolutions of 200 to 400 micrometers and slice thickness of 0.5 to 1.0 mm can be achieved.[9] It is important to select the proper transducer that optimizes resolution while enabling sufficient depth penetration. Lower-frequency transducers have poorer resolution but allow for scanning of deeper tissues, while higher-frequency transducers have better resolution but poorer penetration and thus are limited to evaluation of more superficial tissues. To illustrate this point, in the setting of a TKA, a high-frequency transducer (10 MHz or greater) should be use to evaluate the patellar or quadriceps tendons, while a lower-frequency transducer (7 MHz or lower) should be used to search for fluid collections deep in the calf or thigh, especially in a large patient.[9]

It is possible to evaluate the intra-articular structures of a TKA with US. Bone, metal, polyethylene, and joint fluid each have characteristic ultrasound appearances.[10] Where the modality really excels, however, is in the evaluation of periarticular soft tissues. US is also excellent for detecting effusions and extra-articular fluid collections such as abscesses and bursitis. Because it allows real-time, dynamic imaging, US is ideal for localization and guidance of needle placement during aspiration of fluid collections, and also during biopsies of synovium and soft tissue masses. Also, symptomatic popliteal cysts in patients with TKAs may be aspirated under US guidance. Extended-field-of-view imaging is a newer function that allows imaging over a large anatomic region, which is advantageous in the evaluation of a total joint replacement.[10]

Computed Tomography

Although computed tomography (CT) shares with conventional radiography and fluoroscopy the same basic physics of detection of x-rays transmitted through a patient, CT is much more sensitive to small differences in densities of tissues. Thus, it depicts soft tissues as well as bone much more effectively. CT also allows for evaluation of structures in 3 dimensions through acquisition of numerous thin contiguous slices. Through reformatting, which has been hugely improved by the advent of first helical CT then multidetector CT, it is possible to produce images in any plane desired that are of a quality equal or nearly equal to the images in the plane of original acquisition.

In the past, CT was considered to be of limited utility in the setting of metallic orthopedic hardware. This is due to the *beam-hardening* star artifacts produced when the metal severely attenuates the x-ray beam, resulting in incomplete projection data. As CT hardware has improved (primarily in the form of multidetector CT) and as reformatting software has also been perfected, it has become possible to substantially minimize these artifacts.

Multidetector CT (MDCT) allows for the use of very high photon techniques, which helps to overcome the severe attenuation of the x-ray beam by the metal. Also, very thin overlapping slices can be obtained and reconstructed into thicker slices. The process of reformatting (typically producing sagittal or coronal images from the original axial data), which is greatly facilitated by MDCT, also results in reduction in the metal artifact. The "soft tissue" or smooth reconstruction filter (rather than the typical "bone" or edge-enhancing filter) and wide windows (3000 to 4000 Houndsfield units) when viewing images also serves to diminish metal artifacts. The increasing use of titanium in orthopedic implants has been helpful, too, because titanium has a relatively low x-ray attenuation coefficient, which results in less beam-hardening artifact.[11] Unicondylar prostheses are particularly amenable to evaluation by CT, as the lesser volume of metal results in less artifact than does the greater volume of metal in a TKA.

One important drawback of CT is the relatively high radiation dose to the patient. Doses are generally increased with the MDCT techniques designed to reduce metal artifacts. This is somewhat offset by the fact that the tissues in the extremities are relatively insensitive to radiation, and the dosage to more radiation-sensitive central organs from scattered radiation during an extremity CT is quite small. Nevertheless, caution should be exercised in using these techniques on younger patients and on anatomy nearer to radiosensitive organs (i.e., a scan of the hips, in which the gonads and axial skeleton could receive significant radiation).

Berger and Rubash have described a CT protocol for evaluation of component malrotation prior to revision surgery.[12] The patient is positioned supine, with the knee in full extension. The scan plane is perpendicular to the mechanical axis of the knee, as determined by an AP scout view. Then, a lateral scout view is obtained, and scanning is performed perpendicular to the long axis of the femur, then perpendicular to the long axis of the tibia (achieved by tilting the gantry). Next, 1.5-mm-thick slices are obtained at 4 locations: through the epicondylar axis of the femur, through the tibial tubercle, through the top of the tibial plateau, and through the tibial component itself. The rotation of the femoral component is determined by measuring the posterior condylar angle (the angle subtended by the surgical epicondylar axis and the posterior condylar line). The rotation of the tibial component is measured by comparing the AP axis of the tibial plateau with the position of the tibial tubercle.

CT Arthrography

At our institution, it is becoming more and more common to evaluate TKAs with the combination of a conventional aspiration arthrogram with computed tomography. Joint aspiration and intra-articular contrast administration are performed under fluoroscopy, and then the patient is sent immediately to the CT scanner. Metal artifact reduction techniques and multiplanar reformatting are used. Although this technique is not yet

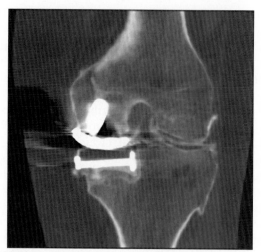

FIGURE 4-1. CT Arthrogram of a knee with a medial unicondylar prosthesis. Note the minimal artifact produced by the metallic hardware on this reformatted image in the coronal plane. This technique affords excellent visualization of the bone beneath the metal components, as well as the native lateral compartment. Note the clearly defined intact body of the lateral meniscus. A small region of osteolysis is evident in the medial femoral condyle. The vague linear lucency beneath the tibial tray is nonspecific, as no contrast tracks into it.

well studied, it seems likely that CT arthrography will eventually be proven to be significantly more sensitive and specific for loosening and osteolysis than conventional arthrography alone (Figure 4-1).

Magnetic Resonance Imaging

In the past, MRI was considered to be of little value in patients with metallic implants. This is because of the severe artifacts that are produced by metals with ferromagnetic properties, of which most orthopedic implants have consisted in the past. Significant strides have been made in recent years in reducing these artifacts, so that MRI in patients with orthopedic implants such as TKAs is now more useful. Knees with unicondylar prostheses are particularly amenable to evaluation by MRI, as the smaller volume of metal results in less artifact than in a TKA, and the structures of the native compartments of the joint are readily evaluated.

MRI differs from radiography, fluoroscopy, and CT in that it does not involve ionizing radiation. Instead, it employs a very strong magnetic field and radiofrequency signals to produce images. Radiofrequency waves are a type of electromagnetic radiation, but because they are of an energy that does not result in ionization, they do not have the harmful effects of x-rays.

MRI shares with CT the advantage of being able to depict structures in 3 dimensions via acquisition of thin

contiguous slices. With MRI, however, it is possible to produce images of the same quality in virtually any plane. Perhaps the greatest advantage of MRI is the much greater contrast that can be obtained between different types of soft tissues than can be obtained with CT. It is because of this advantage in contrast resolution that MRI is generally much better than CT at depicting the anatomy of musculoskeletal soft tissue structures and is generally much more sensitive to soft tissue pathologies than CT. One caveat is that cortical bone and soft tissue calcifications are better evaluated by CT than by MRI because they contain essentially no hydrogen atoms that can be magnetized. Also, CT can achieve better spatial resolution than MRI, which is also advantageous in the evaluation of small calcifications and fine osseous detail.

Several strategies have been developed in recent years to minimize artifacts from metallic implants, resulting in improved depiction of the periprosthetic structures. These include relatively minor changes to imaging sequences on commercially available MR software such as orienting the frequency-encoding gradient along the long axis of the prosthesis, using fast spin-echo sequences, using three-dimensional acquisitions and thin sections, using high image matrix size (e.g. 512×512) increasing receiver bandwidth, and reducing interecho spacing. Use of inversion recovery fat suppression (STIR) results in less artifact than frequency-selective fat suppression.[11,13,14]

These improvements allow the routine visualization of both intracapsular and extracapsular components of joint arthroplasty.[13] Sofka, Potter, and Figge have shown the usefulness of MRI in influencing clinical management of patients with painful TKA by revealing tendon tears, polyethylene granulomatosis, ligament tears, and unexpected inflammatory synovitis in patients with normal radiographs.[15] Olsen et al. have developed a metal artifact reduction sequence (MARS) that uses some of the previously described techniques as well as *view angle tilting* to significantly improve visualization of periprosthetic bone and soft tissue structures in TKA patients. This is achieved without an increase in imaging time.[16] These advantages do not imply that MRI should replace radiographs as the first-line modality for imaging of the symptomatic TKA. Rather, MRI is now a much more helpful second- or third-line modality to be used when radiographs are negative or have findings of uncertain significance. Also, it should be emphasized that these artifact reduction techniques do not allow evaluation of the metallic components themselves, but rather allow improved evaluation of the soft tissues and bone marrow adjacent to the prostheses.

RADIOLOGICAL FINDINGS OF TKA COMPLICATIONS

Instability (Joint)

Asymmetric widening of the prosthetic joint space suggests ligamentous imbalance and varus-valgus instability.[17] Flexion instability in the anterior-posterior plane can result in acute posterior dislocation (Figure 4-2), which is more common in posterior stabilized prostheses.[1] Symptomatic instability occurs in less than 1% to 2% of patients after primary TKA, but it is one of the more frequent underlying causes of failure, accounting for 10% to 20% of all revisions.[1]

Component Malposition/Malalignment

Evaluation of TKA alignment is important because of the direct relationships between malalignment, loosening, and instability. Both implant alignment and bony alignment must be evaluated to distinguish ligamentous instability from implant malpositioning. This is generally done with weightbearing radiographs.

The mechanical axis should pass through the center or just medial to the center of the prosthetic knee with both components perpendicular to it. The femoral com-

ponent should be within 4 to 11 degrees of valgus, with 7 degrees generally optimal.[1,17–19] On the lateral view, the posterior flange of the femoral component should be parallel or nearly parallel to the long axis of the femur and the femoral component outline should match the outline of the original bone.[17,18] Notching of the anterior femoral cortex can be seen when the femoral component is undersized. This predisposes to fracture. The posterior aspect of the anterior flange should be parallel to and flush with the anterior femoral cortex.[17]

The tibial prosthesis should be aligned perpendicular to the tibial shaft on the AP view. Varus malalignment of the tibial component has been identified as a risk factor for prosthesis loosening.[1] On the lateral view, the position of the tibial component should be either central or posterior relative to the center of the tibial shaft. The plateau should be parallel to the ground or slope downward no more than 10 degrees on the lateral view.[17,18] Overhang of the tibial component can result in bursitis, especially anteriorly.[17]

It has been reported that optimal TKA results are achieved when the joint line is altered 8 mm or less and the patellar height (as measured from the distal point on the femoral articular surface to the inferior pole) is 10 to 30 mm.[18,20] The AP thickness of the patellar implant should not exceed the thickness of the original patella, as increased retinacular pressure may lead to pain and maltracking. Patellar tracking can be grossly assessed on tangential patellar views with the knee in 30 to 40 degrees of flexion.[17] On this view, patellar tilt is assessed as the angle between a line along the anterior aspect of the femoral condyles and a line along the patellar component cement-bone interface.

Component malrotation can lead to rotational instability.[12] Berger and Rubash describe a method of evaluating component malrotation prior to revision surgery using CT. The rotation of the femoral component is evaluated using the posterior condylar angle. The normal posterior condylar angle for men is 0.3 degrees (+/− 1.2 degrees) and 3.5 degrees (+/− 1.2 degrees) for women. The rotation of the tibial component is determined using the tibial tubercle orientation. The normal rotation value for the tibial component is 18 degrees (+/− 2.6 degrees) of internal rotation from the tip of the tibial tubercle. When femoral and tibial rotations were combined, patients without patellofemoral symptoms all had TKAs with mild degrees of combined external rotation (0 to 10 degrees), while patients with patellofemoral problems all had TKAs with combined internal rotation. The degree of internal rotation correlated directly with the severity of patellofemoral complication.[12]

FIGURE 4-2. Tibiofemoral dislocation. Lateral radiograph shows posterior tibial dislocation.

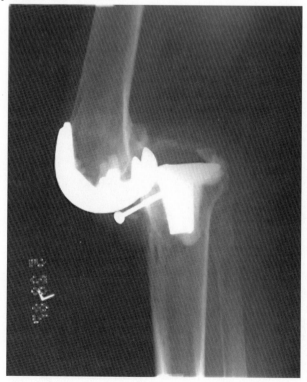

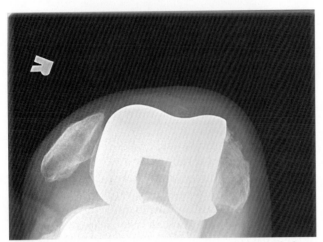

FIGURE 4-3. Patellar dislocation. *Sunrise view* radiograph shows lateral dislocation of a nonresurfaced patella.

Extensor Mechanism Complications

Patellofemoral complications are the most common postoperative problems associated with the current generation of TKAs and are the most common reason for revision surgery.[12] Patellar tilt and patellar subluxation are commonly seen on tangential (*sunrise*) views. These findings are often due to a tight lateral retinaculum, but a search should also be made for radiographic clues indicating component malrotation, valgus alignment, or oversizing of either the femoral or tibial component in the AP dimension—all of which can also lead to patellar tilt, subluxation, and even dislocation (Figure 4-3). Patellar tilt and subluxation also tend to result in more rapid polyethylene wear, which can lead to particle disease and even metallosis if the components are metal backed.[17]

The polyethylene portion of the patellar component has been reported to come loose from its metal backing. The dense synovial linear opacities of metallosis may be apparent in this situation.[21] The radiolucent polyethylene component often is displaced inferiorly into the region of Hoffa's fat pad, but may be difficult to identify on routine radiographs. Adequate visualization may require soft tissue radiographic techniques, CT, or arthrography[21] (See Figure 4-4). Displacement of the metal backing and polyethylene together, which results from fracture of fixation pegs,[17,18] is easily identified. A displaced patellar component may result in abrasion and rupture of the quadriceps or patellar tendons.[18]

FIGURE 4-4. Patellar component dislocation. (A) Lateral radiograph (-) lucent polyethylene component with its dense metallic backing displaced into the suprapatellar pouch. (B) Lateral view from air arthrogram better displays the dislocated component and confirms its intra-articular position. Air was used as a contrast agent due to the patient's history of severe allergic reaction to iodinated contrast.

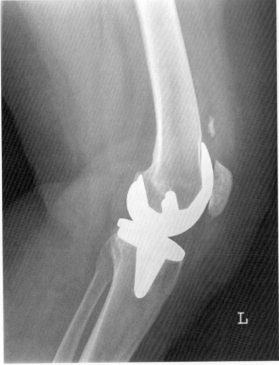

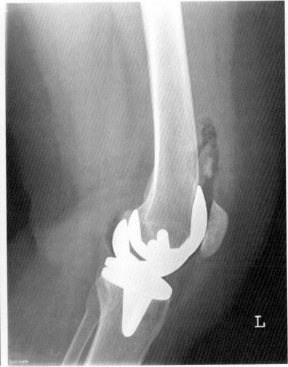

A   B

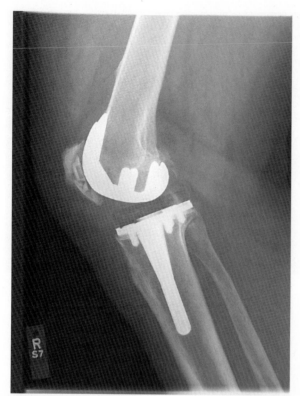

FIGURE 4-5. Patellar fracture. Lateral radiograph shows slightly displaced transverse fracture through the midpatella.

Patellar stress fractures are not uncommon,[18] as the process of patellar resurfacing results in a thinned patella that may be devascularized and that has stress risers in peg holes[21] (Figure 4-5). Patellar component fractures may also be seen. These occur almost exclusively in metal-backed protheses.[18]

Rupture of the quadriceps or patellar tendon results in abnormal position of the patella (low and high, respectively) and localized soft tissue swelling with obscuration of fat planes. A wavy or buckled appearance of the soft tissues in the region of the tendon is sometimes seen. An abnormally low patella (patella infera) can also occur with an intact quadriceps tendon after TKA, due to fibrosis and scar contracture in Hoffa's fat pad. An abnormally high patella (patella alta) with an intact patellar tendon is much less likely. [17]

Stress Shielding

Ideally, a prosthetic joint component would carry stress and distribute it to the underlying bone in a manner identical to the original bone. The mechanical properties of the prosthetic components are different than the original bone, however, resulting in altered distribution of forces to underlying bone. Bone is formed and retained along the lines of stress in that bone. Thus, bone resorption

occurs in areas that no longer receive as much stress after joint replacement. This is called *stress shielding*. On radiographs, this is evident as rarefaction of trabeculae, or localized osteopenia. This must be differentiated from osteolysis, which causes focal complete destruction of bone. Progressive bone loss due to stress shielding is one of the primary causes of loosening and one of the limiting factors in the life span of a joint prosthesis. Stress shielding occurs in all knees in which the femoral component has an anterior femoral flange.[19]

Polyethylene Wear

The posteromedial aspect of the tibial component and the patellar component are most frequently involved in polyethylene wear,[17] which is most prevalent in prostheses with metal backing.[17,18] Wear should be suspected when radiographs show narrowing of prosthetic joint spaces on weightbearing views. When wear is asymmetric, varus or valgus deformity or patellar tilt results. Polyethylene fragments may be shed into the joint. It is important to look for loose intra-articular, porous-coating beads on radiographs, because they can lead to an accelerated type of wear, called *third-body wear*. Annual weightbearing films are recommended to detect subclinical wear in TKAs, especially for prostheses with metal backing.[17] Early detection may allow simple exchange of the polyethylene liner before irreversible damage to the metal tray occurs.[22]

Using ultrasound, it is possible to detect polyethylene wear directly by measuring the thickness of the polyethylene tibial tray.[23] The joint effusion and synovitis that can result from polyethylene wear are also detectable with ultrasound. The effusion appears completely black (hypoechoic), while synovitis is manifested as fronds or nodules of intermediate echogenicity projecting into the joint fluid. This is most readily visualized in the suprapatellar pouch.[10] It is also possible to directly evaluate the tibial tray with ultrasound, enabling detection of polyethylene wear and the fractures of the tray that can result.[10]

Particle Disease/Osteolysis

Osteolysis is a general term that simply means destruction of bone. In the setting of joint replacement, however, the term is used more specifically to describe bone destruction due to the presence of particulate debris, and is thus also called *particle disease*. Sources of particles are polyethylene surface wear, cement, and metal.[19] Debris of a critical size triggers an inflammatory reaction with macrophages and foreign body giant cells, which results in osteolysis. When severe, the loss of bone from osteolysis can result in component loosening.

Osteolysis is manifested on radiographs and on CT as focal periprosthetic areas of marked lucency due to com-

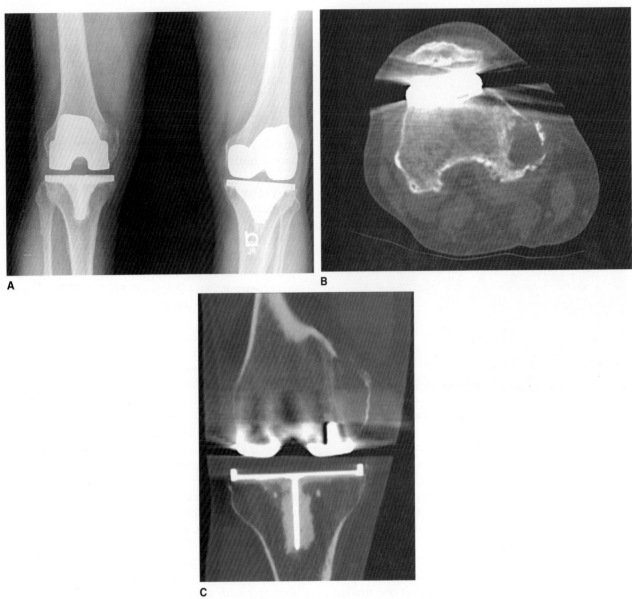

FIGURE 4-6. Osteolysis. (A) AP standing radiograph of both knees shows a focal, well-defined region of lucency/bone destruction in the medial femoral condyle, with an apparent break in the overlying cortex suggesting a pathologic fracture. (B and C) Axial and coronal reformatted CT images allow determination of the volume of osteolysis and confirm the presence of a pathologic fracture. Note the minimal artifact produced by the metallic hardware on this multidetector study using artifact reduction techniques.

plete loss of trabeculae (Figure 4-6). The reduction in metal artifacts and the improved ability to reformat high-quality multiplanar images made possible by multidetector CT have resulted in CT becoming a valuable tool for the detection and quantification of osteolysis. Puri et al. showed helical CT with metal artifact minimization to be more sensitive than radiographs for identifying and quan-

tifying osteolysis after total hip arthroplasty.[24] Work by Seitz et al. indicates that CT is similarly advantageous in the evaluation of osteolysis in the knee.[25] On sonographic images, osteolysis can be appreciated as focal loss of the normal bright, hyperechoic line of cortical bone, with an underlying hypoechoic, cystlike erosion.[10] The MRI appearance of osteolysis has been described as focal periprosthetic intraosseous masses with low T1 signal and heterogeneous, predominantly low to intermediate T2 signal. With IV contrast, these masses show peripheral enhancement and some irregular internal enhancement.[14]

Metal Synovitis/Metallosis

Metallosis can occur in TKAs when the polyethylene separates from the metal backing of the patellar component.[19] Metallosis can also occur when polyethylene wear is so severe that there is metal-on-metal contact. A dense synovial *metal line* seen on radiographs is pathognomonic. A dense joint effusion and/or synovitis are always present (Figure 4-7).[17]

Quale et al. described 5 patients with titanium-induced arthropathy associated with polyethylene-metal separation after total joint replacement (3 hips, 2 knees). Radiographs revealed abnormal position of the metal components in all patients and opaque curvilinear peri-articular deposits in 4 of them. Arthropathy caused by deposition of small titanium particles from metal friction (in the absence of interposed polyethylene) was pathologically proven to correspond to the periarticular opacities.[21]

FIGURE 4-7. Metallosis. Lateral radiograph shows a very dense joint effusion, evident both in the suprapatellar pouch and posteriorly, in this knee with a unicondylar prosthesis. Note the markedly narrowed joint space and the jagged anterior edge of the tibial component, indicating severe polyethylene wear, component fracture, and metal-to-metal contact.

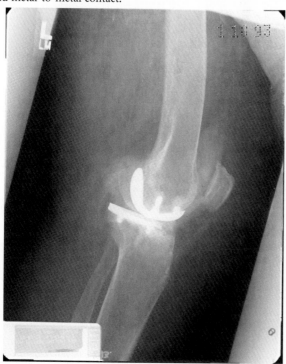

Infection

The rate of infection following primary total knee arthroplasty is between 0.5%[26] and 2% and increases to 5% after revision surgery.[27] Being able to differentiate loosening from infection is vitally important, since a noninfected prosthesis can be removed and replaced in a single procedure. A patient with an infected prosthesis must undergo several months of antibiotic therapy between resection of the prosthesis and revision.

Radiographs may be normal in the setting of infection. Alternatively, serial radiographs may demonstrate progressive periprosthetic radiolucency. Lucencies may also occur in the absence of infection and are often absent in the early stages of infection.[28] Extensive periosteal new bone formation and osteolysis are suggestive but not diagnostic of infection[17] (See Figure 4-8A).

Joint aspiration is the most useful confirmatory procedure. Sensitivity and specificity have been reported to be 67% and 95.6%, respectively—and even as high as 100% in a series of 43 knees reported by Duff et al.[29] Levitsky et al. concluded in 1991 that preoperative joint aspiration is the most useful single test in the workup of a painful total joint arthroplasty.[28] It should be noted, however, that the data from which this conclusion was drawn did not include comparison with the WBC scan–sulfur colloid marrow scan combination, which now shows the best accuracy of all radionuclide scans.

Arthrographic features that suggest infection include extension of contrast between the cement/bone or prosthetic/bone interface, filling of peri-articular cavities or sinus tracts, and lymphatic opacification[30] (Figures 4.9 and 4.10). It is important to be aware that tracking of contrast underneath the tibial tray can be seen as a *normal variant* and does not necessarily indicate loosening or infection. Tracking of contrast around the tibial pegs is always abnormal, however. Also important is that lymphatic opacification is not specific for loosening or infection, as it can occur in the setting of a small joint capacity and distension with contrast. Synovitis may also predispose to lymphatic opacification.[30]

Bone scan uptake patterns around knee prostheses are, unfortunately, more variable than those around hip prostheses. Many asymptomatic patients show persistent periprosthetic uptake for several years after TKR. The natural course of a TKA is to show mildly to moderately increased uptake for years, and normal scans are unusual.[8] Bone graft material may result in increased blastic activity and, thus, prolonged uptake on bone scans. Also, when infection is present, there is no diagnostic pattern of uptake.[31] If a bone scan is negative, infection can be confidently ruled out. For this reason, some believe that the bone scan is useful as an initial screening test, because of its high negative predictive value.

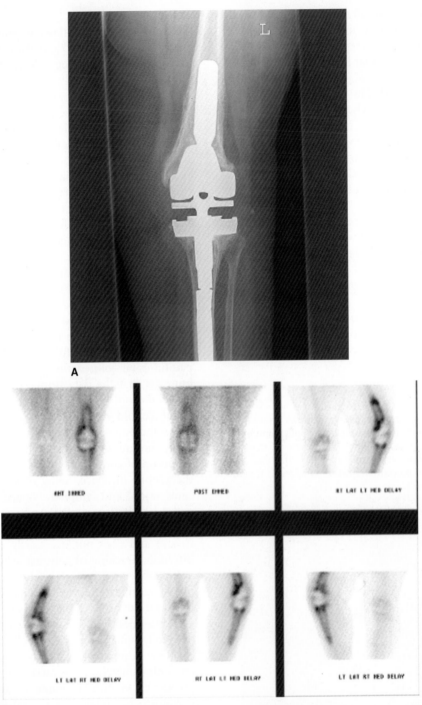

FIGURE 4-8. Chronic osteomyelitis. (A) AP radiograph of a revision TKA complicated by chronic osteomyelitis (culture-proven coagulase negative *Staphylococcus* infection). Note the wide lucencies at bone-metal interfaces about both the tibial and femoral components and also periostitis, which is most evident at the medial femoral metaphysis. (B–D) Three-phase bone scan of the same patient as in A. (B) anterior images of both knees from the first (blood flow) phase show diffusely increased activity about the left knee. (C) Anterior image of both knees from the second (blood pool) phase shows increased activity better localized to the bone of the tibia and femur about the prosthetic components. (D) Anterior whole body image from the third (delayed) phase shows well-defined intense activity in the same distribution as in the second phase.

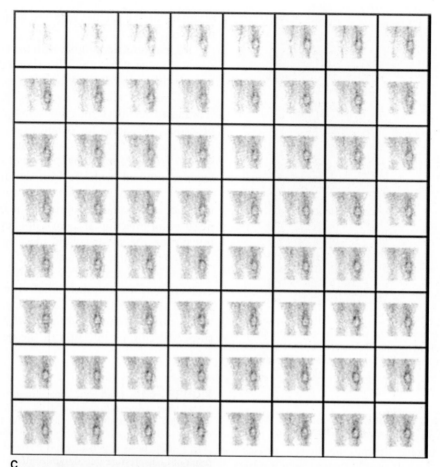

C

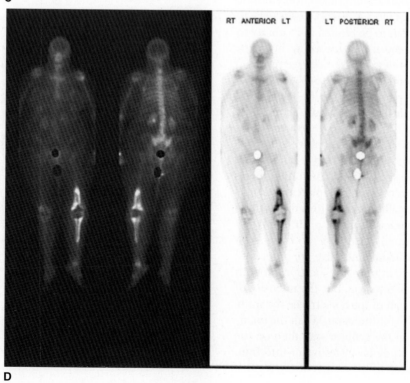

D

FIGURE 4-8. (continued)

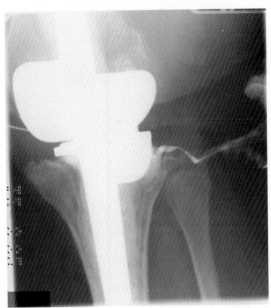

FIGURE 4-9. Infected TKA with sinus tract. AP oblique image from knee arthrogram shows a lateral sinus tract extending from the joint to the skin, opacified by contrast material introduced into the joint via a needle in the medial aspect of the patellofemoral compartment.

Three-phase bone scans should theoretically be more accurate than single-phase scans, as the hyperemia that produces increased uptake during the first 2 phases (blood-flow and blood-pool) should theoretically not be present in loosening (See Figures 4-8B–D). Levitsky et al. found the 3-phase bone scan to be limited in its ability to discern between infection and aseptic loosening, however, due to unacceptably high rates of false-negative results.[28] Accuracies for 3-phase bone scans are 50% to 70%.[31] Increased uptake in all 3 phases can also be seen in the setting of acute heterotopic bone formation, acute stress fractures, noninfectious inflammatory arthropathies, neuropathic arthropathy, and the reparative phase of avascular necrosis. Tonakie et al. state that 3-phase bone scans do little to improve the accuracy of routine bone scanning for diagnosing infected joint replacements.[8]

The combination of a gallium scan with a three-phase bone scan improves accuracy to 70% to 80%.[31] When gallium images are normal, regardless of bone scan uptake, the study is considered negative for infection. Similarly, if there is uptake in the same location on both the bone scan and the gallium scan, but the intensity of the gallium uptake is less that of the bone tracer, the study is considered to be negative for infection. When the intensity of uptake is greater on the gallium scan than on the bone scan, however, the study is suggestive of infection. The study is also considered to be positive if the regions of uptake on the gallium scan and bone scan are not spatially congruent.[31]

The radionuclide studies with the best-reported accuracies (75% to 95%) are WBC (labeled leukocyte) scans paired with either 3-phase bone scans or Tc-99m sulfur colloid marrow scans.[17] Love et al. stated in 2001 that "combined leukocyte-marrow scintigraphy remains the procedure of choice for diagnosis of the infected joint replacement."[31] They based this opinion on accuracies of 90% or greater reported by Palestro et al. for In-111 WBC scans combined with Tc-99m sulfur colloid marrow imaging.[32] When uptake on both studies is of similar intensity and spatially congruent, the study is considered negative for infection. If there is uptake on the WBC scan, but not on the sulfur colloid marrow scan, the study is considered positive for infection.[31]

FDG PET appears to be a promising technique for the evaluation of musculoskeletal infections. De Winter et al. in 2001 showed FDG PET to have sensitivity, specificity, and accuracy of 100%, 86%, and 93% for patients with suspected chronic infection of the peripheral skeleton.[2]

FIGURE 4-10. Lymphatic opacification. This lateral image from a knee arthrogram shows opacification of popliteal fossa lymphatics by contrast material injected into the joint space. This finding is suggestive of loosening and/or infection, but is nonspecific, as it can be seen with any type of synovitis and can also be the result of high-pressure injection of contrast into a joint with small capacity.

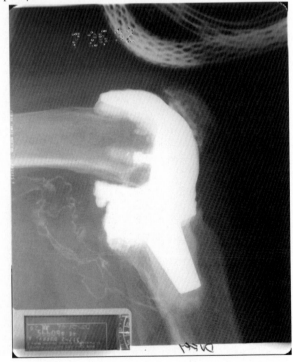

In a series of 22 patients with 29 metallic orthopedic implants for trauma (not joint replacements), Schiesser et al. demonstrated sensitivity, specificity, and accuracy of 100%, 93.3%, and 97%, respectively.[3] In the study by De Winter, FDG PET performed well in identifying infection in the small subgroup of patients with joint prostheses— 8 true-positive, 8 true-negative, and only one false-positive result. Of these 17 patients, seven had TKAs. The one false-positive result was in a TKA with aseptic loosening.[2] Other authors have found FDG PET to be disappointing in its ability to distinguish between aseptic loosening and infection.[31] Thus, further studies are necessary, but it is conceivable that FDG PET will play a significant role in the workup of the painful TKA in the future.

Ultrasound is useful when periarticular fluid collections are suspected as a manifestation of an infected prosthesis. Such collections will be completely black (hypoechoic) if simple, or of heterogeneous echogenicity if complex. Complex fluid collections can be differentiated from normal soft tissues by fluidlike motion of echoes when compression is applied and released with the transducer, and by mass effect on adjacent normal structures. It should be emphasized that although infected fluid collections tend to be complex, the fact that a collection is complex does not necessarily imply infection. Ultrasound is very useful in guiding percutaneous needle aspiration of fluid collections for decompression and for microbiological evaluation.

CT and MRI are also capable of depicting periprosthetic fluid collections, especially when metal artifact reduction techniques are used. Fluid collections that show a peripherally enhancing rim following intravenous contrast and that appear to communicate with the joint replacement are highly suspicious for infection, but cannot be differentiated from noninfected postsurgical collections in the recently postoperative period. It is technically more challenging to aspirate fluid collections under MRI guidance than under ultrasound guidance.

Loosening

TKA component loosening can occur as a consequence of bone loss from stress shielding. It can also occur due to infection or osteolysis from particulate debris. Some authors state that loosening in TKAs is most common in the femoral component,[33] while others[18,19] believe that it is more common on the tibial side. This discrepancy seems to be based on whether one considers subsidence to be a type of loosening. The tibial component often subsides, usually on the medial side, which results in a shift of the tibial component into varus angulation.[1,19] This is especially prevalent in uncemented tibial components.[17]

The fibular head can be used as a bony landmark to aid in detection of tibial component subsidence.

Radiographic criteria for loosening include a wide (greater than 2mm) or progressively enlarging cement-bone or metal-cement lucent line, component migration, collapse of underlying trabecular bone with subsidence of the component, cement fractures, and changes in the degree of knee angulation on weightbearing views[17,18] (Figures 4-11 and 4-12). It should be emphasized that a lucent zone of 1 to 2mm between cement and bone is considered normal and is likely due to contraction of the cement.[18,33] When a lucent line progressively widens on subsequent radiographs true loosening can be diagnosed.[33] With uncemented prostheses, the finding of displaced porous-coating beads (bead shedding) also indicates loosening.[17] Loosening is more difficult to detect in the femoral component, because on the AP view the component obscures the prosthetic-bone interfaces. The x-ray beam must be perpendicular to the cement-bone interface for the thin radiolucent lines to be detectable. Positioning is therefore crucial and some investigators have recommended the use of fluoroscopically guided

FIGURE 4-11. Loosening. Lateral radiograph shows a wide lucency surrounding the stem of the tibial component and borderline-width lucencies under the tibial tray. Note also the large joint effusion evident in the suprapatellar pouch and posteriorly. Cultures of aspirated joint fluid were negative.

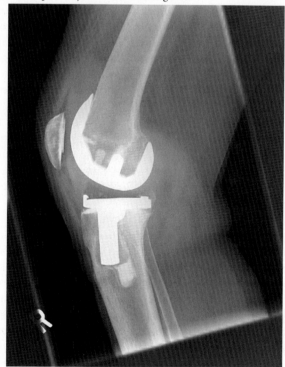

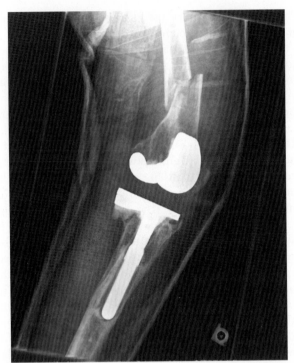

FIGURE 4-12. Periprosthetic fracture and loosening. AP radiograph shows an angulated, displaced fracture through the femoral metaphysis just proximal to the femoral component. Note also the wide lucencies about the stem and underneath the tray of the tibial component, indicative of loosening.

radiographs.[6] In both cemented and uncemented prostheses, the radiolucent zones are often bordered by a thin layer of lamellar bone resulting from stress remodeling. When this *neocortex* is absent, failure of the prosthesis is more likely.[17] The Knee Society Evaluation/Scoring Zone System may be used to describe, document, and follow periprosthetic radiolucent lines.[34]

Fluoroscopic push-pull maneuvers can be used to document gross loosening. In equivocal cases, arthrographic evaluation can be helpful. Aspiration of joint fluid for cultures should be performed first, then contrast is injected. Tracking of contrast into and along periprosthetic lucencies indicates loosening.

Bone scans are less helpful in evaluating for loosening in TKAs than in total hip arthroplasties. This is because the natural course of the TKA is to show mildly to moderately increased uptake for many years.[35] Intense focal uptake after more than 6 months postoperatively suggests loosening or infection,[17] but false-positive rates are high (up to 72%).[36] Sequential bone scans showing increasing radiotracer uptake are also suggestive of loosening, but are not diagnostic, as wide variability in uptake has been shown in asymptomatic patients followed with sequential scans.[36]

Periprosthetic Stress/Insufficiency Fracture

Periprosthetic fractures are uncommon, but occur most frequently in patients with rheumatoid arthritis.[19] They are most common in the distal femur. Notching of the anterior femoral cortex during resurfacing and osteoporosis are risk factors. Stress fractures can occur anywhere in the lower extremity and pelvis after TKA, due to increased activity[17] (See Figure 4-12).

Nondisplaced periprosthetic fractures that may be occult on radiographs (and even on CT) may be identifiable with MRI, especially when recently developed metal artifact reduction techniques are used. Such fractures appear as linear low T1, high T2 signal abnormalities, with variable amounts of surrounding high T2 signal marrow edema.

Bursitis and Tendon Pathology

Pain from soft tissue pathologies such as tendinitis, tendon tear, bursitis, or distended popliteal cysts can mimic a loosened or infected joint. The patellar and quadriceps tendons are well suited to evaluation by ultrasound. Normal tendons appear hyperechoic and show a fibrillar echotexture when imaged perpendicular to the ultrasound beam. Tendinitis is manifested as thickening and heterogeneous hypoechogenicity, with loss of the normal fibrillar appearance.[9,10] Tendon tears are also readily identified with ultrasound. Complete tears manifest as fluid-filled gaps extending all the way through the substance of the tendon, often with retraction of the torn ends of the tendon. Partial tears can manifest either as fluid-filled gaps that do not extend through the entire substance of the tendon or as longitudinal clefts along the long axis of the tendon.[9]

Tendinitis and tendon tears may also be detected with MRI, especially when metal artifact reduction sequences are used. Tendinitis and partial tears can be difficult to differentiate, as both can appear as tendon thickening and increased proton density and increased T2 signal within the tendon substance. In chronic partial tendon tears, the tendon is often thinned but of normal low proton density and T2 signal. Complete tendon tears often show retraction of the torn ends with a gap filled with high T2 signal fluid or heterogeneous signal blood products.[37]

Popliteal (Baker's) cysts and other extra-articular fluid collections, such as bursitis, hematoma, and soft tissue abscess, are detected by ultrasound (Figure 4-13) and also often by MRI. Such collections can be aspirated under ultrasound guidance for symptomatic relief and microbiological analysis. Corticosteroids and anesthetics may be injected into the cyst or bursa under ultrasound guidance following aspiration.

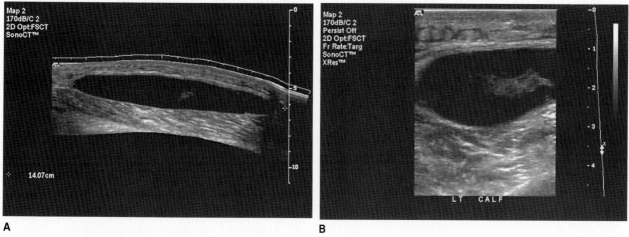

FIGURE 4-13. Hematoma. (A) Sagittal extended field-of-view ultrasound image of an intermuscular hematoma between the soleus and gastrocnemius muscles in a patient who recently underwent TKA. The hematoma is largely anechoic, but a small amount of clot is evident centrally. (B) Magnified field of view showing the characteristic heterogeneously hyperechoic clot centrally within the hematoma.

REFERENCES

1. Clarke HD, Scott WN. Knee axial instability. *Orthop Clin North Am.* 2001;32(4):627–637.

2. De Winter F, Van De Wiele C, Vogelars D, De Smet K, Verdonk R, Dierckx RA. Fluorine-18 fluorodeoxyglucose-positron emission tomography: a highly accurate imaging modality for the diagnosis of chronic musculoskeletal infections. *J Bone Joint Surg.* 2001;83-A(5):651–660.

3. Schiesser M, Stumpe KDM, Trentz O, Kossman T, von Schulthess GK. Detection of metallic implant associated infection with FCD PET in patients with trauma: correlation with microbiologic results. *Radiology.* 2003;226(2):391–398.

4. Goergen TG, Dalinka MK, Alazraki, et al. *American College of Radiology ACR Appropriateness Criteria: Evaluation of the Patient with Painful Hip or Knee Arthroplasty.* Reston, VA: ACR; 1999.

5. Lonner JH, Laird MT, Stuchin SA. Effect of rotation and knee flexion on radiographic alignment in total knee arthroplasties. *Clin Orthop.* 1996;331:102–106.

6. Fehring TK, McAvoy G. Fluoroscopic evaluation of the painful total knee arthroplasty. *Clin Orthop.* 1996;331:226–233.

7. Telepak RJ. Nuclear medicine. In: Brant WE, Helms CA, eds. *Fundamentals of Diagnostic Radiology.* Philadelphia: Lippincott, Williams & Wilkins; 1999.

8. Tonakie AWJ, Wahl R. Nuclear medicine imaging. In: Freiberg AA, ed. *The Radiology of Orthopedic Implants: An Atlas of Techniques and Assessment.* St. Louis: Mosby, Inc.; 2001:199–211.

9. Jacobson JA, Lax MJ. Musculoskeletal sonography of the postoperative orthopedic patient. *Semin Musculoskeletal Radiol.* 2002;6(1):67–77.

10. Adler RS. Ultrasound of joint replacements. In: Freiberg AA, ed. *The Radiology of Orthopedic Implants: An Atlas of Techniques and Assessment.* St. Louis: Mosby, Inc.; 2001: 183–197.

11. White LM, Buckwalter KA. Technical considerations: CT and MR imaging in the postoperative orthopedic patient. *Semin Musculoskeletal Radiol.* 2002;6(1):5–17.

12. Berger RA, Rubash HE. Rotational instability and malrotation after total knee arthroplasty. *Orthop Clin North Am.* 2001;32(4):639–647.

13. Sofka CM, Potter HG. MR imaging of joint arthroplasty. *Semin Musculoskeletal Radiol.* 2002;6(1):79–85.

14. White LM, Kim JK, Mehta M, et al. Complications of total hip arthroplasty: MR imaging—initial experience. *Radiology.* 2000;215(1):254–262.

15. Sofka CM, Potter HG, Figge M. Magnetic resonance imaging of total knee arthroplasty: findings, techniques, optimization and clinical relevance. *Radiology.* 2000;217: S576.

16. Olsen RV, Munk PL, Lee MJ, et al. Metal artifact reduction sequence: early clinical applications. *Radiographics.* 2000; 20:699–712.

17. Allen AM, Ward WG, Pope TL. Imaging of the total knee arthroplasty. *Radiol Clin North Am.* 1995;33(2):289–303.

18. Weissman BN, Sledge CB. *Orthopedic Radiology.* Philadelphia: W.B. Saunders; 1986.

19. Manaster BJ. Orthopedic hardware: arthroplasties. Lecture given at the Armed Forces Institute of Pathology, Walter Reed Medical Center, Washington, D.C. May, 2001.

20. Figge HE III, Goldberg VM, Heiple KG, et al. The influence of tibial-patellofemoral location on function of the knee in patients with the posterior stabilized condylar knee prosthesis. *J Bone Joint Surg Am.* 1986;68:1035–1040.

21. Quale JL, Murphey MD, Huntrakoon M, Reckling FW, Neff JR. Titanium-induced arthropathy associated with polyethylene-metal separation after total joint replacement. *Radiology.* 1992;182:855–858.

22. Engh GA, Dwyer KA, Hanes CK. Polyethylene wear of metal-backed tibial components in total and unicompartmental knee prostheses. *J Bone Joint Surg Br.* 1992;74:9–17.

23. Yashar AA, Adler RS, Grady-Benson JC, et al. An ultrasound method to evaluate polyethylene component wear in total knee replacement arthroplasty. *Am J Orthop.* 1996;25(10): 702–704.

24. Puri L, Wixson RL, Stern SH, et al. Use of helical computed tomography for the assessment of acetabular osteolysis after total hip arthroplasty. *J Bone Joint Surg Am.* 2002;84-A(4): 609–614.

25. Seitz P, Ruegsegger P, Gschwend N, Dubs L. Changes in local bone density after knee arthroplasty. the use of quantitiative computed tomography. *J Bone Joint Surg Br.* 1987; 69(3): 407–411.

26. Rand JA. The future of knee joint replacement. In: Morrey BF, ed. *Joint Replacement Arthroplasty.* New York: Churchill Livingstone; 1991:1127–1129.

27. Hanssen AD, Rand JA. Evaluation and treatment of infection at the site of a total hip or knee arthroplasty. *J Bone Joint Surg Am.* 1998;80:910–922.

28. Levitsky AL, Hozack WJ, Balderston RA, et al. Evaluation of the painful prosthetic joint—relative value of bone scan, sedimentation rate, and joint aspiration. *J Arthroplasty.* 1991; 6(3):237–244.

29. Duff PD, Lachiewicz PF, Kelley SS. Aspiration of the knee joint before revision arthroplasty. *Clin Orthop.* 1996; 331: 132–139.

30. Kwon DS, Newman JS, Newberg AH. Musculoskeletal imaging and interventions. In: Freiberg AA, ed. *The Radiology of Orthopedic Implants: An Atlas of Techniques and Assessment.* St. Louis: Mosby, Inc.; 2001:1–18.

31. Love C, Tomas MB, Marwin SE, et al. Role of nuclear medicine in diagnosis of the infected joint replacement. *Radiographics.* 2001;21:1229–1238.

32. Palestro CJ, Swyer AJ, Kim CK, Goldsmith SJ. Infected knee prostheses: diagnosis with In-111 leukocyte, Tc-99m sulfur colloid, and Tc-99m MDP imaging. *Radiology.* 1991;179: 645–648.

33. Griffiths HJ. Imaging of orthopedic hardware—orthopedic complications. *Radiol Clin North Am.* 1995;33(2):401–410.

34. Ewald FC. The Knee Society total knee arthroplasty roentgenographic evaluation and scoring system. *Clin Orthop.* 1989;248:9–12.

35. Duus BR, Boeckstyns, Stadeager C. The natural course of radionuclide bone scanning in the evaluation of total knee replacement—2 year prospective study. *Clin Radiol.* 1990; 41:341–343.

36. Hoffman AA, Wyatt RWB, Daniels AU, et al. Bone scans after total knee arthroplasty in asymptomatic patients—cemented versus cementless. *Clin Orthop.* 1990;251: 183–188.

37. Kaplan PA, Helms CA, Dussault R, et al. Tendons and muscles. In: Kaplan PA, Helms CA, Dussault R, et al., eds. *Musculoskeletal MRI.* Philadelphia: W.B. Saunders; 2001: 55–87.

PART II

General Principles of
Revision Surgery

CHAPTER 5

Skin Exposure Issues

Ginger E. Holt and Douglas A. Dennis

Primary wound healing is critical for the success of any total knee arthroplasty (TKA). Wound healing problems following TKA are infrequent, but can be a harbinger of devastating results. Delays in wound healing risk infection and implant failure, and can ultimately result in amputation.[1] Wound problems are minimized by proper selection of skin incisions, understanding vascular anatomy and patient risk factors, and using operative techniques that protect the soft tissues. When wound complications do arise, prompt management is imperative. Special attention is required in revision TKA procedures due to prior surgical incisions.

PATIENT RISK FACTORS

Numerous reports suggest an increased incidence of wound healing difficulties in patients who chronically use steroids[2–11] (Table 5.1). Corticosteroid use has been shown to decrease fibroblast proliferation, which is necessary for wound healing.[5] Chronic corticosteroid use also reduces collagenase clearance from the healing wound, which results in diminished collagen accumulation at the wound healing site and a subsequent decrease in wound tensile strength.[4,10,11] An increased incidence of wound complications in patients with rheumatoid arthritis (RA) has been well documented. Although the specific cause of this association is not known, it may be related to the increased long-term use of corticosteroids in many of these patients.[12–17]

Patients with substantial obesity demonstrate increased wound complication rates.[7,16,18–21] Extreme obesity can create exposure difficulties in TKA, necessitating more vigorous retraction of skin flaps and the subsequent risk of soft tissue devascularization. Additionally, in heavier patients with a thick adipose layer, the skin is less adherent to its underlying vascular supply, which increases the risk of separation of the dermis from the subcutaneous layer during skin retraction.[2]

The damaging effects of cigarette smoking have been well documented and are related to the systemic vasoconstriction resulting from nicotine use.[22–28] Smoking has been found to be the single most important risk factor for the development of postoperative complications relating to wound healing.[27] The proposed mechanism is that nicotine changes skin homeostasis by directly affecting dermal fibroblasts through a specific nicotinergic pathway.[28]

While the exact relationship remains unclear, the increased frequency of wound problems in patients with diabetes mellitus may be secondary to delayed collagen synthesis and delayed wound tensile strength. Early capillary ingrowth into the healing wound is also reduced.[2,20,29–31] Use of high-dose nonsteroidal anti-inflammatory drugs (NSAIDs) inhibits the acute inflammatory response, which is an important step in the early phases of wound healing. Inhibition of this early, acute inflammatory response may exacerbate wound healing difficulties.[32] Patients on chemotherapy may be similarly at risk for delayed wound healing. The routine need to discontinue methotrexate in preoperative patients with RA remains unclear. Bridges and associates[33] found a slight increase in the incidence of infection in 10 patients treated with methotrexate when compared with patients with RA in whom methotrexate had been discontinued more than 1 month preoperatively. Other larger comparison studies have demonstrated no increase in wound healing complications with continuance of methotrexate perioperatively in patients with RA.[34,35]

Adequate hydration is necessary for satisfactory wound healing. Hypovolemia can delay wound healing due to reduced oxygen delivery to the healing soft tissues.[2]

TABLE 5.1. Patient Risk Factors for Problems with Wound Healing.

Steroid use
Rheumatoid arthritis
Extreme obesity
Cigarette smoking
Diabetes mellitus
High-dose nonsteroidal anti-inflammatory drug use
Chemotherapy
Methotrexate use
Inadequate hydration
Hypovolemia
Reduced transcutaneous oxygen levels
Irradiated skin
Scarring from previous burns

Reduction in transcutaneous oxygen levels has been documented to increase wound healing complications following lateral retinacular release in TKA[36] and to decrease wound healing after soft tissue flap transfers.[37] Use of continuous passive motion (CPM) beyond 40 degrees has been shown to reduce transcutaneous oxygen tension measured in the healing wound edges, especially during the 3 days following TKA. CPM should be limited to less than 40 degrees during the early postoperative period if the risk of skin necrosis is substantial.[38,39] Additional risk factors for wound complications following TKA include those knees in which the anterior skin has previously been irradiated or undergone scarring from previous burns.

WOUND COMPLICATION MANAGEMENT

Various types of wound complications can occur, including prolonged postoperative drainage, superficial soft tissue necrosis, and full-thickness soft tissue necrosis, in which the prosthetic components are usually exposed. All 3 types of wound problems require immediate attention, as delay in treatment risks deep infection and subsequent failure of the TKA.

Prolonged Serous Drainage

If the TKA wound is chronically draining, but does not exhibit substantial erythema or purulence, immobilization and local wound care can be pursued. In the authors' experience, if drainage persists beyond 5 to 7 days despite immobilization, elevation, and local wound care, spontaneous cessation of drainage is unlikely and surgical debridement is indicated. Subcutaneous hematomas or large intra-articular hemarthroses are commonly encountered in cases of persistent wound drainage.

Hematomas threaten the wound integrity by increasing soft tissue tension, releasing toxic breakdown products of hemoglobin, and serving as a healthy medium for bacterial growth.[2]

Scientific data are lacking to clearly support surgical drainage rather than observation of the nondraining hematoma. We recommend treating the nondraining hematoma through close observation as long as no signs of impending skin necrosis from excessive soft tissue tension are present. An additional consideration for surgical drainage is a large hematoma that substantially limits knee range of motion. Drainage procedures should be performed in the operative theater with perioperative antibiotic therapy.

The incidence of prolonged drainage in patients who eventually develop culture-proven infected TKA ranges from 17% to 50%.[40–42] Weiss and Krackow,[40] in a retrospective review of 597 TKAs, identified 8 patients (1.3%) with persistent wound drainage. All were treated with surgical irrigation, debridement, and parenteral antibiotics. All cases healed without infection despite the fact that 2 patients (25%) had positive cultures at the time of irrigation and debridement. The authors suggest that prompt surgical management in these cases may prevent chronic drainage problems from becoming established infections.

Superficial Soft Tissue Necrosis

Necrotic tissue generally requires surgical debridement. Small necrotic areas less than 3 cm in diameter may heal with local wound care or delayed secondary closure.[9] Larger areas of superficial necrosis should be debrided and covered with split-thickness skin grafting or fasciocutaneous flaps.[43–45] Vacuum-assisted wound closure (VAC) may be used following debridement to reduce the size of the initial wound, allowing for later skin grafting while suppressing bacterial overgrowth.[46] In a comparison of VAC versus saline dressing changes, Joseph et al.[47] found that the negative pressure of the VAC facilitated reparative granulation tissue instead of fibrosis, which was found in the beds of wounds treated with traditional dressing changes. The improvement in measured wound depth reduction (66% for VAC versus 20% for saline dressings) significantly improved the rate of healing in VAC-treated wounds. It is important to point out that VAC is used as an adjunct to wound debridement and not as a substitute.

Full-Thickness Soft Tissue Necrosis

Full thickness soft tissue necrosis is usually associated with exposed prosthetic components and requires immediate, aggressive debridement. Simple secondary closure procedures are often unsuccessful, and some type of flap reconstruction is usually required. Various types of flaps

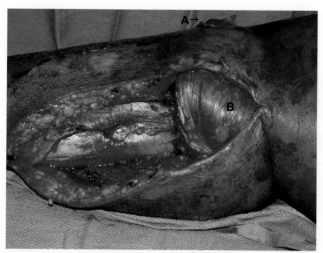

FIGURE 5-1. Obese patient with chronic inferior wound drainage and skin breakdown 3 × 3 cm in dimension over the exposed patellar tendon (A) requiring rotational gastrocnemius flap (B) and skin grafting. (Courtesy of Bruce Shack, MD.)

have been used, including cutaneous,[48] fasciocutaneous,[43,44] myocutaneous,[48–54] and myotendinous.[55] Bengston and associates[49] reported on the treatment of 10 TKAs with full-thickness skin loss and exposed prosthetic components. Delayed closure failed in 6 of 6 cases in which it was attempted. Split-thickness skin grafting failed in both cases in which it was attempted. In contrast, coverage with gastrocnemius myocutaneous flaps proved successful and was recommended as the treatment of choice in these cases. Gerwin et al.[56] reviewed 12 patients

with full-thickness skin necrosis and exposed prostheses, 6 of whom had positive deep cultures. All patients were treated with aggressive debridement and closure with medial gastrocnemius myocutaneous flaps. Eleven of 12 patients (92%) obtained excellent results, with ten (82%) retaining their components or having a successful reimplantation. Nahabedian et al.[57] reported an 83% success rate in salvaging TKAs with wound breakdown with medial gastrocnemius flaps. Adam et al.[58] presented a 76% success rate in preserving TKAs with exposed components due to wound breakdown with myocutaneous flaps, but the functional results were not as good as compared with knees that healed with primary wound healing, stressing once again the importance of preoperative assessment and intraoperative techniques to minimize wound complications from occurring.

The medial head of the gastrocnemius muscle is often the preferred flap for reconstruction[57] (Figure 5-1). It is both larger and 2 to 3 cm longer than the lateral gastrocnemius muscle. Furthermore, because it does not have to traverse the fibula, it has a larger arc of motion. It provides excellent soft tissue coverage in the region of the patella and tibial tubercle, the area where the incidence of skin necrosis is the highest (Figure 5-2A, B). Free myocutaneous flaps may be used,[2,59] but they are reserved for cases with full-thickness necrosis that cannot be covered with other local flap reconstructions (Figure 5-3A, B). In cases in which tendinous structures are compromised by infection or debridement, myotendinous gastrocnemius flaps can be used.[55] This flap uses the superficial layer of the Achilles tendon with the deep

FIGURE 5-2. (A) Nonhealing anterior knee wound following TKA requiring a medial myocutaneous rotational gastrocnemius flap. (A) primary closure of myocutaneous gastrocnemius harvest site. (B) Myocutaneous gastrocnemius flap. Knee wound following rotation and closure of the medial myocutaneous gastrocnemius flap. (Courtesy of Bruce Shack, MD.)

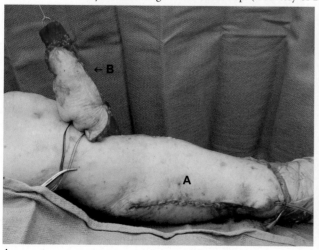

A

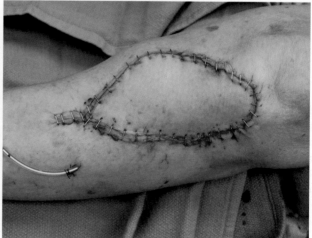

B

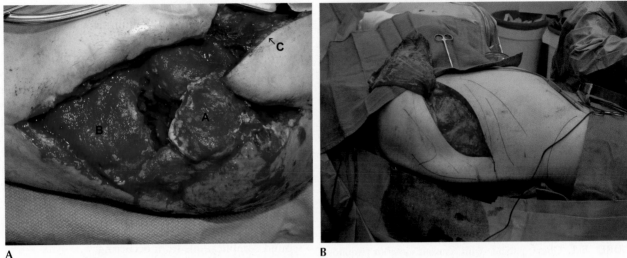

FIGURE 5-3. (A) Nonhealing anterior knee wound with methicillin-resistant *Staphylococcus aureus* (MRSA) infection in a diabetic patient who has a failed rotational gastrocnemius flap, a local rotational flap skin grafting, and aggressive dressing changes following resection arthroplasty and cement spacer. A free latissimus flap was used for coverage. (A) patella. (B) patellar tendon covered by granulation tissue from dressing changes. (C) incision for vascular anastomosis. (B) Harevesting of the free latissimus flap. A myocutaneous flap was not incorporated. The latissimus was transferred and covered with a skin graft. (Courtesy of Bruce Shack, MD.)

aponeurotic layer of the gastrocnemius to reconstruct tendon defects.

Antibiotic Use

Parenteral antibiotics are often required in cases with persistent drainage and wound necrosis, but they should not be used indiscriminately. Unnecessary use of antibiotics risks alteration of bacterial flora and sensitivities, should deep infection occur.[2] Joint aspiration for culture is suggested before initiation of antibiotic therapy to maximize culture results. Cultures of superficial drainage are often spurious, with little correlation with deep infecting organisms.[2,9,60]

VASCULAR ANATOMY

The blood supply to the soft tissues of the anterior aspect of the knee is random, receiving contributions from multiple vessels.[2,61–66] This blood supply arises predominantly from the terminal branches of the peripatellar anastomotic arterial ring. This anastomotic ring has numerous contributing arterial branches, including the medial and lateral superior geniculate arteries, the supreme geniculate artery, the anterior tibial recurrent artery, and a branch of the profunda femoris artery (Figure 5-4). In contrast to the skin circulation of the thigh proximal to the knee, there is no underlying muscle or intermuscular septa directly anterior to the knee to provide a direct

pathway for arterial perforators.[2,63] Skin circulation in this area is dependent on the dermal plexus, which originates directly from arterioles traveling within the subcutaneous fascia. Any surgical dissection performed superficial to this subcutaneous fascia disrupts the arterial supply to the skin and increases the possibility of skin necrosis. Elevation of skin flaps about the anterior aspect of the knee requires dissection deep to the subcutaneous fascia to preserve the perforating arteriolar network between the subcutaneous fascia and dermal plexus.[2]

SKIN INCISION

Analysis of vascular anatomy about the knee suggests that choice of a midline skin incision is less disruptive to the arterial network.[2] Medial peripatellar skin incisions are undesirable because they create a large, laterally based skin flap, which has been associated with higher wound complication rates.[2] Transcutaneous oxygen measurements, both before and after skin incisions about the knee, have demonstrated reduced oxygenation of the lateral skin region.[67,68] The further medially the skin incision is made, the larger the lateral skin flap. A larger lateral skin flap has a lower oxygen tension, which increases the risk of wound complications. Placement of the skin incision slightly lateral to the midline assists in eversion of the patella, particularly in obese patients in whom a large and bulky lateral skin flap resists patellar eversion.

Use of previous skin incisions is generally recommended. Although it is usually safe to ignore previous short medial or lateral peripatellar incisions, one should be wary of wide scars with thin or absent subcutaneous tissues, as damage to the underlying dermal plexus is likely, increasing the risk of wound necrosis.[2] Problems with placement of a longitudinal incision crossing a transverse incision previously used for high tibial osteotomy are uncommon.[69,70]

If long parallel skin incisions exist, choice of the lateralmost skin incision is favorable to avoid a large lateral skin flap that has previously been compromised at the time of the initial lateral skin incision. In complex situations, such as knees with multiple incisions or previously burned or irradiated skin, plastic surgical consultation is wise, both for the configuration of the preferred skin incision, as well as for consideration of preoperative muscle flap procedures if the risk of skin necrosis is substantial. In selected complex situations, wound complications can be reduced by using a staged technique. A *pre-revision*

FIGURE 5-4. Diagram demonstrating the extraosseous peripatellar anastomotic ring supplied by six main arteries. ATR, anterior tibial recurrent; LIG, lateral inferior genicular; LSG, lateral superior genicular; MIG, medial inferior genicular; MSG, medial superior genicular; SG, supreme genicular.

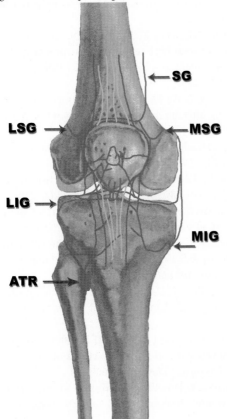

skin incision to the depth of the subcutaneous fascial layer is made and then closed. If this incision heals without difficulty, one can later proceed with TKA with much greater confidence. This does not take into account the substantial dissection that occurs with a TKA, and caution is still warranted, with careful intraoperative and postoperative management of the soft tissues.[71]

Another complicating factor in choosing a skin incision follows previous muscle flap procedures. Knowledge of the prior surgical procedures is imperative before proceeding with surgical intervention. Consultation with a plastic surgeon is also recommended. Care must be exercised not to disrupt the vascular pedicle of the flap or portions of the muscular flap itself.

Soft tissue expansion techniques have been used successfully in cases of contracted soft tissues from previous skin incisions, burns, or irradiation.[71–77] Success has also been described for tissue expansion before primary TKA, conversion of arthrodesis, reimplantation following infection, and revision TKA.[71,72–80] These techniques involve implantation, usually subcutaneously, of an expandable reservoir, into which saline can be intermittently injected to expand the surface area of the skin. Studies have shown that while epidermal thickness is maintained, dermal thinning occurs, and overall dermal collagen synthesis is increased. Complications with soft tissue expansion have been minimal and include hematoma formation, reservoir deflation, infection, and skin necrosis from vigorous tissue expansion.

Manifold et al.[71] reported on the long-term results of 27 patients (29 knees) who underwent preoperative tissue expansion. At a mean follow-up of 34 months, the average Knee Society score was 83.7. One major wound complication required abandonment of the planned TKA. Minor wound complications were cited for 6 of the 29 expansion procedures and 5 of the subsequent TKAs.

Disadvantages of soft tissue expansion include the requirement for additional surgical procedures and the time required for expansion, which is approximately 3 to 6 weeks.

TECHNICAL FACTORS

A thorough preoperative vascular examination of the limb is necessary to minimize the risk of wound healing difficulties. The skin incision for TKA should be of adequate length to avoid excessive tension on the wound edges, particularly when the knee is positioned in extremes of flexion. Gentle retraction of the skin edges is necessary to avoid disruption of perforating arterioles originating in the subcutaneous fascial layer. It is best not to undermine large areas of skin. If undermining skin flaps is required, it must be done in the subfascial plane to preserve the blood supply to the skin, which originates in the dermal plexus.[2,63] Numerous studies have demonstrated that a lateral retinacular release decreases lateral skin oxygenation and increases the subsequent risk of wound complications.[3,36,81,82] If a lateral retinacular release is required, attempts should be made to preserve the lateral superior geniculate artery. Meticulous wound hemostasis is paramount to avoid postoperative hematoma formation. Routine use of suction drainage reduces pain and postoperative hematoma formation. Wound closure without tension is imperative in minimizing the risk of skin necrosis.

SUMMARY

Wound problems are a dreaded complication following TKA, and all measures should be taken to avoid them. Preventative measures include proper choice of the skin incision, gentle handling of the soft tissues, meticulous hemostasis, and wound closure without excessive tension. Should persistent wound drainage or soft tissue necrosis occur, early intervention is imperative, because delay risks deep infection and ultimate failure of the TKA. Cases associated with full-thickness soft tissue necrosis often require transfer of well-vascularized tissue, such as a medial gastrocnemius myocutaneous flap reconstruction.

REFERENCES

1. Poss R, Thornhill TS, Ewald FC, et al. Factors influencing the incidence and outcome of infection following total joint arthroplasty. *Clin Orthop.* 1984;182:117–126.
2. Klein NE, Cox CV. Wound problems in total knee arthroplasty. In: Fu FH, Harner CD, Vince KG, et al., eds. *Knee Surgery.* Vol 2. Baltimore: Williams & Wilkins; 1994: 1539–1552.
3. Scuderi G, Scharf SC, Meltzer LP, et al. The relationship of lateral releases to patella viability in total knee arthroplasty. *J Arthroplasty.* 1987;2:209–214.
4. Craig SM. Soft tissue considerations. In: Scott WN, ed. *Total Knee Revision Arthroplasty.* Orlando, FL: Grune & Stratton; 1987:99–112.
5. Green JP. Steroid therapy and wound healing in surgical patients. *Br J Surg.* 1965;52:523–525.
6. McNamara JJ, Lamborn PJ, Mills D, et al. Effect of short-term pharmacologic doses of adrenocorticosteroid therapy on wound healing. *Ann Surg.* 1969;170: 199–202.
7. Nelson CL. Prevention of sepsis. *Clin Orthop.* 1987;222: 66–72.
8. Petty W, Bryan RS, Coventry MB, Peterson LF. Infection after total knee arthroplasty. *Orthop Clin North Am.* 1975; 6:1005–1014.
9. Sculco TP. Local wound complications after total knee arthroplasty. In: Ranawat CS, ed. *Total Condylar Knee Arthroplasty: Technique, Results, and Complications.* New York: Springer-Verlag; 1985:194–196.
10. Wahl LM. Hormonal regulation of macrophage collagenase activity. *Biochem Biophys Res Commun.* 1977; 74:838–845.
11. Werb Z. Biochemical actions of glucocorticoids on macrophages in culture: Specific inhibition of elastase, collagenase, and plasminogen activator secretion and effects on other metabolic functions. *J Exp Med.* 1978;147: 1695–1712.
12. D'Ambrosia RD, Shoji H, Heater R. Secondarily infected total joint replacements by hematogenous spread. *J Bone Joint Surg.* 1976;58A:450–453.
13. Garner RW, Mowat AG, Hazelman BL. Wound healing after operations on patients with rheumatoid arthritis. *J Bone Joint Surg.* 1973;55B:134–144.
14. Grogan TJ, Dorey F, Rollins J, et al. Deep sepsis following total knee arthroplasty: ten year experience at the University of California at Los Angeles Medical Center. *J Bone Joint Surg.* 1986;68A:226–234.
15. Thomas BJ, Moreland JR, Amstutz HC. Infection after total joint arthroplasty from distal extremity sepsis. *Clin Orthop.* 1983;181:121–125.
16. Wilson MG, Kelley K, Thornhill TS. Infection as a complication of total knee replacement arthroplasty: Risk factors and treatment in sixty-seven cases. *J Bone Joint Surg.* 1990; 72A:878–883.
17. Wong RY, Lotke PA, Ecker ML. Factors influencing wound healing after total knee arthroplasty. *Orthop Trans.* 1986; 10:497.
18. Garcia Hidalgo L. Dermatological complications of obesity. *Am J Clin Dermatol.* 2002;3(7):497–506.
19. Cruse PJ, Foord R. A five-year prospective study of 23 649 surgical wounds. *Arch Surg.* 1973;107:206–210.
20. Ecker ML, Lotke PA. Postoperative care of the total knee patient. *Orthop Clin North Am.* 1989;20:55–62.
21. Dickhaut SC, DeLee JC, Page CP. Nutritional Status: Importance in predicting wound-healing after amputation. *J Bone Joint Surg.* 1984;66A:71–75.
22. Craig S, Rees TD. The effects of smoking on experimental skin flaps in hamsters. *Plast Reconstr Surg.* 1985;75: 842–846.
23. Benowitz NL, Kuyt F, Jacob III P. Influence of nicotine on cardiovascular and hormonal effects of cigarette smoking. *Clin Pharmacol Ther.* 1984;36:74–81.
24. Mosely LH, Finseth F, Goody M. Nicotine and its effect on wound healing. *Plast Reconstr Surg.* 1978;61:570–575.

25. Rees TD, Liverett DM, Guy CL. The effect of cigarette smoking on skin-flap survival in the face lift patient. *Plast Reconstr Surg.* 1984;73:911–915.

26. Kaufman T, Eichenlaub EH, Levin M, et al. Tobacco smoking: impairment of experimental flap survival. *Ann Plast Surg.* 1984;13:468–472.

27. Moller AM, Pederson T, Villebro N, et al. effect of smoking on early complications after elective orthopaedic surgery. *J Bone Joint Surg.* 2003;85B:178–181.

28. Arredondo J, Hall LL, Ndoye A, et al. Central role of fibroblast alpha 3 nicotinic acetylcholine receptor in mediating cutaneous effects of nicotine. *Lab Invest.* 2003;83(2): 207–225.

29. Goodson III WH, Hunt TK. Studies of wound healing in experimental diabetes mellitus. *J Surg Res.* 1977;22: 221–227.

30. Goodson III WH, Hunt TK. Wound healing and the diabetic patient. *Surg Gynecol Obstet.* 1979;149:600–608.

31. McMurry Jr JF. Wound healing with diabetes mellitus: Better glucose control for better wound healing in diabetes. *Surg Clin North Am.* 1984;64:769–788.

32. McGrath MH. The effect of prostaglandin inhibitors on wound contraction and the myofibroblast. *Plast Reconstr Surg.* 1982;69:74–85.

33. Bridges SL Jr, Lopez Mendez A, Tracy I, et al. Should methotrexate be discontinued prior to total joint arthroplasty in rheumatoid arthritis patients? *Arthritis Rheum.* 1989;32(suppl 4):543.

34. Kasden ML, June L. Postoperative results of rheumatoid arthritis patients on methotrexate at the time of reconstructive surgery of the hand. *Orthopaedics.* 1993;16: 1233–1235.

35. Perhala RS, Wilke WS, Clough JD, et al. Local infectious complications following large joint replacement in rheumatoid arthritis patients treated with methotrexate. *Arthritis Rheum.* 1991;34:146–152.

36. Johnson DP, Eastwood DM. Lateral patellar release in knee arthroplasty: Effect on wound healing. *J Arthroplasty.* 1992; 7(suppl):427–431.

37. Achauer BM, Black KS, Litke DK. Transcutaneous PO$_2$ in flaps: A new method of survival prediction. *Plas Reconstr Surg.* 1980;65:738–745.

38. Goletz TH, Henry JH. Continuous passive motion after total knee arthroplasty. *South Med J.* 1986;79: 1116–1120.

39. Johnson DP. The effect of continuous passive motion on wound-healing and joint mobility after knee arthroplasty. *J Bone Joint Surg.* 1990;72A:421–426.

40. Weiss AP, Krackow KA. Persistent wound drainage after primary total knee arthroplasty. *J Arthroplasty.* 1993;8: 285–289.

41. Bengston S, Knutson K, Lidgren L. Treatment of infected knee arthroplasty. *Clin Orthop.* 1989;245:173–178.

42. Insall J, Aglietti P. A five to seven-year followup of unicondylar arthroplasty. *J Bone Joint Surg.* 1989;245:173–178.

43. Hallock GG. Salvage of total knee arthroplasty with local fasciocutaneous flaps. *J Bone Joint Surg.* 1990;72A: 1236–1239.

44. Lewis Jr VL, Mossie RD, Stulberg DS, et al. The fasciocutaneous flap: A conservative approach to the exposed knee joint. *Plast Reconstr Surg.* 1990;85:252–257.

45. Ries MD. Skin necrosis after total knee arthroplasty. *J Arthroplasty.* 2002;17(4 suppl 1):74–77.

46. Webb LX. New Techniques in wound management: vacuum-assisted wound closure. *J Am Acad Orthop Surg.* 2002;10(5):303–311.

47. Joseph E, Hamori CA, Bergman S, et al. A prospective randomized trial of vacuum assisted closure versus standard therapy of chronic nonhealing wounds. *Wounds.* 2000;12: 60–67.

48. Lian G, Cracchiolo III A, Lesavoy M. Treatment of major wound necrosis following total knee arthroplasty. *J Arthroplasty.* 1989;4(suppl):S23–S32.

49. Bengston S, Carlsson A, Relander M, et al. Treatment of the exposed knee prosthesis. *Acta Orthop Scand.* 1987;58: 662–665.

50. Eckardt JJ, Lesavoy MA, Dubrow TJ, et al. Exposed endoprosthesis: management protocol using muscle and myocutaneous flap coverage. *Clin Orthop.* 1990;251:220–229.

51. Greenberg B, LaRossa D, Lotke PA, et al. Salvage of jeopardized total knee prosthesis: The role of the gastrocnemius muscle flap. *Plast Reconstr Surg.* 1989;83:85–89,97–99.

52. Hemphill ES, Ebert FR, Muench AG. The medial gastrocnemius flap in the treatment of wound complications following total knee arthroplasty. *Orthopaedics.* 1992;15: 477–480.

53. Salibian AH, Anzel SH. Salvage of an infected total knee prosthesis with medial and lateral gastrocnemius muscle flaps: a case report. *J Bone Joint Surg.* 1983;65A:681–684.

54. Sanders R, O'Neill T. The gastrocnemius myocutaneous flap used as a cover for the exposed knee prosthesis. *J Bone Joint Surg.* 1981;63B:383–386.

55. Rhomberg M, Schwabegger AH, Ninkovic M, et al. Gastrocnemius myotendinous flap for patellar or quadriceps tendon repair, or both. *Clin Orthop.* 2000;377:152–160.

56. Gerwin M, Rothaus KO, Windsor RE, et al. Gastrocnemius muscle flap coverage of exposed or infected knee prostheses. *Clin Orthop.* 1993;286:64–70.

57. Nahabedian MY, Orlando JC, Delanois RE, et al. Salvage procedures for complex soft tissue defects of the knee. *Clin Orthop.* 1998;356:119–124.

58. Adam RF, Watson SB, Jarratt JW, et al. Outcome after flap cover for exposed total knee arthroplasties: a report of 25 cases. *J Bone Joint Surg.* 1994;76B:750–753.

59. Gordon L, Levinsohn DG. Versatility of the latissimus and serratus anterior muscle transplants in providing cover for

exposed hardware and endoprostheses. *Orthop Trans.* 1992; 16:68.

60. Insall J, Scott WN, Ranawat CS. The total condylar knee prosthesis: a report of two hundred and twenty cases. *J Bone Joint Surg.* 1979;61A:173–180.

61. Müller W, ed. *The Knee: Form, Function, and Ligament Reconstruction.* Berlin: Springer-Verlag; 1983:158–167.

62. Scapinelli R. Studies on the vasculature of the human knee joint. *Acta Anat.* 1968;70:305–331.

63. Craig SM. Soft tissue consideration in the failed total knee arthroplasty. In: Scott WN, ed. *The Knee.* Vol 2. St. Louis, MO: Mosby Year Book; 1994:1279–1295.

64. Abbott LC, Carpenter WF. Surgical approaches to the knee joint. *J Bone Joint Surg.* 1945;27:277–310.

65. Björkström S, Goldie IF. A study of the arterial supply of the patella in the normal state, on chondromalacia patellae and in osteoarthrosis. *Acta Orthop Scand.* 1980;51: 63–70.

66. Waisbrod H, Treiman N. Intra-osseous venography in patellofemoral disorders: a preliminary report. *J Bone Joint Surg.* 1980;62B:454–456.

67. Johnson DP. Midline or parapatellar incision for knee arthroplasty: A comparative study of wound viability. *J Bone Joint Surg.* 1988;70B:656–658.

68. Johnson DP, Houghton TA, Radford P. Anterior midline or medial parapatellar incision for arthroplasty of the knee: a comparative study. *J Bone Joint Surg.* 1986;68B:812–814.

69. Ecker ML, Lotke PA. Wound healing complications. In: Rand JA, ed. *Total Knee Arthroplasty.* New York: Raven Press; 1993:403–407.

70. Windsor RE, Insall JN, Vince KG. Technical consideration of total knee arthroplasty after proximal tibial osteotomy. *J Bone Joint Surg.* 1988;70A:547–555.

71. Manifold SG, Cushner FD, Craig-Scott S, Scott WN. Long-term results of total knee arthroplasty after the use of soft tissue expanders. *Clin Orthop.* 2000;380:133–139.

72. Mahomed N, McKee N, Soloman P, et al. Soft-tissue expansion before total knee arthroplasty in arthrodesed joints: a report of two cases. *J Bone Joint Surg.* 1994;76B:88–90.

73. Argenta LC, Marks MW, Pasyk KA. Advances in tissue expansion. *Clin Plast Surg.* 1985;12:159–171.

74. Manders EK, Oaks TE, Au VK, et al. Soft-tissue expansion in the lower extremities. *Plast Reconstr Surg.* 1988;81: 208–219.

75. Manders EK, Schenden MJ, Furrey JA, et al. Soft-tissue expansion: concepts and complications. *Plast Reconstr Surg.* 1984;74:493–507.

76. Radovan C. Tissue expansion in soft-tissue reconstruction. *Plast Reconstr Surg.* 1984;74:482–492.

77. Riederman R, Noyes FR. Soft tissue skin expansion of contracted tissues prior to knee surgery. *Am J Knee Surg.* 1991; 4:195–198.

78. Namba RS, Diao E. Tissue expansion for staged reimplantation of infected total knee arthroplasty. *J Arthroplasty.* 1997;12:471–474.

79. Santore RF, Kaufman D, Robbins AJ, Dabezies Jr EJ. Tissue expansion prior to revision total knee arthroplasty. *J Arthroplasty.* 1997;12:475–478.

80. Rand JA, Ries MD, Landis GH, et al. Intraoperative assessment in revision total knee arthroplasty. *J Bone Joint Surg.* 2003;85A(Suppl 1):526–537.

81. Clayton ML, Thirupathi R. Patellar complications after total condylar arthroplasty. *Clin Orthop.* 1982;170:152–155.

82. Kayler DE, Lyttle D. Surgical interruption of patellar blood supply by total knee arthroplasty. *Clin Orthop.* 1988;229: 221–227.

CHAPTER 6

Exposure Options for Revision Total Knee Arthroplasty

Gerard A. Engh

A well-planned surgical approach is crucial to avoid damaging important structures in a knee already compromised by previous surgery. With previous knee surgery, the skin may have become densely scarred into the deep fascial layers or even to the underlying bone. This scarring may be the effect of multiple incisions, draining sinuses, or old skin sloughs. As a result, exposure in revision knee arthroplasty is particularly difficult secondary to a loss of tissue elasticity and the overall thickening of the capsular envelope that surrounds the knee.

To achieve a safe and satisfactory exposure for revision surgery, the surgeon must give special consideration to any condition that has resulted in a restricted arc of knee motion (less than 90 degrees of flexion). A loss in the elasticity of the extensor mechanism, a common sequel to the development of arthritis, may be exacerbated with total knee arthroplasty failure. Patients lose flexibility secondary to guarding from the pain of arthritis, and they may lose additional motion in response to postsurgical pain following their index arthroplasty. With limited knee flexion, stretching of the knee structures such as the capsule and the soft tissue envelope does not occur. The elasticity of the soft tissue structures is lost. Pain associated with failure of the prosthesis often results in further loss of knee motion, as does the trauma of multiple revision operations. In addition, the biologic response to infection, particulate debris, and the soft tissue trauma associated with knee instability further compromise tissue compliance.

Multiple exposure options exist for the stiff and badly scarred knee. Wide exposure through a full incision reduces surgical time and enhances component removal, soft tissue balancing, bone reconstruction with allografts or augments, and reimplantation of long-stemmed revision components. By properly selecting and implementing the exposure method, the surgeon can avoid the devastating complications of wound slough and/or iatrogenic knee instability. It is most important that the ligamentous support to both the tibiofemoral and patellofemoral articulations is not compromised. Instability of either the tibiofemoral or patellofemoral joint dooms the revision arthroplasty to failure.

Patients at increased risk for wound healing complications include immunocompromised individuals, such as those with rheumatoid arthritis, systemic lupus erythematosus, and vasculitis, as well as patients on immunosuppressive drugs and corticosteroids. These patients are prone not only to wound healing problems, but because of the friable nature of their skin, they are also prone to skin sloughs from manual pressure or vigorous skin retraction. Often, the epidermal layer is thin with poor elasticity that makes skin closure difficult. Extra caution is warranted throughout the surgical procedure to protect the epithelial barrier from external insults.

All patients are at increased risk of infection with revision total knee arthroplasty. The risk of deep infection in revision surgery often is reported as 3 to 4 times greater than with primary total knee surgery. The increased risk is a combination of the poorly vascularized tissue often encountered with multiple operations, the increased operative time for revision surgery, prior wound healing problems, and the increased age and poorer metabolic state of this patient population. The risk of infection is even greater in diabetic patients and those immunocompromised either by disease or medication.

PREOPERATIVE ASSESSMENT

A medical history should be obtained that includes details of any previous surgery on the knee, any wound problems or wound drainage, and the use of antibiotics. If there was a wound healing problem, it is important to note if there was a secondary wound exploration and closure. If so, what was the length of time between the primary and secondary surgical procedure? It is important to inquire when knee stiffness began and what method of management (i.e., manipulation, arthroscopy, or additional surgery) was employed to try to restore motion. The medical history should also include information concerning systemic diseases such as diabetes, rheumatoid arthritis, and other connective tissue disorders. The use of corticosteroids and antimetabolites, including drugs such as methotrexate and Embryl, should be documented.

The range of motion, the degree of fixed flexion contracture, and the maximum active and passive knee flexion should be documented carefully with a goniometer. The knee should be checked for an extension lag. The mobility of the patella in the coronal plane, or the lack of mobility, is indicative of the degree of scarring of the extensor mechanism. The location of the patella is important, as patella baja makes dislocation of the patella more difficult at the time of surgery.

Careful selection of previous skin incisions is essential to avoid skin necrosis. During physical examination, the surgeon must carefully inspect all scars, noting their location and proximity to the incisions that may be needed for revision total knee arthroplasty. The surgeon should identify and document the location of the most recently used incision and the history of wound healing with surgery through that incision. If no incision is amenable for use in the revision surgery, the surgeon must thoroughly examine the quality of skin over the front of the knee and carefully consider the need to cross or incorporate previous skin incisions. Particular attention should be directed toward the general health of the skin and the pliability of the wound edges and subcutaneous tissue beneath the soft tissue envelope of the knee. Finally, to avoid last-minute decisions, the surgeon should clearly outline the surgical approach in the preoperative office notes. Using these notes, the surgeon can implement this plan on the day of surgery.

Plastic surgery consultation should be considered if the soft tissue envelope is scarred to an extent that wound breakdown is anticipated and other options have been exhausted. Although tissue expansion or use of a sham incision are often carried out by plastic surgeons, many orthopedic surgeons prefer to do these procedures themselves, as they have the best understanding of their requirements relative to the skin and soft tissues for wound closure.

If a draining sinus with deep infection is present, satisfactory wound closure must be obtained with the first stage of a two-stage revision. When necessary, pedicle flaps should be placed at the time the failed, infected implant is removed. However, when a pedicle flap is present, the bulk of the pedicle flap may compromise subsequent surgical exposure. The flap may require mobilization; this should be considered when planning the surgical approach for the revision procedure.

Preoperative radiographs are useful in determining if there is a bone block restricting knee flexion. In most instances, 14-inch × 17-inch radiographs provide satisfactory visualization of the knee components. The lateral radiograph is particularly helpful in identifying posterior osteophytes or heterotopic bone that may block flexion, and in determining the location of the patella. An Insall-Salvati ratio of less than 1 indicates a shortened patellar tendon that will make patellar displacement difficult. The anteroposterior (AP) radiograph is useful in identifying capsular ossification, periosteal new bone formation, and component subsidence. Full limb (51-inch) standing radiographs of the extremity may be required to evaluate the quality of fixation and the location of the femoral and tibial stems. The surgeon should pay particular attention to the fixation of the tibial stem. In some circumstances, a tibial tubercle osteotomy is necessary to access a well-fixed tibial stem. Given a well-fixed femoral stem, it may be necessary to breach the anterior femoral cortex to access the stem-cement interface.

SHAM INCISIONS AND TISSUE EXPANDERS

Two surgical options used to minimize the risk of wound healing complications with revision procedures are sham incisions and tissue expanders. Both options improve the circulation and compliance of the skin coverage of the knee.

A sham incision extending to the level of the deep joint capsule serves 3 purposes. First, densely scarred skin margins can be mobilized. Second, the sham incision enhances collateral circulation within the skin. Third, since the joint capsule is not breached, this incision should not lead to a periprosthetic knee infection even if wound breakdown occurs. In addition, the surgeon gains confidence that revision surgery without wound breakdown is feasible without the need for pedicle flaps or tissue expanders.

Tissue expansion is a viable method of creating abundant skin for satisfactory wound closure when the elasticity of the integument has been lost. Tissue expansion is indicated whenever prior incisions have created areas of immobile, adherent, and relatively thin skin and subcutaneous tissue (Figure 6-1). Either single or multiple expanders can be used. With tissue expansion, the surgeon can, on average, achieve a 3- to 5-cm increase in

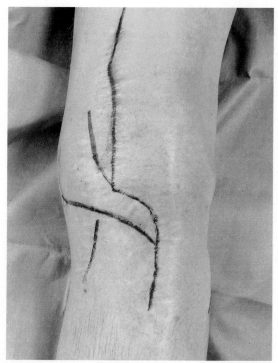

FIGURE 6-1. Multiple previous scars are outlined with a marking pencil. The skin and subcutaneous tissues adhere at the apex of the interconnecting scars. A decision was made to use tissue expanders preoperatively because of the multiple scars and loss of skin elasticity.

the circumference of the extremity by injecting approximately 300 mL of sterile saline into the expanders over a 6- to 10-week time interval (Figure 6-2). The average volume of saline injected at each weekly visit is 10% of the volume of the expander, but can be greater, as long as there is prompt capillary refill and the patient experiences no additional discomfort (Figure 6-3).

Tissue expansion actually produces additional skin with new epithelial cells. Although relatively thin, the new skin is highly vascular. When the older, relatively avascularized tissue is excised at the time of revision surgery, the new skin provides healthy and pliable tissue ideal for wound coverage and skin closure.[1]

The tissue expanders are removed through the incision used for revision total knee arthroplasty (Figure 6-4). A portion of this same incision was used to initially insert the tissue expanders.

PRINCIPLES OF SKIN INCISIONS

Whenever multiple prior incisions are present, the most lateral longitudinal skin incision appropriate for revision total knee arthroplasty should be used. However, the most recent skin incision should be considered, if such an incision had been used for prior revision surgery and had healed without complications. If no prior incision is positioned such that it can be used for the revision surgery, the operation can be performed safely through a new skin incision, as long as a bridge of skin maintains an adequate blood supply to the tissue. To preserve an adequate blood supply and prevent marginal skin necrosis, a distance of at least one-half the length of the planned incision must be maintained between an old skin incision and the new incision (Figure 6-5).

In some instances it may be necessary to incorporate a prior incision or to cross an old transverse skin incision. As a rule, any new incision should intersect an old incision at a right angle as much as possible. A new incision should not engage an old incision at an acute angle, as the thin peninsula of skin isolated between the two incisions is susceptible to skin necrosis.

FIGURE 6-2. Tissue expanders are inserted through the upper end of the incision that will be used for the revision total knee arthroplasty surgical procedure. The locations of the ports for saline injection are outlined as circles. Each of the two subcutaneous expanders were filled initially with 30 mL of saline.

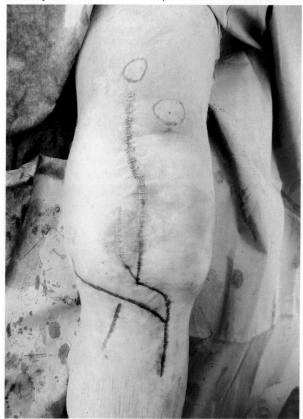

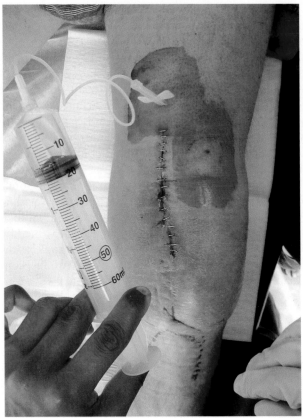

FIGURE 6-3. Tissue expansion is performed in the office 10 days after the placement of inflatable bladders using a 23-gauge butterfly needle. The tissues are expanded to approximately 10% of their volume or until skin blanching or discomfort is encountered.

FIGURE 6-4. The two bladders, *in situ* for 6 weeks, are removed at the time of total knee arthroplasty. Note the location of the bladders between the subcutaneous tissue and the joint capsule.

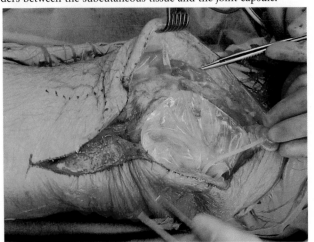

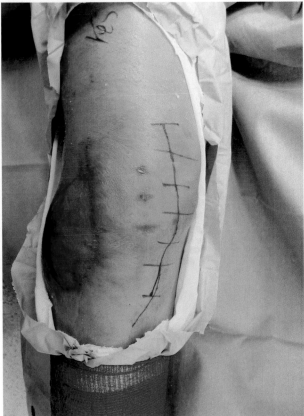

FIGURE 6-5. After revision arthroplasty for infection and placement of a lateral gastrocnemius pedicle flap, this incision is displaced to the medial side of the midline to preserve a skin bridge at least two times the length of the planned longitudinal incision.

SYSTEMATIC SURGICAL APPROACH FOR THE STIFF KNEE

As with any knee arthroplasty, a sound recommendation is to insert a pin through the medial third of the tibial tubercle to protect the patellar tendon from avulsion (Figure 6-6). The pin should be directed into the lateral tibial plateau to avoid interference with preparation of the tibia for a stemmed revision component. When the patellar tendon avulses from the tubercle, the avulsion occurs directly at the level of tendon attachment to bone. The tendon does not rupture in its midsubstance. A pin prevents the tendon from pulling away from its bony insertion with patellar eversion and dislocation.

A modification of the routine surgical approach to total knee arthroplasty is indicated for knees with less than 90 degrees of knee flexion. To provide safe and satisfactory exposure for the stiff knee, a number of steps should be completed in a logical and sequential manner to further enhance exposure.

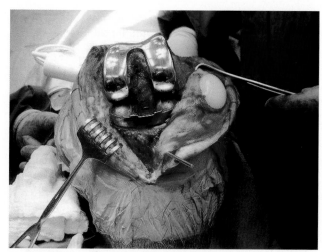

FIGURE 6-6. A pin placed in the tibial tubercle protects the patellar tendon from avulsion at its insertion.

Skin Incision

The skin is easiest to incise with the knee in flexion, as there is tension on the tissue and the elasticity of the skin provides unassisted skin retraction. The incision must be long enough to avoid vigorous skin retraction during the surgical procedure. Do not compromise surgical exposure by attempting revision surgery through a short skin incision. The incision must be at least 8 to 10 inches in length, directly through the skin and subcutaneous tissue, and centered, as much as possible, along the medial border of the patella and patellar tendon. A skin incision that extends beyond any prior skin incisions permits access to normal tissue planes. Areas of normal tissue are needed to identify the correct tissue plane for deeper tissue dissection into the adjacent scar tissue. Avoid large tissue flaps, if possible. If the skin adheres to deep fascial structures, it must be freed to allow retraction of the underlying tissues.

Capsular Incision

The capsular incision is also easiest to perform with the knee in flexion. The capsule can be opened in one of two manners: along the medial border of the patella and extended both proximally and distally, or at the proximal end of the skin incision along the medial border of the quadriceps tendon and then extended distal to the medial border of the tibial tubercle. Although most incisions are made along the medial border of the quadriceps tendon, an alternative in the stiff knee is to drift laterally through a portion of the quadriceps tendon as the incision progresses proximally. Detaching part of the quadriceps tendon in an oblique fashion from its insertion to the patella enhances eversion and lateral displacement of the patella. Such an approach has been referred to as the *wan-dering resident's approach* (Figure 6-7), implying a limited appreciation of anatomy by junior residents as they develop their surgical skills with simple primary knee arthroplasty procedures. In essence, a limited quadriceps snip has been performed and is acceptable as long as the incision across the quadriceps tendon is well above the patella. An alternative incision is the direct midline capsular incision as described by Insall, in which the extensor retinaculum is peeled from the medial side of the patella.[2] This approach also detaches the medial part of the quadriceps tendon from the patella and thereby aids in displacing the patella. In most revision cases, approaches such as a midvastus or subvastus incision should be avoided because exposure of the knee is compromised.

Restoring the Synovial Recesses over the Femoral Condyles

Next, attention is directed to the suprapatellar region. In most revision cases, adhesions have formed not only beneath the quadriceps tendon but also between capsular layers over the medial and lateral femoral condyles. These adhesions limit surgical exposure, as the superficial tissue layers cannot fall away from the femur when the knee is brought into deep flexion. The quadriceps expansion, including both the vastus medialis and lateralis, should be freed completely from adhesions to the underlying femur

FIGURE 6-7. The wandering resident's approach.

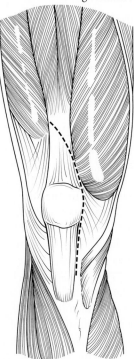

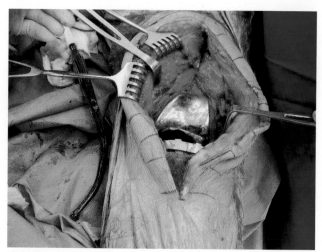

FIGURE 6-8. The synovial recesses are opened, elevating the vastus medialis from adhesions to the medial femoral condyle.

(Figure 6-8). These adhesions should be divided with sharp dissection or with a cautery. The tissue dissection should continue over the epicondyles, staying superficial to the collateral ligaments. This is more difficult in the lateral gutter, as the patella is difficult to displace laterally at this stage of the surgical procedure. To allow lateral displacement or dislocation of the patella and gain access to the region over the lateral femoral condyle, the knee is placed in full extension or even hyperextension. In addition, a lateral retinacular release may improve exposure of the lateral compartment for opening the lateral synovial recess.

In knees with extensive scarring, as after implantation of a cement spacer for infection, the capsular layers have become exceedingly thick. The sheer bulk of tissue limits the surgical exposure. In such knees, it is often necessary to debulk the capsular envelope before the lateral recesses about the femoral condyles can be exposed.

Lateral Retinacular Release

In most cases, performing a lateral retinacular release improves the surgical exposure and allows the patella to be everted and displaced. A lateral retinacular release can be performed either from the outside in, or from the inside out. In some instances, a thin layer of synovium can be preserved when performing the release from outside in. In either instance, this release should be approximately 2 to 3 cm lateral to the patella. The release should extend to, or above, the level of the vastus lateralis insertion to the quadriceps tendon and distal to the border of the tibia. With a lateral retinacular release, the superior lateral genicular artery is encountered but often is hard to identify at the inferior margin of the vastus lateralis. To preserve blood supply to the patella, an attempt to preserve this vessel is indicated. In many instances, the vessel is

stretched, cut, or torn with the lateral retinacular release. If this is the case, the vessel should be cauterized.

Dissection of the Joint Capsule

The capsular incision is extended distally, opening the joint capsule medial to the patella and patellar tendon and ending at the inferior margin of the tibial flare. The incision should leave a small border of capsular tissue on the medial side of the patellar tendon to permit capsular closure without placing sutures directly into the patellar tendon. The capsular incision ends just proximal to the pes anserine insertion. The medial joint capsule then is elevated from the medial tibial flare at least to the midline of the tibia. This layer of tissue can be released with a cautery or elevator, or with sharp dissection. The sleeve of tissue must remain intact. The tissue layer of the deep medial collateral ligament is thin and can be avulsed easily from the tibial flare. An avulsion of this thin capsular layer creates medial laxity of the knee.

Detaching the medial capsule from the anterior one-half of the metaphyseal flare allows the tibia to sublux forward from under the medial femoral condyle in primary knee arthroplasty cases. With the more extensive scarring present with revision cases, the capsule may need to be released around to the posterior corner of the medial tibial plateau. This step is especially necessary if a stemmed tibial component is being revised.

Patellar Displacement and Dislocation

The aforementioned steps should be completed before any attempt to flex the knee and displace the patella. A pin should have been placed in the medial third of the patellar tendon insertion to the tibial tubercle to protect the patellar tendon before dislocating the patella (See Figure 6-6). To allow full exposure of the tibiofemoral joint, the patella can be dislocated in one of two ways. Traditionally, while keeping a watchful eye on the patellar tendon insertion, the patella is everted and dislocated as the knee is brought into flexion. The knee should be flexed slowly as the tibia is externally rotated to reduce stress on the patellar tendon. If flexion is blocked or the patellar tendon insertion is in jeopardy, then alternative steps should be taken to relax the extensor mechanism.

Fehring et al. describe an alternative method for dislocating the patella that inverts rather than everts the patella.[3] In essence, the patella is slid laterally over the side of the lateral femoral condyle. A bent Homan retractor holds the patella lateral to the distal femur. Exposure of the proximal tibia is slightly compromised. The authors advocate making an anteromedial to posterolateral tibial cut with an extramedullary guide, or if the incision does not provide adequate exposure for the tibial cut, using an intramedullary guide as is used traditionally with revision total knee arthroplasty instrumentation. This method of exposure was used in 95% of the revision cases in the study by Fehring et al. without a single case of patellar tendon avulsion.

Patella baja makes displacement or dislocation of the patella difficult. A shortened patellar tendon does not allow enough excursion of the patella to move it lateral to the tibial plateau. Whenever patella baja is compromising the surgical exposure, a tibial tubercle osteotomy should be considered to improve surgical exposure of the proximal tibia.

Patellar Tendon Scar

A routine finding in revision total knee arthroplasty is a dense layer of scar that forms beneath the extensor mechanism. The tissue that develops around the patella is a distinct layer of fibrous tissue that engulfs the margins of the patellar implant. A similar dense layer of scar forms along the entire course of the patellar tendon, from the patella to the tibial tubercle. This layer limits the elasticity of the extensor mechanism. The patellar tendon scar should be excised to restore the pliability of the patellar tendon. Often, a layer of fat is still present beneath this layer of scar, making it relatively easy to remove the scar and not violate the deeper layer of the patellar tendon.

OPTIONS FOR MANAGING THE EXTENSOR MECHANISM

Whenever the knee lacks 90 degrees of flexion, the extensor mechanism is at risk of avulsion or rupture when vigorous efforts are made to retract the patella to achieve exposure. If the extensor mechanism is not relaxed, avulsion of the patellar tendon at its insertion to the tibial tubercle may occur, as this is the weakest point of this structure. Avulsion or rupture of the patellar tendon that occurs intraoperatively is a difficult complication to manage. Direct suture repair or staple repair has a high rate of failure.[4] Repair with augmentation, such as with a semitendinosus graft, requires postoperative knee immobilization.[5] Although the extensor mechanism can be stabilized, immobilization of an already stiff knee is likely to result in less than satisfactory knee motion with the revision total knee arthroplasty.

Relaxing tension from the extensor mechanism should not be an afterthought performed only after struggling with a difficult surgical exposure. Methods of relaxing tension include quadriceps snip, quadriceps (patellar) turndown, and a tibial tubercle osteotomy. Each of the 3 options has advantages and disadvantages; thus, the decision of which adjunct procedure to use should be thoroughly considered in the preoperative planning and carried out strategically during the surgical exposure. This planning process is guided somewhat by the location of

the patella. When patella baja is present, a distal release with an extended tibial tubercle osteotomy should be considered. In severe patella baja, no amount of proximal release may be sufficient to translate the patella lateral to the tibial plateau. In addition, the osteotomized tubercle can be translated as much as 2 cm proximally, which improves both range of motion and patellar impingement against the tibial component. When the patella is in a normal or elevated position, the scarring that limits knee motion is most severe in the quadriceps tendon proximal to the patella. A proximal release provides direct access to the scarred area and is more likely to aid in the recovery of knee motion. In a study by Barrack et al., patients who underwent a full quadriceps turndown were compared with a group of patients managed with tibial tubercle osteotomies.[6] The group of patients who had quadriceps turndown had a significantly greater increase in the arc of motion.

Quadriceps Snip

A quadriceps snip is the most widely used method for relaxing and protecting the extensor mechanism with revision total knee arthroplasty[7] (Figure 6-9). John Insall is generally credited with describing and recommending this technique. Originally, Insall referred to this as a *rectus snip*. This term may better describe the actual surgical technique of sharply dividing the rectus tendon at or near its musculotendinous junction.

FIGURE 6-9. The quadriceps snip.

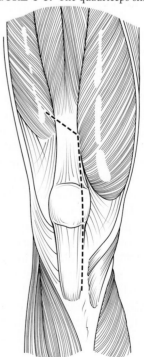

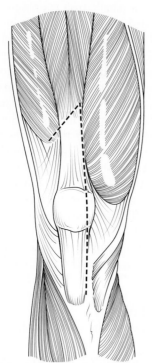

FIGURE 6-10. The V-Y quadricepsplasty.

The most important consideration with a quadriceps snip is to divide the tendon at its proximal end. This is to avoid devascularization of the patella, and more importantly, to allow direct repair of the vastus medialis into the quadriceps tendon and the quadriceps expansion distal to the location of the snip.

Technique The technique currently recommended is to open the capsule of the knee with a medial parapatellar or midline capsular incision. Next, the junction of the rectus femoris with the quadriceps tendon is identified. The tendon is then divided obliquely at a 45-degree angle, which is parallel to the direction of the vastus lateralis muscle fibers. As a rule, the tendon is divided in its entirety. At the end of the procedure, no attempt is made to reattach the rectus muscle to the quadriceps tendon. No modification of postoperative rehabilitation is necessary. Although recovery of full quadriceps function may be delayed, good return of function is realized.

Insall originally performed the quadriceps snip with a transverse incision across the quadriceps tendon. An advantage to a 45-degree oblique incision through the tendon is to maintain, in its entirety, the insertion of the vastus lateralis to the quadriceps tendon. The intact *vastus lateralis bridge*, as this is called, preserves blood supply to the quadriceps tendon and the patella, and it keeps a part of the extensor mechanism intact.

Scott and Siliski modified this technique by dividing the quadriceps tendon obliquely but downward and distally.[8] The authors termed this a *V-Y quadricepsplasty* (Figure 6-10), pointing out the advantage of preserving the superior lateral geniculate artery. They also pointed out that the length of the incision into the lateral retinaculum could be titrated and, if necessary, converted to a full quadriceps turndown if exposure is inadequate with division of the quadriceps tendon alone.

Quadriceps Turndown

A quadriceps turndown is a feasible option but should be reserved only for the most severely ankylosed knees (Figure 6-11). In such knees, scarring can be so extensive in the lateral gutter, capsule, and vastus lateralis as to prohibit knee flexion even with a full quadriceps release. Before converting a quadriceps snip to a full quadriceps turndown, a full lateral retinacular release should be performed. The lateral retinacular release may be enough to allow knee flexion. However, if knee flexion remains limited following a lateral retinacular release, a decision must be made either to proceed with a full turndown or to combine a tibial tubercle osteotomy with a quadriceps snip. The determining factor is whether the pathology prohibiting flexion is mostly adhesions in the lateral gutter or adhesions distal and posterior to the patellar tendon.

In 1943, Coonse and Adams originally described a quadriceps turndown as an inverted V-incision with

FIGURE 6-11. The quadriceps turndown.

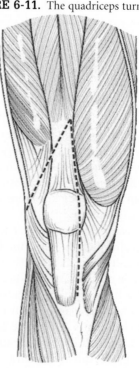

the capsule and quadriceps tendon turned distally on a broad-based flap to preserve vascularity.[9] Insall modified this approach to adopt this technique at any stage of knee surgery when a medial exposure places undue tension on the patellar ligament insertion to the tibial tubercle. Insall renamed this modification *patellar turndown approach.*[2]

Technique A straight midline or standard medial parapatellar approach is made. A second incision made at a 45-degree acute angle from the apex of the quadriceps tendon is extended distally through the vastus lateralis and iliotibial tract. The base of the capsular incision should be broad, with the apex at the proximal end of the quadriceps tendon. To avoid devascularization of the patella, the inferior lateral genicular artery should be preserved, along with the vessels within the remaining fat pad attached to the inferior pole of the patella.

The apex of the quadriceps tendon must be repaired along with the entire medial arthrotomy. If necessary to achieve correct patellar tracking, the lateral retinaculum can be left open as a lateral retinacular release. The patient should be immobilized in extension for at least 2 weeks and then limited to flexion beyond 60 degrees for the next 6 weeks. Most patients have an extension lag that, as a rule, resolves within 6 months.

Tibial Tubercle Osteotomy

In 1983, Dolin originally introduced the use of a tibial tubercle osteotomy in total knee arthroplasty[10] (Figure 6-12). A longitudinal osteotomy 4.5 cm in length was made along the medial border of the tibial tubercle. The tibial tubercle and attached tendon were then flipped laterally, leaving the lateral soft tissues and a small bone bridge to act as an osteoperiosteal flap. To repair the osteotomy, a 36-mm cortical screw was passed through a drill hole (approximately 4.5 mm) in the tibial tubercle and anchored into a threaded hole in the underlying bone cement. Dolin reported no complications with this technique used in the knees of 30 patients, including 4 knees with advancement or relocation to optimize extensor mechanism balance. However, Wolff et al. reported a high incidence of fixation failure with tibial tubercle osteotomy in knees in which the tubercle fragment was short and fixed with screws.[11]

Whiteside subsequently modified and popularized Dolin's technique.[12] He recognized the advantages of an extended tubercle osteotomy and fixation with wires instead of screws. He also noted that a tibial tubercle osteotomy provided excellent exposure by laterally displacing the tibial tubercle along with the patellar tendon and patella. An extended tibial tubercle osteotomy was used in a series of 136 total knee arthroplasties that included 76 revision procedures. The postoperative reha-

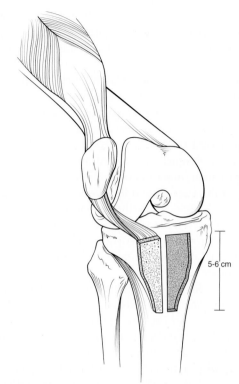

FIGURE 6-12. The tibial tubercle osteotomy.

bilitation was not modified. With the use of wire, the potential for loss of fixation was reduced. Only 2 proximal tubercle avulsion fractures occurred, but these fractures did not widely separate or result in quadriceps dysfunction. Whiteside did report three cases of tibial fracture and subsequently made further modifications to his surgical technique.

Technique The tibial tubercle osteotomy, as described by Whiteside, should be 6 to 8 cm in length. The corners of the osteotomy are marked and drilled with a 1/8-inch drill. The tibial metaphyseal cortex is then opened with an oscillating saw along the length of the osteotomy. The width of the osteotomy should be at least the full width, but preferably 1.5 times the width of the tibial tubercle. The proximal transverse cut is made in an oblique upward manner to provide a ledge on the fragment of bone to prevent proximal migration of the osteotomized tubercle after reduction of the osteotomy. The distal transverse bone cut is made at a 45-degree angle from the longitudinal cut. The lateral metaphyseal cortex is then perforated with a 1-inch-wide, curved osteotome along the length of the planned osteotomy. The osteotomized fragment is hinged laterally, maintaining all of the soft tissue attachments. If the soft tissue attachments to the tubercle are maintained, the tubercle usually will not displace proximally. To allow full eversion of the tibial tubercle, the more proximal capsular and soft tissue attachments located just lateral of the tibial plateau and more proximally along the lateral border of the patellar tendon must be released.

Rigid fixation of the tibial tubercle to the tibia is essential to restore knee flexion in the early postoperative interval. The use of 3 wires (16-gauge or stronger) passed through drill holes in the tubercle and medial tibial cortex is the preferred method of fixation. The drill holes are placed at an obliquely downward angle to minimize the risk of proximal migration of the tibial tubercle. Range of motion in the knee should be passively tested to be sure the fixation is rigid. To further enhance fixation, cortical or cancellous screws can be placed, or a cerclage wire can be passed through both cortices. The long stem of a revision tibial component may have to be negotiated to accommodate screw fixation.

Exposure for revision surgery is optimal with a tibial tubercle osteotomy. The extensor muscles, including the rectus femoris, are not compromised, allowing for a quicker and more complete recovery of extensor mechanism function as compared with a quadriceps snip. However, with a tubercle osteotomy, bone bleeding is increased and the soft tissue coverage over the tibial tubercle is often only skin, with no substantial subcutaneous tissue. Postoperative wound drainage from this area can lead to sinus tract formation and the potential for deep infection. An additional risk associated with a tibial tubercle osteotomy is that fixation can be lost and/or fracture of either the tubercle fragment or the tibia can occur. As previously mentioned, Whiteside reported 3 tibial shaft fractures from a group of 136 total knee arthroplasties managed with an extended tibial tubercle osteotomy. Ritter et al. reported 2 tibial shaft fractures from 9 revision total knee arthroplasties managed with a 10-cm-long extended tibial tubercle osteotomy.[13]

ALTERNATIVE TECHNIQUES FOR ACHIEVING SURGICAL EXPOSURE

Situations may present that require more radical maneuvers to achieve adequate exposure in the most difficult revision cases. Three techniques should be considered when scarring and ankylosis are extensive and of long-standing duration. These are the femoral peel, epicondylar osteotomy, and quadriceps myocutaneous flap.

Femoral Peel

In 1988, Windsor and Insall described a technique called a *femoral peel*.[14] Much as its name implies, a femoral peel releases all of the soft tissues subperiosteally from the distal end of the femur. In essence, a femoral peel skeletonizes the distal femur. A femoral peel is necessary when the extent of scar tissue formation is so robust that even after removing the block to knee flexion from the extensor mechanism the knee still cannot be adequately flexed to proceed with revision knee surgery.

In knees without extensive scarring, stripping the collateral ligaments and all capsular structures from the femur would create marked knee instability. However, when the capsular envelope is extensively scarred and thickened, stability is restored at the end of the revision arthroplasty by simply reapproximating the medial parapatellar incision. The inelastic quality of the soft tissue envelope provides satisfactory stability to the knee even though the bony attachments of the collateral and capsular ligaments have been sacrificed. In effect, the situation that calls for the surgeon to perform a femoral peel also makes this procedure a viable option.

In knees that have lost flexibility, the synovial pouch and capsular recesses in the posterior fossas are often obliterated on both the medial and lateral sides. In addition, osteophytes and foreign bodies from implant delamination and wear may interfere with knee flexion. From an anterior approach to the knee, it is surgically impossible to remove this block to flexion. Often, the surgeon has released the soft tissue attachments around the medial side of the knee completely and still cannot achieve enough knee flexion to proceed with the revision surgery. Thus, the decision to perform a femoral peel usually is not planned but becomes necessary in the course of a revision total knee arthroplasty.

Technique In most instances, the femoral peel involves only detaching the collaterals and capsular structures from the medial femoral condyle. This can be accomplished either with sharp dissection with a scalpel or with a cautery. Once the capsule is dissected free from the medial femoral condyle, the knee loses stability in flexion and the scarred capsular structures blocking flexion can be excised from the medial side.

In the most severe cases the distal femur is fully skeletonized on both the medial and lateral sides. The femur is herniated, so to speak, through its soft tissue investment. The femoral peel is relatively safe as long as the tissue dissection is close to bone. Often after completing a femoral peel, the hypertrophic scar needs to be excised from the posterior fossa to allow knee flexion. After the hypertrophic capsule and scar are removed, a relatively thin and pliable layer of posterior capsule is still present and can be identified by placing the knee in full extension and distracting the tibia away from the femur.

No attempt is made to reattach the collateral ligaments to the femoral condyles. With the knee in full extension, stability of the knee is usually excellent even before capsular repair. When the patella is reduced and the repairs of the extensor retinaculum and wound closure are complete, the knee is stable in flexion.

No clinical studies have reported results with knee arthroplasty using the femoral peel. The extensive soft tissue dissection may devascularize the distal end of the femur. Thus, caution is recommended with this procedure.

Medial Epicondylar Osteotomy

Epicondylar osteotomy is another valuable method of enhancing exposure in both total knee arthroplasty and revision knee arthroplasty.[15] Much like a femoral peel, an epicondylar osteotomy provides exposure of the posterior compartments of the knee by destabilizing the knee in flexion. Instead of sharply releasing all the soft tissues including the collateral ligaments from the condyles, an epicondylar osteotomy detaches the epicondyle with a large fragment of bone that can be reattached to restore stability after the revision components have been implanted. In this regard, an epicondylar osteotomy is somewhat similar to a tibial tubercle osteotomy; one end of a stabilizing structure is released temporarily to allow access for revision surgery and the structure is then repaired to reestablish stability. In most instances, the osteotomy involves only the medial epicondyle. With the medial epicondyle detached, the knee is unstable medially in flexion and the knee hinges open laterally with the extensor mechanism and tibia externally rotated. An osteotomy of both femoral epicondyles is indicated in 2 scenarios. The first is in the conversion of a knee fusion to a total knee arthroplasty, and the second is when a full distal femoral allograft is used in the composite reconstruction of a failed total knee arthroplasty. In both instances, the reattached epicondyles restore stability in flexion so effectively that even varus-valgus or constrained condylar components have not been necessary.

The epicondylar osteotomy does not rely on a densely scarred soft tissue envelope to provide stability. Therefore, an epicondylar osteotomy is indicated when knee flexion is blocked, yet the collateral ligaments and capsular tissues are not a thickened sleeve of hypertrophic fascial tissue. The decision between an osteotomy and a femoral peel is dictated by the character of the tissue that is encountered during the revision surgical exposure.

Technique The epicondylar osteotomy is performed with the knee at 90 degrees of knee flexion. Osteophytes are removed from the margins of the medial femoral condyle. A 1.5-inch osteotome is placed in the long axis of the femur just lateral to the origin of the medial collateral ligament (Figure 6-13). By palpating the epicondyle proximally, the adductor magnus tendon is

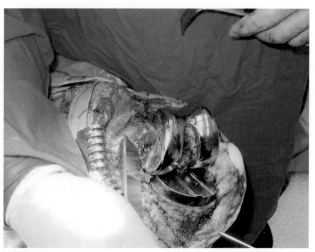

FIGURE 6-13. A medial epicondylar osteotomy is performed with a $1^{1}/_{2}$-inch osteotome.

located. The osteotome is advanced so as to exit above the adductor tendon. This ensures that the adductor tendon as well as the collateral ligaments are fully released with the osteotomized bone fragment. A fragment of bone approximately 4 cm in diameter and 1 cm thick is detached from the epicondyle. A cortical bridge of bone should remain at the junction of the osteotomized epicondyle and the anterior femoral resection for the revision knee implant. This bridge is used for anchoring repair sutures to reattach the epicondyle at the end of the procedure.

The wafer of bone is detached and hinged posteriorly with the large osteotome. This provides direct visualization of the posterior capsule (Figure 6-14). The posterior

FIGURE 6-14. Following the epicondylar osteotomy, the tibia is easily rotated away from the medial femoral condyle and the posterior fossa is exposed.

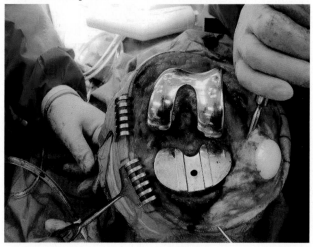

capsule is released directly from the back of the femur with a cautery while the knee is in flexion and hinged open laterally. Hypertrophic capsule osteophytes and foreign bodies are easily visualized and removed to further enhance exposure. The tissue can be dissected across the entire posterior compartment of the knee. The tibia falls back underneath the femur only when exuberant soft tissue has been removed, restoring a semblance of posterior recesses to the knee.

Detaching the medial epicondyle in continuity with the adductor tendon does not create knee instability in extension. In fact, with the knee in extension, the knee often is still unbalanced. If the knee failed in a varus attitude, the medial side remains too tight. A similar situation can be encountered with a femoral peel. In such a situation, further release of the medial soft tissue sleeve is indicated to restore a balanced extension gap. This can be accomplished either by conventional stripping of the collaterals from the tibial metaphysis, or by selectively detaching contracted portions of the medial collateral ligament from the inferior aspect of the medial epicondyle.

After the revision is complete, the epicondylar fragment of bone is repaired with heavy nonabsorbable or slowly absorbable (No. 2 or heavier) sutures placed through the epicondyle and adjacent medial femoral condyle. The cortical bridge at the anteromedial border of the knee is used to anchor these sutures. A heavy-gauge needle is passed through the epicondyle and then under the cortical bridge in a figure-of-eight or mattress fashion. A minimum of 3 sutures are necessary for the repair. Like the osteotomy, the repair is performed with the knee at 90 degrees flexion, recognizing that stability in flexion is being restored with the final components in place. The epicondyle may be positioned posteriorly because of scar tissue. If this occurs, a release of this tissue from the posterior border of the epicondyle is necessary to allow the epicondyle to reposition to a satisfactory location. Some of the epicondylar wafer may overhang the condyle. In this case, the overhanging bone may need to be trimmed back to avoid impinging with the prosthesis.

Osteotomy of the lateral femoral epicondyle also is performed with the knee in 90-degree flexion. The fragment of bone is usually 3 cm in diameter. There is no tendon that inserts into the lateral epicondyle from the proximal end; therefore, stability can be lost in both flexion and extension, even though the iliotibial band provides some stability in extension. The lateral epicondyle can be reattached with heavy nonabsorbable or slowly absorbable sutures. Cancellous lag screws also may be used if the revision prosthesis does not preclude the placement and stability of the screws. If screws are used, the drill hole in the epicondylar fragment should be slightly oversized to avoid fragmentation of the epicondyle when the screw is inserted.

Quadriceps Myocutaneous Flap

Kerry et al. described a technique for tumor resection and insertion of a prosthesis in which a U-shaped myocutaneous flap based on the quadriceps muscle is used in the surgical approach.[16] Medial and lateral longitudinal incisions are made along the line of the femoral shaft and joined by a transverse anterior incision. Next, the extensor mechanism is divided, either by a turndown through the quadriceps tendon, or a turn-up through the tibial tubercle. The quadriceps muscle remains attached to both the deep fascia and skin, thereby preserving the blood supply to the soft tissues while exposing the entire distal end of the femur. The entire quadriceps muscle is raised from the lateral intermuscular septum and from the medial side along the adductor tendons. This approach, as reported by the authors, is used for tumor resections as well as in the insertion of a revision, tumor, or custom total knee prosthesis. Wound healing was not a problem in the report of 13 cases with follow-up of 1 to 13 years.

Revision total knee arthroplasty surgery in knees with severe ankylosis is the most challenging of surgical procedures for the arthroplasty surgeon. Although we have tried to cover principles and describe techniques, no amount of preparation can substitute for experience with these difficult cases. The surgeon needs to gain experience with cases of mild to moderate complexity before undertaking the most difficult procedures.

REFERENCES

1. Gold DA, Scott SC, Scott WN. Soft tissue expansion prior to arthroplasty in the multiply operated knee. *J Arthroplasty.* 1996;11(5):512–521.
2. Insall JN. *Surgical Approaches to the Knee.* New York: Churchill-Livingstone; 1984:41–54.
3. Fehring TK, Odum S, Griffin WL, Mason JB. Patella inversion method for exposure in revision total knee arthroplasty. *J Arthroplasty.* 2002;17(1):101–104.
4. Rand JA, Morrey BF, Bryan RS. Patellar tendon rupture after total knee arthroplasty. *Clin Orthop.* 1989;244:233–238.
5. Cadambi A, Engh GA. Use of a semitendinosus tendon autogenous graft for rupture of the patellar ligament after total knee arthroplasty. a report of seven cases. J Bone Joint Surg. 1992;74A(7):974–979.
6. Barrack RE, Smith P, Munn B, et al. Comparison of surgical approaches in total knee arthroplasty. *Clin Orthop.* 1988;356:16–21.

7. Garvin KL, Scuderi G, Insall JN. Evolution of the quadriceps snip. *Clin Orthop.* 1995;321:131–137.

8. Scott RD, Siliski JM. The use of a modified V-Y quadricepsplasty during total knee replacement to gain exposure and improve knee flexion in the ankylosed knee. *Orthopedics.* 1985;8:45–48.

9. Coonse K, Adams JD. A new operative approach to the knee joint. *Surg Gynecol Obstet.* 1943;77:344.

10. Dolin MG. Osteotomy of the tibial tubercle in total knee replacement. *J Bone Joint Surg.* 1983;65-A:704–706.

11. Wolff AM, Hungerford DS, Krakow KA, Jacobs MA. Osteotomy of the tibial tubercle during total knee replacement. *J Bone Joint Surg.* 1989;71A:848–852.

12. Whiteside LA. Exposure in difficult total knee arthroplasty using tibial tubercle osteotomy. *Clin Orthop.* 1995;321:32–35.

13. Ritter MA, Carr K, Keating M, Faris, PM, Meding JB. Tibial shaft fracture following tibial tubercle osteotomy. *J Arthroplasty.* 1996;11(1):117–119.

14. Windsor RE, Insall JN. Exposure in revision total knee arthroplasty: the femoral peel. *Tech Orthop.* 1988;3:1–4.

15. Engh GA. Medial epicondylar osteotomy: a technique used with primary and revision total knee arthroplasty to improve surgical exposure and correct varus deformity. *Instr Course Lect.* 1999;48:153–156.

16. Kerry RM, Masri BA, Beauchamp CP, Duncan CP. The quadriceps myocutaneous flap for operation on the distal femur. *J Bone Joint Surg.* 1999;81B(3):485–487.

CHAPTER 7

Removal of the Femoral and Tibial Components for Revision Total Knee Arthroplasty

Daniel J. Berry

The importance of implant removal in revision knee arthroplasty frequently is overlooked as the surgeon concentrates on the planned reconstructive phase of the operation.[1] However, safe and effective implant removal is important for several reasons. First, implant removal can be a time-consuming process, particularly if the surgeon is not familiar with optimal techniques or if the surgeon does not have optimal tools available for the purpose. Second, severe bone loss or bone fracture can occur during implant removal. Marked unnecessary bone loss has a substantial negative impact on the type and quality of the reconstruction that subsequently can be performed. Methods of safe implant removal have advanced dramatically over the last decade, and in most cases today, implants can be removed efficiently and with relatively little bone loss.

TOOLS FOR IMPLANT REMOVAL

Tools available for implant removal include hand instruments, power instruments, and ultrasonic instruments. In addition, certain implant-specific instruments are helpful to disassemble or extract certain implant designs.

Hand Instruments

Osteotomes Osteotomes can be used to divide implant-cement interfaces and implant-bone interfaces. Stacked osteotomes can be used to lever implants away from underlying bone or cement. When bone beneath the implant is soft, it is important to be careful that osteotomes do not crush the underlying bone. When an osteotome is used to remove cemented implants, keeping the osteotome at the implant-cement interface rather than the cement-bone interface is preferable.

Gigli Saws Gigli saws can be used to cut beneath implants in areas that are inaccessible to power saws.[2] However, Gigli saws can migrate, and most surgeons have found that they tend to remove more bone than hand saws for applications such as removal of the femoral component.

Punches Punches are useful to disimpact well-fixed implants from the bone.

Power Instruments

Power Saws Power saws can very effectively divide the implant-bone interfaces of uncemented implants. Thin saw blades remove less bone, but can also wander into healthy bone.

Power Burs Thin-profile cutting burs can divide interfaces that are not easily accessible to power saws.

Metal Cutting Instruments Metal cutting instruments can cut away portions of well-fixed metal implants, thereby allowing access to otherwise inaccessible interfaces. For example, a metal cutting instrument can be used to remove a portion of a femoral or tibial component to allow access to a well-fixed underlying stem.

Ultrasonic Instruments

Ultrasonic instruments can be very useful to divide metal-cement and cement-bone interfaces. Special ultrasonic cutting tips are available that allow the metal-cement interface to be divided effectively.[3–5]

STRATEGIES FOR IMPLANT REMOVAL

Exposure

Adequate exposure is essential for safe implant removal. A safe path to disrupt implant interfaces must be gained and soft tissues, especially the extensor mechanism, popliteal vascular structures, and the collateral ligaments must be protected. A safe trajectory for implant extraction, particularly for the tibial component, also must be gained, while protecting the remaining bone from damage.

Loose Implants Loose implants typically can be removed with little difficulty, once adequate exposure has been achieved. As implants are removed, care should be taken that surrounding soft tissue and bony structures are not damaged. Loose, uncemented implants may have fibrous fixation that allows micromotion but does not allow easy extraction. The fibrous tissue usually can be disrupted with an osteotome, following which the loose implant is easier to remove.

Well-Fixed Cemented Implants For well-fixed cemented implants, it is desirable to remove the metal implant from the cement mantle and leave the cement mantle behind (Figure 7-1). Subsequently, the cement can be removed under direct vision with hand or power instruments, thereby minimizing bone loss. Implants with a smooth surface typically can be debonded from the underlying cement without difficulty. For implants that are well bonded to the cement, more aggressive means of cutting the implant free of the cement with saws,

FIGURE 7-1. Disrupting the cement-metal interface of a femoral component with an osteotome. The goal is to debond the implant from the cement first, then to remove remaining cement after the metal implant has been removed.

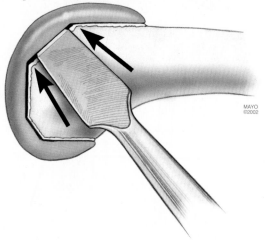

osteotomes, or ultrasonic instruments sometimes are necessary.

Well-Fixed Uncemented Implants For well-fixed uncemented implants, the implant-bone interface should be divided before extraction is attempted, otherwise substantial bone loss can result if the bone is pulled away with the implant. The bone-implant interface is best divided sharply with a power saw, Gigli saw, osteotomes, or thin high-speed cutting tools.

Order of Implant Removal An orderly process of implant removal reduces the likelihood of associated complications. In most cases the preferred sequence of implant removal, after gaining knee exposure, is: (A) removal of the tibial polyethylene insert; (B) removal of the femoral component; (C) removal of the tibial component; and (D) removal of the patellar component. This order of implant removal provides successively better exposure for removal of each subsequent implant. Removal of the tibial insert facilitates exposure of the femoral component because knee flexion is easier, and removal of the femoral component provides better access to the posterior aspect of the tibial component, facilitating its safe removal.

METHODS TO REMOVE EACH IMPLANT

Removal of the Tibial Polyethylene Insert

The tibial polyethylene insert, whether modular or non-modular, usually can be disengaged from the underlying metal tibial tray. Removal of the tibial polyethylene insert creates a space that allows easier exposure of the remaining implants and sometimes can reduce the amount of dissection required to gain access to the tibial and femoral components. Removal of the polyethylene insert of most modular knees (and even nonmodular knees) can be achieved by levering the tibial insert out of the tray with an osteotome. Many manufacturers also have implant-specific tools to remove the modular polyethylene from the tibial tray. The surgeon should be aware that special screws or pins may secure the tibial insert to the tray; having manufacturer-specific screwdrivers or pin-grasping instruments available is helpful. When difficulty is encountered removing the tibial polyethylene from the tray, an osteotome or saw can be used to divide the tibial polyethylene, after which it can be removed from the metal tray.

Removal of the Femoral Component

Removal of the femoral component begins by dividing the implant-cement interface (for cemented implants) or the implant-bone interface (for uncemented implants). For cemented implants, the best instruments are osteotomes or ultrasonic instruments, and for uncemented implants the best instruments are power saws, thin osteotomes, or thin high-speed cutting instruments. The anterior flange interface, distal interface, and chamfer interfaces usually all can be accessed without difficulty. Fixation pegs at the distal interface may impede access to a small central part of that interface. Narrow osteotomes or saws can be used to work along the chamfer interfaces or in the narrow spaces between fixation pegs of the distal interface. It is best to work from both the medial and lateral sides of the implant separately; this reduces the distance that the sharp instruments travel while out of sight beneath the implant, and thus reduces the likelihood of the instrument wandering away from the implant and creating excessive bone loss. The posterior condylar interfaces are hardest to access, but often there is osteolysis or little fixation at this interface. Dividing this interface is best done with special angled osteotomes, a thin saw, or a Gigli saw. Once the implant interfaces are divided, the femoral component may be removed with a company-specific or generic extractor that grasps the femoral implant and allows extraction with a slap hammer. Alternatively the implant can be tapped off of the femur gently using a metal punch against the anterior flange of the implant.

Posterior stabilized implants with a closed posterior cam box present interfaces that are difficult to access. Special care needs to be taken to remove these implants gently to avoid fracturing a condyle away from the femur.

Removal of the Tibial Component

Most tibial components can be removed by passing a saw or osteotome beneath the tibial tray, then levering the tibial component away from underlying bone. As is the case for femoral components, cemented implants usually can be removed by passing an osteotome between the implant and the cement. When the metal implant is roughened, porous coated or precoated, the cement may not readily separate from the metal. In this circumstance the cement can be divided with a saw or ultrasonic instruments to facilitate implant removal. Uncemented implants usually can be removed by dividing the bone-implant interface with a saw. When pegs, central stems, or keels prevent the surgeon from passing instruments from anterior to posterior, to divide posterior interfaces of the tibial implant, good medial exposure with external tibial rotation often allows instruments to be passed in a medial to lateral direction posterior to the pegs or keel. Care should be taken to protect soft tissues in the popliteal fossa area.

Once the proximal tibial interface is divided the tibial implant usually can be removed by using stacked osteotomes (Figure 7-2) to lever the tibial implant out of the tibia or by using a manufacturer specific or generic tibial implant extractor to pull the implant out of the tibia. During this process, the knee needs to be hyperflexed and the tibia translated anteriorly to avoid impingement of the tibial tray against the femoral condyle during extraction. The surgeon needs to be careful to avoid avulsion of the patellar tendon insertion at the tibial tubercle during this exposure. When extraction is difficult, a punch can be inserted beneath the tibial tray to drive it out of the tibia with a hammer. To gain purchase on the tray with a punch, a small medial or lateral hole in the tibial metaphyseal bone may be made that allows the punch to be directed perpendicularly against the tibial tray (Figure 7-3).

The surgeon should be cautious not to exert excessive force when trying to remove a tibial tray with a well-fixed keel or stem. At times the interface between the stem and the tibia needs to be accessed directly and divided before

FIGURE 7-2. Stacked osteotomes are used to lever a tibial component away from the bone. Care must be taken to avoid crushing underlying bone. The broadest osteotome is placed nearest the bone.

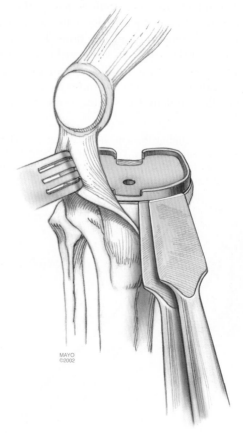

MAYO
©2002

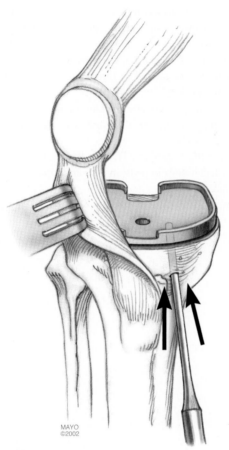

FIGURE 7-3. A punch used to disimpact a tibial component through a small hole drilled in the metaphysis.

the tray is removed. This technique is discussed in the following section.

Well-fixed, all-polyethylene implants can be removed easily by using a saw to cut through the inferior aspect of the tray at the bone-cement interface, thereby providing the surgeon with direct access to remaining cement and the keel. The keel can be removed by using a thin bur to cut the cement-implant interface.

Removal of Implants with Stems

Uncemented Stems Most implants with uncemented stems can be extracted using the same methods discussed previously for condylar implants. Most long uncemented knee implant stems are smooth or fluted with smooth surfaces and are not biologically fixed in the metaphysis or diaphysis. Therefore, once the condylar interfaces are divided, the implant with the stem attached can be driven out of the bone. Well-fixed roughened or porous stems are more difficult to remove. Thin high-speed cutting tools can be used to divide the metal-bone interface, or trephines designed to remove well-fixed total hip arthro-

plasty stems can be used to cut the stem free of bone. Initial removal of the condylar portion of the implant, discussed below, may be required to access the stem.

Cemented Stems Well-fixed implants with cemented stems can be very difficult to remove[6] and require an individualized approach that depends on the specific design and patient anatomy. Usually the interfaces of the condylar portion of the tibial or femoral implant are divided and then the implant—with stem attached—is driven out of the remaining cement. When this is not possible, sometimes the condylar portion of the implant can be disassembled from the stem, allowing the stem to be accessed separately. Alternatively, metal cutting instruments can be used to cut the stem, or a portion of the femoral or tibial implant, thereby allowing direct access to the stem (Figure 7-4). Once direct access to the stem has been gained, thin high-speed cutting tools or ultrasonic instruments can be used to divide the cement interface, allowing stem extraction. Some stems have manufacturer-specific threaded

FIGURE 7-4. Gaining access to a well-fixed tibial stem by cutting the metal tray of the tibial component. After the tray is removed, the interface along the stem can be divided.

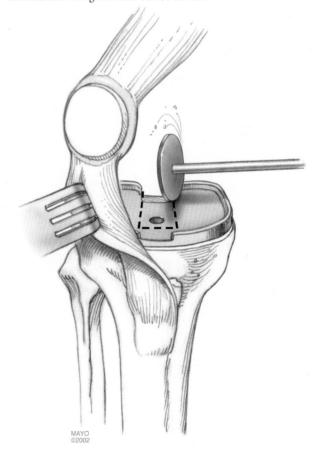

holes in the accessible end that help the surgeon gain purchase for extraction. On rare occasions, an osteotomy of the femur or extended tibial tubercle osteotomy may be needed to remove a very well-fixed stemmed implant.

REFERENCES

1. Berry DJ. Component removal during revision total knee arthroplasty. In: Lotke PA, Garino JP, eds. *Revision Total Knee Arthroplasty.* Philadelphia: Lippincott-Raven Publishers; 1999:187–196.

2. Firestone TP, Krackow KA. Removal of femoral components during revision knee arthroplasty. *J Bone Joint Surg.* 1991;73B:514.

3. Caillouette JT, Gorab RS, Klaspper RC, Anzel SH. Revision arthroplasty facilitated by ultrasonic tool cement removal. *Orthop Rev.* 1991;20:353–440.

4. Klapper RC, Caillouette JT. The use of ultrasonic tools in revision arthroplasty procedures. *Contemp Orthop.* 1990;20:273–278.

5. Klapper RC, Caillouette JT, Callaghan JJ, Hozack WJ. Ultrasonic technology in revision joint arthroplasty. *Clin Orthop.* 1992;285:147–154.

6. Cameron HU. Difficult implant retrieval: a case report. *Can J Surg.* 1989;32:220–221.

CHAPTER 8

Allograft in Revision Total Knee Arthroplasty

J. Craig Morrison and Donald T. Reilly

Some degree of bone loss is present in every failed total knee arthroplasty. In most instances, bone loss is minor and adequate bone stock is available to support primary components. However, certain failure modes lead to more severe bone loss that may affect the structural integrity of revision components. Management of this type of bone loss and the accompanying soft tissue asymmetry is the most challenging aspect of revision total knee arthroplasty. Augmentation with cement, bone graft, and modular or custom components may be needed. Cement is adequate in smaller defects and has been used in larger defects with screws.[1,2] Cement has poor biomechanical properties; therefore, as defects increase in size or complexity, other solutions are necessary. Graft offers intraoperative flexibility and relatively low cost when compared with customs. Autograft is preferred; however, it is usually in short supply in the revision setting. Therefore, allograft is relied on commonly in these situations. Despite its widespread use, good clinical studies are sparse. In this chapter, we delineate the indications and results of allograft in revision total knee arthroplasty.

PREOPERATIVE PLANNING

Modes of Failure

Although cliché, it is true that successful revision surgery begins with careful preoperative planning. It is essential in predicting the severity and location of bone loss. Planning should begin with an understanding of the mode of failure if the factors leading to the primary failure are to be corrected at revision surgery. The most common reasons for knee revision are aseptic loosening, osteolysis, and infection.[3]

Aseptic loosening alone is unlikely to result in massive bone loss unless grossly loose components are neglected.

However, loosening secondary to malalignment from ligament imbalance or component malposition can lead to characteristic deficiencies. This is most commonly seen in a residual varus malalignment that results from a varus tibial cut, an inadequately released medial side, or a combination of both. The tibial plateau collapses on the compression (medial) side, and the tibial component lifts off on the tension (lateral) side (Figure 8-1). Femoral condyles can collapse in the same way, particularly the lateral femoral condyle in an excessively valgus femur.

Although less commonly reported than in total hip arthroplasty, osteolysis from polyethylene debris does occur in cemented and cementless total knee arthroplasties.[4] High contact stresses secondary to poor design or technique can result in large volumes of debris. Regardless of particle size, large particle volume can cause early failure and catastrophic bone loss that is almost always underestimated by plain radiographs. As implant design, technique, and polyethylene quality have improved longevity, there is speculation that osteolysis may become a more common cause of late failure as well.[5] The surgeon should be prepared for major bone loss in a patient with a loose, painful total knee and any hint of cystic changes on x-ray.

Poor implant removal technique at the time of revision surgery is a further cause of bone loss. Patience is the key to removing any implant, well fixed or otherwise. It is imperative for the surgeon to expose the implant-bone interface. In cemented implants, disruption must occur at the implant-cement interface, not the cement-bone interface. Thin osteotomes are useful in this regard; however, one must fight the temptation to lever the implant out, as this may crush the underlying soft cancellous bone. Well-fixed cementless implants are difficult to remove. The use of a Gigli saw beneath the anterior flange and along the

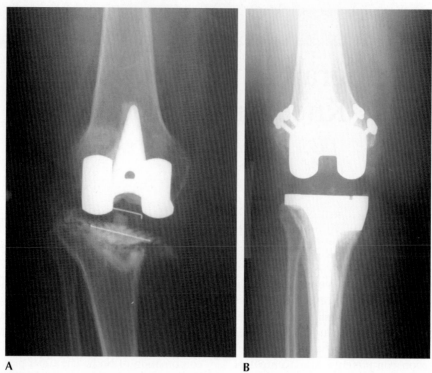

FIGURE 8-1. (A) Radiograph of a failed total knee arthroplasty, demonstrating medial tibial collapse with component liftoff on the lateral side. (B) This knee was reconstructed using a custom tibial component.

posterior condyles, coupled with thin curved osteotomes in the notch is recommended. The use of slap hammers should be avoided until complete implant loosening is confirmed. Ill-advised use of these devices can easily lead to femoral or tibial fractures. In some instances, a condyle or entire distal femur may be removed with the well-fixed implant.[6]

Defect Classification

Assessment of bone deficiency is best done after implant removal and preliminary cuts; however, the surgeon must have a reasonable expectation of the type of bone loss from preoperative x-rays. Several classification systems have been developed in the hip to assist revision surgeons. There has been less emphasis on defect classification in the knee. As in the hip, defects are generally divided into contained or segmental. Contained defects are surrounded by intact bone, whereas segmental defects have no remaining cortex.[7] Segmental defects can be further broken down into circumferential or non-circumferential.[6] Engh and Rubash have both devised classification schemes that attempt to correlate type and severity of defect with a recommended surgical management strategy[3,6] (Tables 8.1 and 8.2). Placement into one of these classification systems preoperatively allows the

surgeon to have appropriate instruments, hardware, and graft on hand to limit intraoperative surprises.

Several options for each category of deficiency are available to the revision surgeon. Cement with or without screws, modular or custom augments, and particulate or bulk graft have all been advocated for certain bone deficiencies.[4,5,8] For any strategy, implant stability on host bone is vital to long-term success. A second goal of revision surgery, namely bone stock restoration, may be accomplished through the use of bone graft. An understanding of the basic science involved in the use of allograft is exceedingly important for the revision surgeon to comprehend. Therefore, a brief review of the biology and biomechanical aspects of allograft is in order.

BASIC SCIENCE OF ALLOGRAFT

Biology

Bone was one of the first tissue transplants performed and remains one of, if not the most, abundant tissues transplanted. Originally, autograft was used to unite fractures and fuse joints. Allograft use increased in prevalence in orthopedic oncology as limb-salvage techniques improved. In revision hip and knee surgery, allograft bone

TABLE 8.1. Anderson Orthopaedic Research Institute Bone Defect Classification Guidelines.

	Preoperative Radiographs	*Surgical Management*
Type 1 defect (intact metaphyseal bone)	A full metaphyseal segment	No augments, structural bone grafts or cement fill >1 cm
Femur	Metaphyseal bone intact distal to the epicondyles	
	No component subsidence or osteolysis	
Tibia	Metaphyseal bone intact above tibial tubercle	
	No component subsidence or osteolysis	
Type 2 defect (damaged metaphyseal bone)	A shortened metaphyseal flare	Joint-line restoration with augments (>4 mm), particulate or chunk bone graft, or >1 cm cement fill; joint-line elevation with a primary component as the revision implant
Femur	Component subsidence or joint-line elevation of the failed component	
	Small osteolytic defects in bone distal to the epicondyles	
Tibia	Component subsidence or position up to or below the tip of the fibular head; a shortened tibial metaphyseal flare	
Type 3 defect (deficient metaphyseal bone)	A deficient metaphyseal segment	A reconstructed condyle or plateau with structural graft or cement, or a custom or hinged component
Femur	Bone damage to or above the level of the epicondyles	
	Component subsidence to the epicondyles	
Tibia	Bone damage or component subsidence to the tibial tubercle	

From Engh, Ammeen,[3] by permission of *Instr Course Lect.*

TABLE 8.2. Massachusetts General Hospital Femoral Defect Classification System for Total Knee Arthroplasty and Treatment Algorithm.

Classification

Minor	Below the level of the epicondyles
	Volume <1 cm^3
	Contained: No cortical bone loss, cancellous defects only
	Uncontained: Cortical loss resulting in an unsupported portion of the implant
Major	Defects are at or above the level of the epicondyles
	Volume >1 cm^3
	Contained: No cortical bone loss, cancellous defects only
	Uncontained: Cortical loss resulting in an unsupported portion of the implant or condylar fracture

Treatment algorithm

Defect Type	*Minor*	*Major*
Contained	Particulate graft	Bulk allograft
	Cement	Femoral head allograft
	Implants: CR or PS +/− stem	Implants: PS with stem, possible Constrained Condylar
Uncontained	Augments	Augments
	Structural graft	Condylar allograft
	Cement or particulate graft if <5 mm fill and varus/valgus stable	Bicondylar allograft
	Implants: PS with stem	Distal femoral allograft
		Implants: Constrained Condylar with long stem or hinged device

From Hoeffel, Rubash,[6] by permission of *Clin Orthop.*

is used when conventional methods of reconstruction are inadequate and because autograft is in short supply. As a tissue, bone has unique properties that are critical for success. *Osteogenesis* is the ability to produce new bone and is accomplished by osteoblasts. Bone proteins, such as bone morphogeneic protein that are a part of the bone matrix, stimulate new bone formation through the recruitment and differentiation of pluripotential mesenchymal stem cells into osteoblasts. This characteristic is known as *osteoinduction*. Lastly, *osteoconduction* is the graft's ability to act as scaffolding for the ingrowth of blood vessels and cells from the host bed. The process known as *creeping substitution* is the gradual resorption and replacement of this scaffolding with host bone. Autograft and fresh allograft possess all of these properties. Fresh allografts, however, are rejected by the host immune system, resulting in complete graft resorption or marked delay in incorporation. Therefore, allograft used in revision joint surgery is processed and possesses the property of osteoconduction only. The success of allograft depends largely on its ability to heal to and incorporate with host bone. Histologically, these events are similar to fracture healing. Inflammation predominates early on. Unlike autograft, in which surviving surface osteoblasts contribute bone, allograft incorporation depends on osteoblasts differentiated from pluripotential cells brought in by vasculature from the host bed. Thus, the process is similar to autograft incorporation, but slower. This early phase is similar for cancellous as well as cortical bone. Creeping substitution characterizes the incorporation of cancellous bone. That is, bone formation and resorption occur concomitantly. Eventually the entire graft may be replaced by host bone. In cortical bone, formation only occurs after resorption. Consequently, the graft is weaker than normal bone for a long period of time and must be protected from excessive loading. In theory, this remodeling process eventually involves the entire structural graft. In reality, these grafts have little biologic activity outside of the graft-host junction.[9]

Although animal studies have supplied most of our knowledge of the basic science of allograft, human retrievals have given the most insight into the biologic behavior of processed allografts in humans. Enneking et al. studied 16 retrieved massive human allografts that had been *in situ* for 4 to 65 months.[10] They demonstrated that union between allograft and host took place slowly at cortical-cortical junctions and more rapidly at cancellous-cancellous junctions. Internal repair was confined to the superficial surfaces and ends of the grafts and had involved only 20% of the graft by 5 years. The deep portions of the graft retained their architecture. Parks and Engh's study of allografts in revision knee arthroplasty retrievals had similar findings with no evidence of revas-

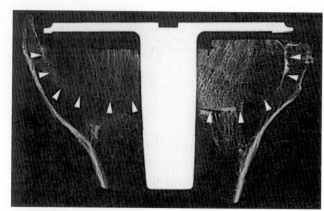

FIGURE 8-2. Slab radiograph showing location and intact structure of two femoral head allografts in the proximal tibia. Note host to graft junction (arrows). (From Parks, Engh,[11] by permission of *Clin Orthop.*)

cularization, resorption, or remodeling beyond the graft-host union[11] (Figures 8-2 and 8-3).

Ultimately, the biology depends greatly on the clinical situation and the type of graft used. As discussed, bone loss in revision surgery can be cavitary or segmental. A cavitary lesion with a well-vascularized bed is ideal for cancellous bone, and complete incorporation is to be expected. With increasing bone loss and decreasing vascularity, a more inconsistent incorporation is to be expected. In contrast, segmental loss requiring large structural allograft relies on cortical-to-cortical contact between host and graft. The majority of the graft is surrounded by soft tissue that is usually avascular scar. Here the allograft can unite to host bone, but there will be little if any internal remodeling of the graft.[10]

FIGURE 8-3. Left to right: live marrow elements, live host bone, dead graft bone, avascular grafted region. The live bone is growing onto the dead graft as if it were a scaffold at the host to graft junction (Stain, hematoxylin and eosin; magnification light microscopy, ×200). (From Parks, Engh,[11] by permission of *Clin Orthop.*)

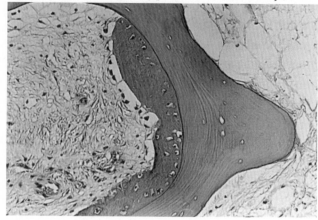

Biomechanics

In reviewing the biology of allografts, we see that union with host bone is the first step toward success. Unfortunately, failure can and does still follow all too often. Fracture of structural allograft is reported to be as high as 16.5%.[12] It goes without saying that the biomechanical behavior of the graft is of critical importance in determining success or failure. The individual factors that influence the physical properties of transplantable bone are analyzed in this section.

The ability of a graft to withstand loads is largely determined by the original properties of the bone at the time of donation. Although supply often limits surgeons' options when choosing donor material, the factors that influence these properties should be known. For instance, bone tissue is strongest in the 20- to 39-year-old age groups and typically weakens thereafter. However, even in the 70- to 79-year-old age group, 70% to 85% of the maximum strength is maintained.[13] The surgeon can more closely control other factors, such as the method of preservation and sterilization.

The more common methods of preserving and storing specimens until they are required for implantation are freezing and freeze-drying. Both alter the immunogenicity of the graft, but freeze-drying has a more substantial effect on the physical properties.[13,14] Freeze-drying causes little change or a slight increase in compressive strength, but lowers the bending and torsional strength substantially.[12,15,16] Cracks have been observed in rehydrated freeze-dried specimens, which might explain the observed reduction in strength.[15] Freezing alone has little if any effect on the physical properties of bone.[15,17] These observations suggest that fresh frozen bone would be best when large torsional and bending loads can be expected. Clinically, this would be seen at the host-graft junction when a whole distal femur was used. Conversely, in a situation in which the graft will see primarily compressive loads, freeze-dried graft should be biomechanically sound. Most cavitary or isolated metaphyseal lesions fall into this category.

Sterilization of a graft prior to implantation can be done either of 2 ways. The grafts can be sterilely harvested and stored, or nonsterile grafts can be secondarily sterilized with high-dose radiation. Radiation below 3 megarads appears to cause little change in bone strength; however, above this level, significant alterations in the physical properties occur, resulting in a decrease in the compressive, bending, and torsional strength of the graft. These effects are magnified when combined with freeze-drying.[16,17]

Once retrieved, preserved, stored, sterilized, and implanted, a bone graft is subjected to load. Bone can fail under the single application of a large load if a fall or some other trauma ensues. However, fatigue failure secondary to repetitive smaller loads is more common with large allografts. Live bone is capable of remodeling when subjected to these loads. Until transplanted bone becomes vascularized it does not have this capability. Because retrieval studies have shown that outside of the host graft junction little remodeling occurs, it is imperative that large allografts be protected with adequate internal fixation to prevent fatigue failure. Intramedullary fixation with stemmed components is preferred over plates and screws because the stress risers made by screw holes weaken the graft, thus increasing the fracture risk.

Disease Transmission

Although extremely rare, transmission of an infectious agent through allograft bone transplantation has received much attention of late. Most of this has centered on transmission of human immunodeficiency virus (HIV). The risk estimate for HIV transmission in 1990 was 1 in 1.6 million.[18,19] With improved screening tools and sterilization methods and stricter donor criteria, this risk may be even less today. More recently the risk of bacterial contamination has emerged. After a Minnesota man died from a *Clostridium* infection 4 days after an osteochondral transplant, the Centers for Disease Control (CDC) uncovered 26 cases of infection from orthopedic allograft transplants. These risks should be considered when counseling patients on surgical options.

Indications and Techniques

Bone deficiency in many revisions is minor and contained. After component removal, bone loss is limited to punctate cancellous defects. Minor defects have been defined differently in terms of size. In general, it is assumed that cancellous metaphyseal bone is in sufficient supply and quality to support primary implants. In these cases, defects can be filled with cement, particulate autograft from bone cuts, or particulate allograft if autograft supply is insufficient. Outcome will be similar regardless of management.

Larger contained defects are commonly seen in failures resulting from polyethylene wear with associated osteolysis and component loosening. In these cases, cancellous metaphyseal bone is insufficient to support a primary component. On the femoral side, an intact rim of metaphyseal cortical bone is invariably present because this bone is stressed by collateral ligament attachments. When the tibial base plate subsides, the resultant defect may depend on the size and position of the base plate in relation to the proximal tibia. Commonly the base plate's perimeter sits just inside the cortical rim of the plateau. When the base plate subsides, an intact cortical rim is left, and a large central, cavitary defect remains after component removal. Although some authors advocate cement fill in these situations, allograft is preferable, because of its potential for incorporation in this setting.[1,2]

Some authors advocate the use of femoral head allografts for these defects.[3,20,21] Attention to detail is critical to success. The surgeon must first prepare the host bone. A clean, vascularized bed is ideal. All cement and fibrous debris should be removed. Sclerotic bone should be removed sufficiently to provide a bleeding bed without compromising structural integrity. Next the graft must be debrided of any cartilage or remaining soft tissue and fashioned to match the host defect as intimately as possible. The use of male and female hemispherical reamers has been described to facilitate this process[21] (Figure 8-4). Alternatively, saws or high-speed burs can be used. The fashioned graft is then placed into the defect. A gentle *press fit* is desirable if possible for additional stability (Figure 8-5). Any gaps between the graft-host junction should be packed with particulate graft (autograft if available). After placement, rigid fixation to host bone should be achieved with K-wires or small fragment screws. Rigid fixation is important for junctional healing, but the minimum amount of fixation necessary should be used to avoid unnecessary stress risers. Next, any protruding

graft should be resected to the level of the previously resected distal femur or proximal tibia. Because these grafts lend structural support to the implant, they must be protected with a load-sharing intramedullary stem. If the previously placed graft encroaches on the stem path it can be fashioned to allow the stem to pass. Often a high-speed bur is preferable to power reamers to allow more control and prevent graft fracture or fixation compromise. Finally, the components are placed. The undersurfaces of the femoral and tibial components should be cemented, as the cancellous allograft surface is excellent for cement interdigitation but has no potential for biologic fixation. The use of a cemented or cementless stem is the surgeon's preference. A cementless stem must be sufficiently long to engage the diaphysis.

Good results have also been published with the use of particulate allograft in these large contained defects.[22] Furthermore, biopsies have confirmed incorporation and revascularization. The downside to particulate graft is its poor load-sharing capability. The surgeon must be confident that the revision component is stable on the intact cortical rim of host bone to avoid asymmetric stress on the implant that may lead to subsidence or component

FIGURE 8-4. (A) Reaming a tibial defect with an acetabular reamer to prepare it for a femoral head allograft. (B) Reaming the femoral head allograft with female hemispheric reamers (Allogrip, DePuy, Warsaw, IN) to remove cartilage and subchondral bone. (C) The arrow indicates the femoral head allograft, which was placed into the proximal tibial defect and cut flush with the proximal tibia. (From Parks, Engh,[11] by permission of *Clin Orthop.*)

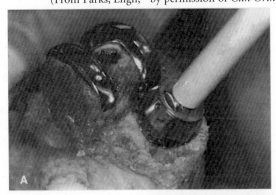
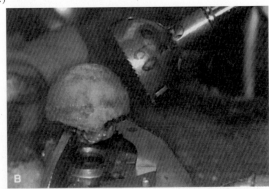
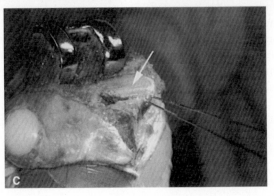

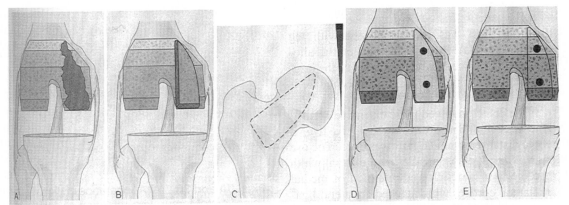

FIGURE 8-5. (A) Typical complex distal femoral condylar deficiency. (B) Appearance of the same deficiency after contouring into geometric configuration. (C) Outline of a femoral head allograft to fit the defect. (D) The deficiency after the placement of the allograft, in which intimate allograft to host bone junction apposition and screw stabilization are shown. (E) The deficiency after bony resection before prosthetic implantation. (From Tsahakis, Beaver, Brick,[20] by permission of *Clin Orthop.*)

fracture. As with structural grafts, an intramedullary stem must be used.

Unlike cavitary, or contained defects, segmental bone loss involves cortical bone that is needed to support implants when the joint line is properly restored. Modular revision implants are well suited to manage these defects if they are not too large.[8,23,24] On the tibial side, wedges or block augments along with intramedullary stems are ideal for defects involving one plateau. In this manner, the implant can be stabilized circumferentially on viable host bone. Unfortunately, tibial augments are not contoured to match the relatively acute flare of the tibial metaphysis. In defects greater than 1 cm there may be significant overhang resulting in medial collateral *tenting* or soft tissue irritation. For reconstruction of defects larger than 1 cm, the surgeon should consider use of a femoral head allograft, partial proximal tibial allograft, or custom augment (Figures 8-1 and 8-6A–D).

FIGURE 8-6. (A and B) Preoperative and postoperative radiographs demonstrating severe proximal tibial bone loss status open reduction internal fixation. (C and D) Five-year postoperative radiographs showing a custom long stem tibial component (Techmedica, Camarillo, CA) and with structural allograft medially.

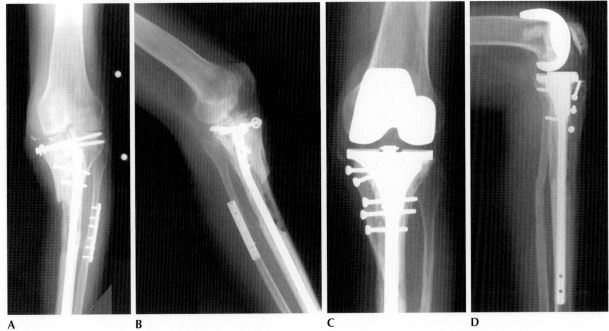

A   B   C   D

If both sides of the plateau are involved, bilateral block augments up to 1 cm are acceptable in helping reestablish the joint line. If larger augments are needed, the surgeon may elect to downsize the tibial base plate up to one size smaller than the femoral component if this will result in stable contact between the smaller augments and host bone. Obviously, this will require a thicker insert, and the revision system must accommodate this. Alternatively, a custom base plate or complete proximal tibial allograft can be used. The real advantage of an allograft is its intraoperative adaptability. In theory, bone stock is reconstituted. This assumption is controversial and not supported by retrieval studies of large structural graft in the hip and knee.[10,11,25] The best one can hope for in this situation is sufficient load-sharing by an intramedullary stem to prevent fatigue failure and ultimately collapse of the allograft. It is essentially an inert implant but with less predictable *in vitro* mechanical characteristics than metal.

The technique for a proximal tibial allograft involves a *back table* arthroplasty. First, the combined thickness of the base plate and allograft must be determined. This composite must restore the joint line when combined with a reasonable range of insert thicknesses. The proximal tibial surface is then resected perpendicular to the host tibial mechanical axis with the proper slope. The graft-host junction is prepared to optimize contact surface area preferably parallel to the proximal surface to decrease shear forces. Internal step cuts further increase contact and enhance rotational stability. Finally, the assembled tibial component is cemented to the allograft and the composite is stabilized to the host with a press-fit stem that engages the tibial diaphysis (Figure 8-7).

Segmental femoral defects should be handled with a similar philosophy. Unlike the tibia, however, in which only one surface must be addressed, the surgeon must adequately reconstruct the distal and posterior surfaces of the femur to obtain symmetric flexion and extension gaps. Modular augments in most revision systems come in sizes up to 12 mm. As long as bone loss is distal to the collateral attachments, augments are sufficient and can even be stacked and cemented together if necessary. Distally, the augments must contact enough host bone to be deemed stable by the operative surgeon. As the trial augment contacts the distal cortical rim during trial femoral insertion, the surgeon must make note of any residual deficiency behind the augment that is now essentially a contained defect. If this residual defect does not jeopardize stability, then cement or morsellized graft can be used. However, if stability may be jeopardized, or the surgeon finds that stem position and femoral component size do not allow the augment to contact the intact cortical rim, then the use of a structural graft as described previously for large contained defects should be added to the construct (Figure 8-8). Furthermore, if this residual

FIGURE 8-7. (A) Failed, infected total knee arthroplasty demonstrating severe tibial and femoral bone loss. (B and C) Postoperative radiographs taken three years after revision using a custom femoral component, custom tibial stem, custom tibial insert, and structural allograft cemented to the tibial and femoral components (Techmedica, Camarillo, CA).

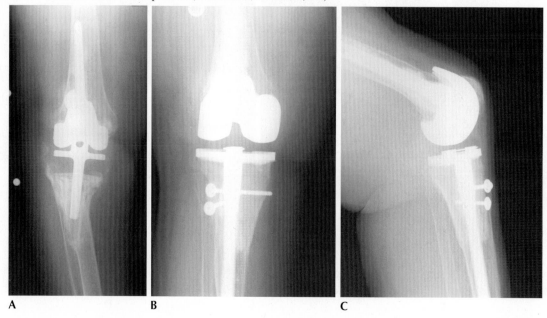

A   B   C

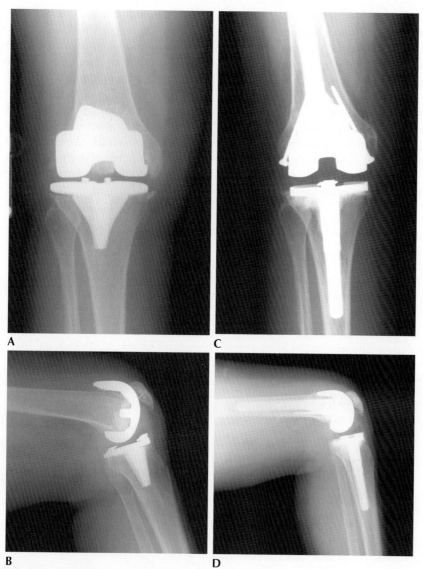

FIGURE 8-8. (A and B) Preoperative radiographs of a failed total knee, demonstrating a loose femoral component and posterior cruciate ligament insufficiency. Although the epicondyles are intact, there is significant cone-shaped bone loss centrally. (C and D) At 4 years postoperatively, the allograft appears to have incorporated nicely.

deficiency is bicondylar, as is seen in the cone-shaped femur, then use of a metaphyseal sleeve augment should be considered. This implant is described in greater detail in the custom chapter and is currently only available with the S-ROM knee system. (DePuy Corporation, a Johnson & Johnson Company, Warsaw, IN).

For bone loss that extends proximally to involve the collateral insertions on the femoral epicondyles, modular augmentation is insufficient. Comminuted supracondylar fractures, neglected femoral subsidence, and revisions for infection account for the majority of these catastrophic scenarios. In these instances, ligamentous stability, as well as component stability must be considered. Options available to the surgeon include segmental replacement with a tumor or custom prosthesis, or reconstruction with a distal femoral allograft. The allograft can be partial or a femoral head if only one condyle is involved, or complete if bicondylar (Figure 8-9A–D). Some authors advocate the use of a highly constrained implant if remaining epicondylar bone is sufficient to allow rigid attachment of the collaterals to the allograft, but use of a rotating hinge may be desirable (Figure 8-10). As in all revisions with significant defects, tightly fitting, long, diaphyseal-filling stems must be used.

FIGURE 8-9. (A) Preparation of the host bed of the lateral femoral condyle (2) with use of an acetabular reamer. *1 = damaged medial femoral condyle, and 3 = tibia.* (B) The femoral-head allograft is prepared with use of a female-type reamer. (C) The femoral head allograft is placed in the prepared host bed and is secured by an interference fit and temporary stabilization with Kirschner wires. (D) The allograft and the bone in the distal part of the femur are resected to allow the revision femoral component with a canal-filling stem to be inserted with cement. (From Engh, Herzwurm, Parks,[21] by permission of *J Bone Joint Surg Am.*)

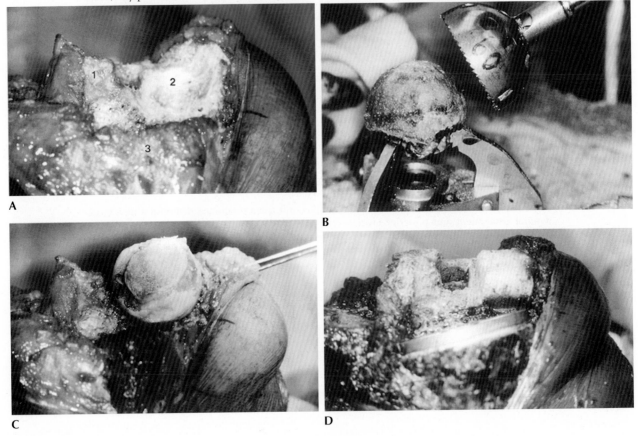

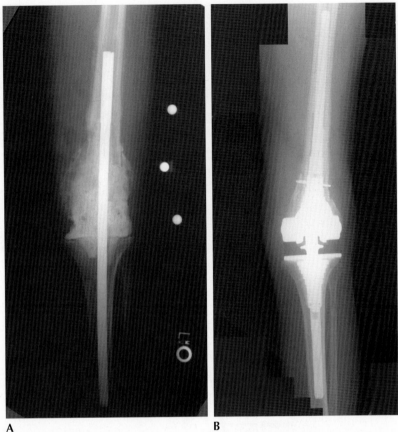

A   **B**

FIGURE 8-10. (A) Preoperative radiograph of a failed total knee status post resection, demonstrating significant femoral and tibial bone loss. (B) This knee was reconstructed using the S-ROM Noiles rotating hinge total knee system (DePuy Orthopaedics, Warsaw, IN).

Clatworthy et al. have elegantly illustrated and described the technique for distal femoral allograft composite reconstruction[26] (Figure 8-11). To ensure proper size, the radiograph of the allograft should be compared with the radiograph of the contralateral knee. They recommend using an allograft smaller than the host bone so that it may be placed within any remaining host cortical shell. As for a proximal tibial allograft, a *back table* arthroplasty is performed after assurance that the graft is the appropriate length to establish the proper joint line. A step-cut junction with host bone is recommended and cerclage wires with strut grafts are preferred over plates and screws to prevent stress risers in the graft (Figure 8-12).

RESULTS

Allograft options include morsellized graft, or structural grafts. Whiteside and Bicalho reviewed their experience with morsellized graft in revision knee arthroplasty.[22] Sixty-two knees required major grafting of the tibia and/or the femur. Major defects were defined as necessitating at least 30 mL of bone graft. Over one-half of the defects required greater than 60 mL of graft. The graft was a combination of fresh frozen cancellous morsels measuring 0.5 to 1.0 cm plus powdered demineralized cancellous bone. The authors emphasized rim fit of the components over at least 25% of the intact cortical rim and press-fit diaphyseal filling stems. All components

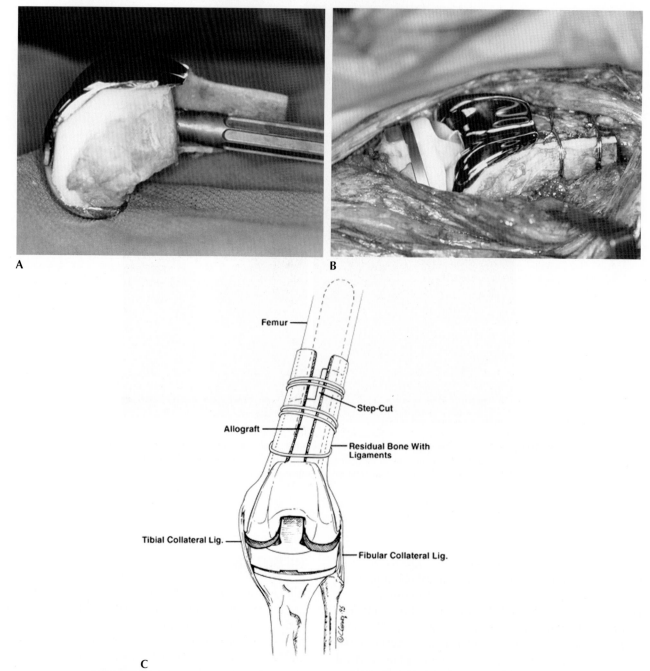

FIGURE 8-11. (A) The component is cemented onto the allograft and cement is inserted up to the level of the step-cut. (B) The distal femoral allograft construct after implantation. (C) The distal femoral allograft construct. (From Clatworthy, Ballance, Brick, et al.,[26] by permission of *J Bone Joint Surg Am.*)

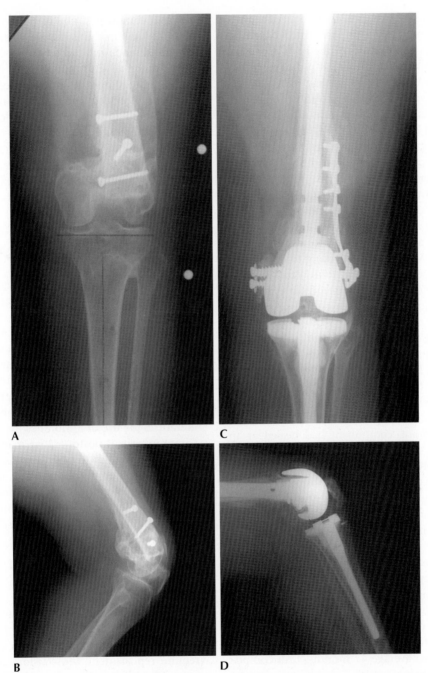

A   C

B   D

FIGURE 8-12. (A and B) Preoperative radiograph of a patient with posttraumatic arthritis with malunion of the distal femur. (C and D) Radiographs at 10 years postoperatively. The knee was reconstructed using structural allograft fixed with a lateral T buttress plate and screws and custom femoral component (Techmedica, Camarillo, CA). Note the fibrous union of the medial epicondyle. Current technique includes a step-cut with cerclage cables rather than overplating.

were cementless. Fourteen knees (22%) underwent revision for various reasons. Two were revised for loosening. All of those revisions had biopsies of the graft between 3 weeks and 37 months. After 1 year, all radiographically visible allografts were said to show healing with a trabecular pattern. Biopsy specimens showed vascular ingrowth and new bone formation. At 37 months, allograft bone was still present, but encased by viable lamellar bone.

Structural bone grafting for segmental, large cavitary, and combined defects has seen promising short- and midterm results. Engh and Parks reviewed the histology and radiographs from seven bulk allografts retrieved from three knees.[11] Five grafts in 2 knees were post-mortem and two grafts in one knee were biopsied at re-revision. Grafts had been in situ for and average of 41 months. All grafts were used to treat T3/F3 lesions according to the Anderson Orthopaedic Research Institute (AORI) classification system. No components were loose and all grafts had healed at the graft-host junction. No grafts had revascularized, resorbed, or remodeled.

Engh et al. also reviewed their midterm clinical results with structural allografts for type III defects.[21] Twenty-nine femoral heads, 5 composite distal femurs, and one composite proximal tibia were used in these reconstructions. At a mean of 50 months, 26 of 30 patients had good or excellent results. Radiographically, all grafts not obscured by the femoral component had healed at an average of 7 months. Three of 4 uncemented components subsided significantly. No cemented components subsided. All stems were uncemented. No revisions were performed for loosening.

Ghazavi et al. followed 30 knees with whole or partial distal femoral or proximal tibia allografts for an average of 50 months.[27] All components were cemented, with uncemented long stems. There were 7 failures. Two of 4 knees revised for septic loosening failed for recurrent infection. One additional failure for infection occurred. Two components loosened, one graft fractured, and one graft-host nonunion occurred. Mow and Wiedel reviewed their results in 13 patients with 15 distal femoral or proximal tibial grafts at an average 47 months.[28] All components were uncemented except for 3 distal femoral and 4 proximal tibias, in which the component was cemented to the allograft only. All grafts healed radiographically. No components loosened or subsided.

Clatworthy et al. reported a series of structural allografts in revision total knee arthroplasty.[26] All defects were large segmental defects defined as loss of supporting cortical rim bone. Defects were further classified as noncircumferential or circumferential. Non-circumferential defects were treated with femoral heads, partial distal femurs, or partial proximal tibias rigidly fixed to host bone. Circumferential deficiencies were managed with allograft composites. The average follow-up of 96 months is the longest in the literature. Fifty-two knees requiring 66 grafts made up the study. Forty-eight of the grafts were whole allograft composites. All components were cemented to allograft, with 39 procedures utilizing press-fit stems. Thirteen knees were considered failures. Five were revised for resorption and loosening. Four knees failed for infection, including one of 6 revised for septic failure. Two knees went on to nonunion with one of these requiring revision. Finally, 2 knees in one patient failed clinically. Overall success was 75%. Graft survival was 92% at 5 years and 79% at 10 years.

POSTOPERATIVE MANAGEMENT

Most of the literature on allografting in revision total knee arthroplasty has focused on radiographic and functional outcomes. Attention to operative technique is stressed and often detailed. Postoperative management, however, is mentioned only in passing. Most surgeons recommend protected weightbearing for a minimum of 6 to 8 weeks. It is probably advisable to extend this until radiographic signs of union at the graft-host interface are present. This could take several months. Although not advocated in the literature, the use of antibiotics for a prolonged time is a common part of postoperative management. Allograft is a nidus for the growth of organisms. Indeed, the infection rate for revisions with allograft is roughly twice that of comparable revision series without allograft.[7,26,28-30] Despite this fact, previous infection is not viewed as an absolute contraindication to the use of allograft.

CONCLUSION

Most defects encountered at the time of revision surgery can be reconstructed with augments and stems available in modern revision systems. Larger defects, however, may require replacement with custom implants or allograft bone. Morsellized allograft is ideal for smaller contained defects and has even been successful in larger defects as long as the component achieves stability on host rim bone.[22] Structural allograft should be considered in large contained, segmental, and combined defects. When circumferential, deficiencies can be reconstructed with whole allograft composites. Medium-term survival is encouraging.[26]

Technique is critical. Rigid fixation between graft and host is essential. Components should be cemented to cut surfaces, as allograft has no biologic potential for ingrowth. Press-fit diaphyseal stems share load to protect grafts, but may allow enough compressive force to promote union. Although radiographic resorption is reported in most series, it is unlikely that grafts revascularize and collapse. Retrieval studies in the knee and hip do not show revascularization or resorption.[10,11,25] Graft collapse is probably due to trabecular fracture and the inability of the graft to repair and remodel. Many acetabular grafts failed early because they were not off loaded. With the use of cages, survival has improved. Likewise, in the knee, stems reduce stress on grafts and protect against early fatigue failure.

REFERENCES

1. Elia EA, Lotke PA. Results of revision total knee arthroplasty associated with significant bone loss. *Clin Orthop.* 1991; 271:114–121.

2. Ritter MA. Screw and cement fixation of large defects in total knee arthroplasty. *J Arthroplasty.* 1986;1:125–129.

3. Engh GA, Ammeen DJ. Bone loss with revision total knee arthroplasty: defect classification and alternatives for reconstruction. *Instr Course Lect.* 1999;48:167–175.

4. Peters PC Jr, Engh GA, Dwyer KA, Vinh TN. Osteolysis after total knee arthroplasty without cement. *J Bone Joint Surg Am.* 1992;74:864–876.

5. Howling GI, Barnett PI, Tipper JL, Stone MH, Fisher J, Ingham E. Quantitative characterization of polyethylene debris isolated from periprosthetic tissue in early failure knee implants and early and late failure Charnley hip implants. *J Biomed Mater Res.* 2001;58:415–420.

6. Hoeffel DP, Rubash HE. Revision total knee arthroplasty: current rationale and techniques for femoral component revision. *Clin Orthop.* 2000;380:116–132.

7. Stockley I, McAuley JP, Gross AE. Allograft reconstruction in total knee arthroplasty. *J Bone Joint Surg Br.* 1992;74: 393–397.

8. Brand MG, Daley RJ, Ewald FC, Scott RD. Tibial tray augmentation with modular metal wedges for tibial bone stock deficiency. *Clin Orthop.* 1989;248:71–79.

9. Garbuz DS, Masri BA, Czitrom AA. Biology of allografting. *Orthop Clin North Am.* 1998;29:199–204.

10. Enneking WF, Mindell ER. Observations on massive retrieved human allografts. *J Bone Joint Surg Am.* 1991;73: 1123–1142.

11. Parks NL, Engh GA. The Ranawat Award. Histology of nine structural bone grafts used in total knee arthroplasty. *Clin Orthop.* 1997;345:17–23.

12. Mankin HJ, Doppelt SH, Sullivan TR, Tomford WW. Osteoarticular and intercalary allograft transplantation in the management of malignant tumors of bone. *Cancer.* 1982; 50:613–660.

13. Pelker RR, Friedlaender GE. Biomechanical aspects of bone autografts and allografts. *Orthop Clin North Am.* 1987;18: 235–239.

14. Friedlaender GE, Strong DM, Sell KW. Studies on the antigenicity of bone. I. Freeze-dried and deep-frozen bone allografts in rabbits. *J Bone Joint Surg Am.* 1976;58: 854–858.

15. Pelker RR, Friedlaender GE, Markham TC, Panjabi MM, Moen CJ. Effects of freezing and freeze-drying on the biomechanical properties of rat bone. *J Orthop Res.* 1984;1: 405–411.

16. Triantafyllou N, Sotiropoulos E, Triantafyllou JN. The mechanical properties of the lyophylized and irradiated bone grafts. *Acta Orthop Belg.* 1975;41(Suppl 1):35–44.

17. Komender A. Influence of preservation on some mechanical properties of human haversian bone. *Mater Med Pol.* 1976;8:13–17.

18. Buck BE, Malinin TI, Brown MD. Bone transplantation and human immunodeficiency virus. an estimate of risk of acquired immunodeficiency syndrome (AIDS). *Clin Orthop.* 1989;240:129–136.

19. Carlson ER, Marx RE, Buck BE. The potential for HIV transmission through allogenic bone. a review of risks and safety. *Oral Surg Oral Med Oral Pathol Oral Radiol Endod.* 1995;80:17–23.

20. Tsahakis PJ, Beaver WB, Brick GW. Technique and results of allograft reconstruction in revision total knee arthroplasty. *Clin Orthop.* 1994;303:86–94.

21. Engh GA, Herzwurm PJ, Parks NL. Treatment of major defects of bone with bulk allografts and stemmed components during total knee arthroplasty. *J Bone Joint Surg Am.* 1997;79:1030–1039.

22. Whiteside LA, Bicalho PS. Radiologic and histologic analysis of morselized allograft in revision total knee replacement. *Clin Orthop.* 1998;357:149–156.

23. Scott RD. Bone loss: prosthetic and augmentation method. *Orthopedics.* 1995;18:923–926.

24. Dennis DA. Repairing minor bone defects: augmentation & autograft. *Orthopedics.* 1998;21:1036–1038.

25. Hooten JP Jr, Engh CA, Heekin RD, Vinh TN. Structural bulk allografts in acetabular reconstruction. Analysis of two grafts retrieved at post-mortem. *J Bone Joint Surg Br.* 1996; 78:270–275.

26. Clatworthy MG, Ballance J, Brick GW, Chandler HP, Gross AE. The use of structural allograft for uncontained defects in revision total knee arthroplasty. a minimum five-year review. *J Bone Joint Surg Am.* 2001;83-A:404–411.

27. Ghazavi MT, Stockley I, Yee G, Davis A, Gross AE. Reconstruction of massive bone defects with allograft in revision total knee arthroplasty. *J Bone Joint Surg Am.* 1997;79: 17–25.

28. Mow CS, Wiedel JD. Revision total knee arthroplasty using the porous-coated anatomic revision prosthesis: six- to twelve-year results. *J Arthroplasty.* 1998;13:681–686.

29. Friedman RJ, Hirst P, Poss R, Kelley K, Sledge CB. Results of revision total knee arthroplasty performed for aseptic loosening. *Clin Orthop.* 1990;255:235–241.

30. Goldberg VM, Figgie MP, Figgie HE III, Sobel M. The results of revision total knee arthroplasty. *Clin Orthop.* 1988; 226:86–92.

CHAPTER 9

Modular Augments in Revision Total Knee Arthroplasty

J. Bohannon Mason

Bone loss and subsequent defects are often encountered in revision total knee arthroplasty and occasionally in primary total knee arthroplasty. The variability in size and location of these defects has led to the development of a multitude of techniques aimed at restoring the physical integrity of the knee and supporting prosthetic replacement. Techniques frequently reviewed in the literature include filling minor defects with cement; augmentation of cement with screws, wires, or mesh; bone grafting; metal augmentation with blocks or wedges; and custom components.

Modularity in total knee systems has earned its acceptance by providing utility in the management of this wide spectrum of bony defects. Consequently, as the array of modular options including offset stems, stem extensions, variable femoral and tibial prosthetic body options, and modular augmentations have evolved, custom implants are now rarely needed. The clinical acceptance of modular metal wedges and blocks is due in large part to their effectiveness in managing the variety of clinical situations that face the knee arthroplasty surgeon.

Bone defects that remain contained by the cortical rim, both in the tibia and in the femur, are generally best managed with bone grafting techniques. A number of authors have reported success using structural as well as morsellized allograft in these contained defects.[1] For very large contained defects, a combination of bulk and morcellized graft may be most appropriate, usually offloaded with extended prosthetic stems.

When the cortical rim of either the distal femur or proximal tibia is breached, the reconstructive options are challenging. In younger patients, structural allograft may be an option for consideration, yet this is tempered by reported problems including host-graft nonunion, disease transmission, and possible late collapse or resorption of the allograft. Indeed, there is a trend in revision centers away from bulk, structural allograft when other options are readily available.

Surgical techniques other than the use of modular or custom implants include shifting of the prosthesis to a region of more supportive host bone stock and/or possibly downsizing the prosthesis. These intraoperative choices represent compromises that may be accompanied by potentially undesirable consequences. On the tibial side, downsizing the tray and shifting away from a compromised cortical rim results in increased unit force transmission across the component to the underlying bone. Reduction of cortical rim contact coupled with an increased reliance on cancellous bone, tray subsidence may result. One clinical study suggests that translation of the tibial tray greater than 4mm may lead to higher component loosening and failure.[2] Downsizing of a femoral component to accommodate anterior or posterior bone loss may inadvertently lead to flexion space instability.

Recognition of the limitations associated with the techniques mentioned previously led to the development of modular metal wedges and block augmentations. The first wedged augmentation of a tibial component was reported by Jeffery et al.[3] The first clinical series reporting use of modular metal wedges for the management of bone deficiency was by Brand et al. in 1989.[4] Modular metal augmentations are now readily incorporated in modern knee reconstruction systems. In this chapter we discuss the relative indications for femoral or tibial augmentations with modular augments, the justification for their use in modern reconstructive surgery, limitations with this approach, and techniques employed.

BONE LOSS: GENERAL CONSIDERATIONS

Bone deficiencies and bone loss are encountered in both primary and revision settings. In a primary knee extreme varus, valgus, or flexion deformities may preoperatively herald the presence of bone defects, which, if ignored, may threaten the component reconstruction. Varus or valgus angulation, in the extreme, can lead to significant bone loss on either the tibial or femoral side of the joint. Although such extreme defects are less commonly encountered in primary knee arthroplasty in clinics today, progressive or rapid bone loss associated with avascular necrosis, neglect, or trauma may result in bone defects that require augmentation. Inflammatory arthropathy, such as rheumatoid arthritis, may result in severe cyst formation and bone loss.

The bone defects seen in revision knee arthroplasty generally occur with component loosening, component removal, or from osteolysis. Several authors have described classification schemes for bone loss about the knee.[5] Deficiencies on the tibial side are typically *central cavitary*, *peripheral*, or a combination. On the femoral side, the loss of structural host bone that requires augmentation is usually distal or posterior (Figure 9-1). Obviously, multiple permutations of any bone loss classification schemes are seen clinically, depending in large part on the mode of failure, the failed component type, and preexisting host bone stock. The most common patterns of bone loss that require modular augmentation include medial tibia in association with varus angulation, lateral tibial augmentation seen with valgus failure, and a

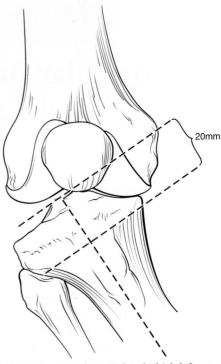

FIGURE 9-2. The size of a peripheral tibial defect can be measured off the reconstructed joint line based on the uninvolved side. (Adapted from Mason and Scott[5] by permission of Lippincott Williams & Wilkins.)

combination of distal and posterior femoral augmentation with component failure.

Preoperative radiographs can help identify patients who may require tibial or femoral augmentation. Brand et al.[4] have proposed a method for estimating tibial defect size based off of preoperative anterior-posterior radiographs. This technique is illustrated in Figure 9-2. A line is drawn down the central axis of the tibia. A perpendicular line is then drawn at the top of the intact tibial plateau. A second perpendicular line is extended to the base of the tibial defect. A differential measurement, corrected for magnification, exceeding 15 mm may require augmentation and should be considered in preoperative planning of the reconstruction.

Estimation of the need for augmentation on the femoral side is slightly more difficult. The 3-dimensional shape of the distal femur captured on 2-dimensional film, along with the metallic bulk of the femoral implant, make visualization of the distal femur difficult. Additionally, the bicondylar overlay on lateral films may lead to underestimation of unicondylar defects. Although oblique x-rays may be of benefit, evolving computed tomography techniques with subtraction algorithms hold great promise for accurate preoperative prediction of bone loss. Addi-

FIGURE 9-1. Modern revision knee systems allow for the use of augments of varying thickness, as here on the posterior and distal femur.

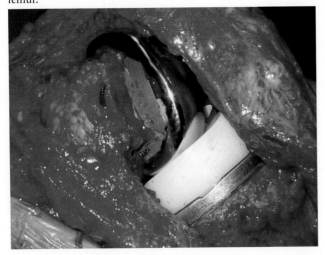

tionally, careful study of the prosthetic design and knowledge of the history of the prosthesis may be of benefit in preoperatively determining the need for femoral augmentation if defects are not obviously apparent.

CLINICAL JUSTIFICATION AND RESULTS USING MODULAR METAL AUGMENTATION

The mechanical strength of augmentation wedges and blocks has been investigated. In vitro studies have focused on two areas of interest.[6] The first is the fixation of the augment to the prosthesis. Most modern designs rely on a screw or snap-lock mechanism, occasionally augmented with cement (Figure 9-3). Older designs relied exclusively on cement fixation of the augment to the prosthesis. All mechanisms of augment fixation have been used successfully in the short term with clinical experience up to 5 years reported. The long-term concerns include loosening, dissociation of the augments, and possible fretting leading to third body wear. Brand et al.[4] reported a revision of a nonmodular tibial tray for polyethylene failure in which they had previously applied a 5 mm wedge with cement for a medial tibial defect. After 5 years *in vivo*, the medial wedge maintained 77% of the sheer strength of control and showed no evidence of corrosion, fretting, or impending failure.

Modular augments used beneath the tibial tray are typically either wedge shaped, which fit above an oblique bone resection, or are blocks. Hemiwedges can be used to fill small peripheral defects, whereas full wedge augments can be used to correct axial alignment beneath the tibial

FIGURE 9-3. Screw-on or snap-fit mechanisms are used for attachment of the augment to the prosthesis in most modern systems.

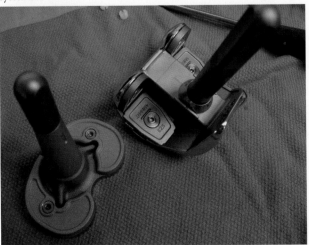

tray or to substitute for more extensive proximal cortical bone loss. Block augments, sometimes referred to as *step wedges*, are employed when bone loss at the cortical rim includes segmented medial (or lateral) bone and supporting anterior or posterior cortical bone at the level of the tray-bone resection.

Fehring et al.[7] found that tensile strain within the cement-bone interface was less with block augments compared with wedges. However, the maximal strain differential between blocks and wedges was only slight, arguing that the augment that best fills the defect should be used.

The long-term results of revision knee arthroplasty with modular augments have not been reported. The first clinical series reporting the use of metal wedges for tibial bone deficiencies was reported by Brand et al.[4] In this series, 22 knees in 20 patients were included. Modular metal wedges used to customize the tibial implant. Three of the 22 knees were revision cases. In each case a small tibial cemented stem extension was employed. Six knees, at average 37 months' follow-up, revealed radiolucent lines beneath the tibial wedge; however, no tibial tray was judged to be loose. Rand[8] reported a series of 28 primary knees at a mean follow-up of 27 months in which defects up to 18 mm were treated. The majority of these were medial bone defects. Clinical scores for all patients were rated as good to excellent despite nonprogressive radiolucent lines beneath 13 of the 28 tibial wedges. In a follow-on study of the same patient cohort, no significant degradation in the radiographic follow-up of the wedges was noted.[9] One patient failed due to patella complications. Despite the use of modular metal augmentations in revision knee reconstruction in multiple clinical series, no other clinical series have focused specifically on the role of modular metal augmentations in the success or failure of the reconstruction.

TIBIAL COMPONENT AUGMENTATION

Modular augmentation represents an attractive option in reconstructive surgery, allowing a surgeon to produce a *custom implant*, reestablish correct component levels with respect to the joint line, maintain or reestablish limb alignment, and adjust soft tissue balance.

Indications

Tibial augmentation with modular metal wedges or blocks is usually applied to defects of 5 to 20 mm in depth, particularly when these defects fail to support more that 25% of the tibial base plate (Figure 9-4). Several factors guide the decision to use modular augments. Since the

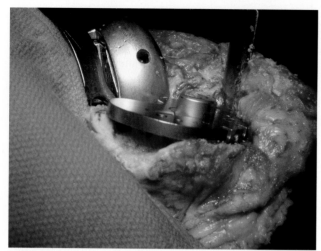

FIGURE 9-4. Uncontained tibial defects such as this medial defect are easily managed with a tibial wedge augment, allowing cortical rim contact with the prosthesis.

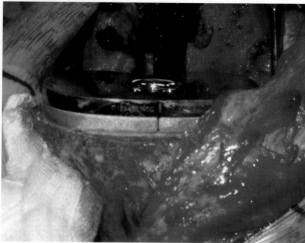

FIGURE 9-5. Tibial bone loss may exceed the height of the modular polyethylene inserts available for a given knee system. In this instance medial and lateral augments are paired to elevate the tibial joint line.

FIGURE 9-6. A full modular wedge augment was used in this patient who had experienced valgus failure of his prior implant. A short stem extension was selected. Despite initial stability, implant loosening occurred at 3-year follow-up. When host bone is significantly compromised to require a tibial augment, a longer stem extension should be considered.

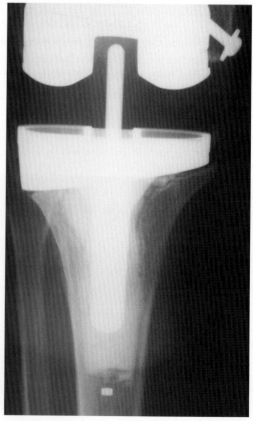

tibial diaphysis tapers distal to the joint line, resection to the supportive tibial host bone requires the use of a smaller base plate or risks overhanging metal, which can be particularly problematic to the patient postoperatively. Tibial defects rectified by downsizing the tibial base plate, with greater resection of bone to the depth of the defect, may limit the opposing femoral component sizing choices. The depth of modular augmentation, too, is limited by several practical considerations. First, most commercially available augments do not taper as the host bone metaphysis does. Larger tibial augments may likewise expose a sharp prosthetic edge at the base of the augment. This modular *overhang* may cause pain and should be avoided if other options for reconstruction are suitable. The depth of a modular augmentation is additionally limited by the extensor mechanism. Resection levels greater than 20 mm below the native joint line place the tibial tubercle and extensor mechanism in jeopardy, particularly if on the lateral side.

Extensive proximal tibial bone loss over both medial and lateral surfaces of the proximal tibia may be handled with thicker polyethylene inserts. However, as the polyethylene insert's thickness increases, the stresses at the insert locking mechanism increase, potentially leading to increased micromotion. This negative biomechanical consequence can be offset by elevating the tibial base plate, and reducing the thickness of the polyethylene insert required. Full tibial base plate augments or bilateral matched medial and lateral augments can be used to raise the tibial tray closer to the native joint line (Figure 9-5). As the tibial base plate is elevated with augments, the stem is effectively shortened, suggesting consideration of a longer stem (Figure 9-6).

Surgical Technique

In reconstructing the deficient proximal tibia with modular augments, the objectives remain restoration of alignment, soft tissue balancing, and a near-anatomic replication of the joint line to restore knee kinematics. In primary and revision knee arthroplasty the initial resection level is selected with optimal preservation of host bone stock. The residual peripheral defects are then assessed. It is important to determine the flexion-extension gap relationship between the femoral and tibial trial components. This is particularly true when trial distal femoral augments are considered, as the tibial resection level equally affects the flexion and extension space. With the trial femoral component in position the knee is brought into full extension and the rotational alignment of the tibial tray relative to the tibial host bone is determined and marked on the proximal tibia. This step is important before preparing the proximal tibia for an augment. The axial rotation of the tibial tray relative to the tibia determines the anterior to posterior (sagittal) orientation of the wedge or block resection. Failure to note this rotational alignment may result in difficulty matching the modular augment to the prepared resection, or inadvertent internal or external rotation of the tibial tray (Figure 9-7).

FIGURE 9-7. It is important to determine the tibial tray rotational alignment prior to resection of the defect. This ensures proper seating of the tibial tray with the augmentation and also ensures the correct rotational relationship to the femoral component. (Adapted from Mason and Scott[5] by permission of Lippincott Williams & Wilkins.)

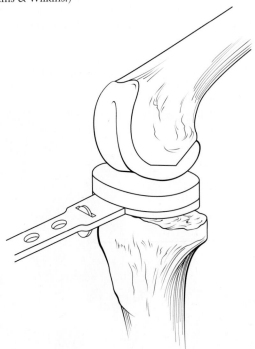

The size of the wedge or block is then determined by measuring the distance between the undersurface of the tibial tray and the depth of the cortical defect. Most revision systems provide resection guides for the various modular components (Figure 9-8). However, in obese patients who require deep resection levels or have lateral defects, these resection guides may be difficult to use and the resection may require free-hand adjustments. A narrow oscillating saw or high-speed bur can be particularly useful in these situations. The selection of a modular augment typically mandates the use of a stem. Consequently, intramedullary alignment systems are most helpful and can prevent errors including medial or lateral displacement of the augment, excessive or reversed slope of the tibial tray, and large errors in axial alignment in the AP plane. Offset stems can be useful in avoiding component overhang.

Estimating the height of the joint line can be difficult in cases with extensive bone loss associated with ligament laxity. Although the kinematic relationship between the femoral and tibial components is most important, the surgeon should strive for accurate joint line restoration. Helpful techniques available to the surgeon include comparing the patella ligament height to the contralateral knee or to the knee prior to reconstruction, as well as radiographically examining the contralateral, uninvolved joint line, and extrapolating the height of the proximal fibula to the native joint line.

Femoral Component Augmentation

The use of modular metal augmentations on the femoral side has received less attention in the literature. Current knee systems include augments of variable thicknesses for the medial and lateral condyles both distally and posteriorly, or in combination. A few systems provide anterior femoral augments. As surgeons become more conscious of soft tissue balance, the role of femoral joint line restoration and correct axial rotation is prioritized. Failure to restore the joint line or properly rotate the components relative to each other can compromise knee kinematics. Knee flexion and patella tracking may be adversely affected.

Rotational alignment is discussed elsewhere in this text. However, modular femoral augments may help facilitate accurate restoration of component rotation. Lateral femoral condylar hypoplasia is often associated with valgus axial alignment. When recognized, lateral condylar hypoplasia is easily managed with posterolateral modular augmentation on the femoral component. Inattention to the relative hypoplasia in this situation may lead to internal rotation of the femoral component, particularly if a posterior condylar referencing system is used. Likewise, a frequently encountered situation in revision arthroplasty

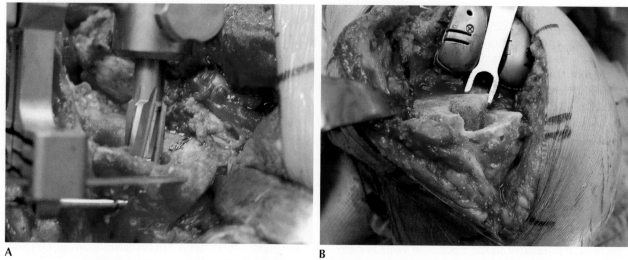

A   B

FIGURE 9-8. (A) Asymmetric tibial bone loss. Note the use of an intramedullary guide and a graduated cutting jig. (B) Resection for modular medial tibial augment.

is the revision of an improperly rotated femoral component. The common error is internal rotation of the femoral component relative to the epicondylar axis. Restoration of proper rotational alignment at revision surgery may require external rotation of the femoral component. The availability of posterior modular augments can be of particular benefit (Figure 9-9). When femoral component failure requires removal of the implant, there is often loss of distal femoral bone.

Additionally, distal resection of bone to achieve a stable bone surface elevates the prosthetic-bone interface. Modular distal femoral augmentation can help reduce this artificial elevation of the joint line. References for femoral joint line mirror the discussions above on tibial joint line restoration. The epicondyle can be used as a relative bony reference point, however, the distance from the epicondyle to the joint line varies from patient to patient.[10] Anterior femoral augments, although less commonly employed, may be of benefit if the prosthetic stem forces the femoral component anteriorly. Anterior-posterior femoral stem translation is available now with most systems. Combined with the flexibility of cementing a smaller diameter femoral stem, it is uncommon that the femoral component cannot be placed flush to the anterior cortex of the femur, obviating the need for space-occupying anterior augments (Figure 9-10).

The modular femoral augments are particularly useful in restoring proper anterior-posterior dimension to the femoral component. As is frequently the case in revision surgery, the flexion space is capacious compared with the extension space. Posterior augmentation of the femoral component allows proper sizing of the prosthesis, maximizing medial-lateral bone coverage and

addressing the extension-flexion mismatch (Figure 9-11). The advantage of modular metal augmentations for the distal femur over solid, nonmodular components is the ability to independently fit defects of each condyle and conserve host bone. The surgical technique for femoral preparation using modular augments is quite simple and familiar to most surgeons. An intramedullary guide is suggested. A stem is recommended when modular augments are employed. As the height of the distal femoral augment increases, the rotational constraint implied by host bone contact within the intracondylar notch region of the component is decreased (Figure 9-12). Many systems allow the use of a constrained condylar designed

FIGURE 9-9. Bone loss is often seen in association with femoral component failure. The posterior femoral condylar bone is particularly susceptible to osteolysis.

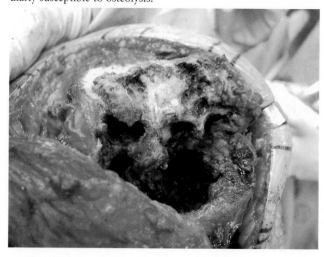

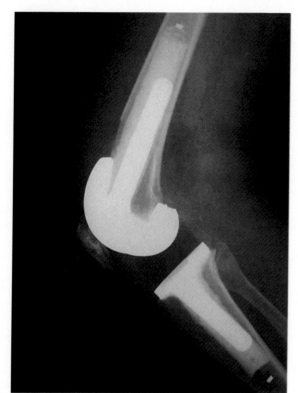

FIGURE 9-10. Modular metal augments can be very helpful in reconstruction of deficient posterior bone loss.

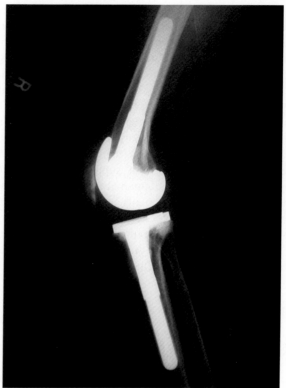

FIGURE 9-11. Posterior modular augments are used to up-size the femoral implant, assisting with flexion space management without affecting the extension space. A cemented stem is intentionally displaced posteriorly, allowing an anterior reference for femoral reconstruction.

knee with cruciate substituting polyethylene inserts. If augments are employed, the extra depth of the box resection of a constrained condylar designed knee provides additional rotational stability to the femoral implant. Additionally, if late ligament instability occurs, the femoral component need not be exchanged to allow use of the condylar constrained tibial insert.

DISCUSSION

Although modular metal augmentation blocks and wedges do not restore host bone stock, properly applied, these augments allow immediate weight bearing and range of motion, transferring loads to intact host bone, while providing durable long-term implant stability.[11] Additionally, the multiple sizes available with modular revision knee systems allow expedient reconstruction at a cost savings compared with custom implants. Recently, modular trabecular metal augments and semicustom trabecular metal augments have become available. These augments offer the same modular benefits of solid metal augments, with the added potential for osteointegration and soft tissue interdigitation.

FIGURE 9-12. Chamfer resections should be assessed and made with the appropriate sized distal femoral augment trial in place. In many revision cases in which distal augments are required, the chamfer resection is minimized. Implanting a condylar constrained femoral housing can increase the rotational stability of the reconstruction.

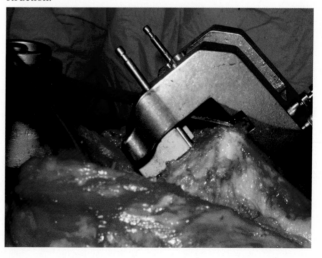

Modular metal wedges allow tremendous intraoperative flexibility in the management of tibial and femoral deficiencies. Load transfer to bone is more evenly distributed by metal augmentation than by other reported techniques of reconstruction of bone defects. Modular augments do circumvent the potential complications associated with bone graft harvest, donor site morbidity, or allograft incorporation. Long-term data regarding the prosthesis–metal augmentation interface with newer snap-fit and screw-fit fixation methods remains to be proven. Current clinical data support the continued application of modular augmentations in revision knee arthroplasty. Modular augments are particularly applicable in revision cases with peripheral cortical defects. Large bone defects that occur in younger patients may still best be managed with bone grafting techniques, which attempt to restore bone stock for potential future surgery.

REFERENCES

1. Gross AE. Cartilage resurfacing. filling defects. *J Arthroplasty.* 2003;18(Suppl 1):14.
2. Lee JG, Keating EM, Ritter MA, Faris PM. Review of the all-polyethylene tibial component in total knee replacement. *Clin Orthop.* 1990;260:87.
3. Jeffery RS, Orton MA, Denham RA. Wedged tibial components for total knee arthroplasty. *J Arthroplasty.* 1994; 9:381.
4. Brand MG, Daley RJ, Ewald FC, et al. Tibial tray augmentation with modular metal wedges for tibial bone stock deficiency. *Clin Orthop.* 1989;248:71.
5. Mason JB, Scott RD. Management of severe bone loss. prosthetic modularity and custom implants. In: Lotke PA, Garino JP, eds. *Revision Total Knee Arthroplasty.* Philadelphia: Lippincott-Raven; 1999:207.
6. Brooks JP, Walker PS, Scott RD. Tibial component fixation in deficient tibial bone stock. *Clin Orthop.* 1984;184:302.
7. Fehring TK, Peindl RD, Humble RS, et al. Modular tibial augmentations in total knee arthroplasty. *Clin Orthop.* 1996;327:207.
8. Rand JA. Bone deficiency in total knee arthroplasty: use of metal wedge augmentation. *Clin Orthop.* 1991;271:63.
9. Pagnano MW, Trousdale RT, Rand JA. Tibial wedge augmentation for bone deficiency in total knee arthroplasty—a follow-up study. *Clin Orthop.* 1995;321:151.
10. Rand JA. Modular augments in revision total knee arthroplasty. *Orthop Clin North Am.* 1998;29:347.
11. Gorlich Y, Lebek S, Reichel H. Substitution of tibial bony defects with allogenic and autogenic cancellous bone: encouraging preliminary results in 18 knee replacements. *Arch Orthop Trauma Surg.* 1999;119:220.

CHAPTER 10

Custom Implants in Revision Total Knee Arthroplasty

J. Craig Morrison, David K. DeBoer, and Michael J. Christie

Revision total knee arthroplasty can be one of the most gratifying procedures performed by a joint replacement surgeon. The painful, unstable failed knee replacement can be made stable and pain-free with careful, well-planned surgery. To be successful, revision knee arthroplasty requires careful preoperative assessment, precise planning, and excellent surgical technique. These principles have been reviewed in great detail in earlier chapters. They should be applied in every revision case no matter the perceived complexity. In complex cases, however, strict adherence to these principles is absolutely necessary for a successful outcome. The goals of revision total knee arthroplasty are the same as in primary total knee replacement: a stable, pain-free knee with functional range of motion to allow locomotion. Several factors contribute to achieving these goals. The patient must have sufficient motor power to support body weight. Knee stability must be achieved through proper soft tissue tensioning or ligament substitution. Knee motion must be sufficient to support the desired function. Finally, implants must achieve stable and durable fixation on the host skeleton. All subsequent function relies on this final tenet. A custom-designed implant makes this possible in the most difficult of cases. In this chapter, we outline the preoperative assessment and surgical planning as they relate to deciding on a custom implant. We review specific cases in which such an implant may be useful.

Custom knee revision implants are used when there are bone deficiencies or anatomic distortions severe enough that modular revision knee systems and simple allografts are insufficient to allow predictable implant stability on viable host bone strong enough to withstand the anticipated loads. Modular augments are too small, offset options for stems are limited, and augmentation with structural allograft is unpredictable and time-consuming to fashion. Extreme failures call for innovative solutions. Custom-designed implants can be used to more predictably solve complex cases with massive bone loss. Critical to the successful use of custom implants is identifying those situations in which their use is necessary, assisting the engineer to correctly size and design the implant, having the instruments necessary for implantation, and creating a backup plan in the unlikely event that the surgical plan must be altered.

A custom implant is designed to fit one particular patient's anatomy. It is designed and manufactured by engineers based on preoperative radiographs, with the design directed by the operative surgeon. In custom total knee arthroplasty, the primary goal is to achieve implant stability on viable host bone. Bone deficiencies are replaced, filled, or bypassed by the metal of the custom implant. The chief alternative to this method of reconstruction, the use of bulk structural allograft, offers several advantages, including its relative economy compared with customs, the ability for the graft to be modified intraoperatively, and the overvalued potential for restoration of bone stock. The disadvantages are formidable and often underappreciated. The graft may fail to heal to the host bone, leading to failure of the implant. Incorporation of large bulk allografts is unpredictable, with failure of the graft due to resorption and fracture proportionate to the length of time implanted. This failure of the graft is a cause for revision, and we find that the graft that remains is often unsuitable to support a new implant. Clatworthy et al. reported on 52 knees with major osseous defects reconstructed with 66 structural allografts at mean follow-up of 97 months.[1] Survivorship of the allograft was 72% at 10 years. Five knees were re-revised for resorption of the graft and 3 additional knees not revised had evidence of graft resorption despite union at the junction.

The operative complexity of the use of allograft should not be understated. Preoperative sizing of the graft is critical. Grafts that are too large or too small significantly complicate reconstruction. There is commonly a mismatch in the canal size; the graft canal too small due to the young age of the donor with the host canal too large due to age and disuse. Shaping allografts and then fixing them to host bone requires significant time under anesthesia and tourniquet. Finally, the potential for disease transmission, while small, is real and not shared with customs.

Rather than accepting the disadvantages of structural allograft, we prefer to replace or bypass major bone deficiencies with custom implants. Depending on the type and severity of bone loss, some or all of the implant may need to be customized. Sometimes this requires the design of a large segmental replacement on either side of the joint. In many cases, however, modular knee systems can be combined with custom modules—a "focused customization," as described by S. David Stulberg (personal communication). In areas in which the standard modules of the revision system are inadequate, a custom module is fabricated. The standard instrumentation can be used, and in many cases trial implants can provide a good idea of implant fit and stability. This provides a wider comfort zone for the surgical team. Using a modular revision system as a foundation, stems can be created that have custom offsets, diameters, lengths, coatings, and locking holes. Likewise, wedges with anatomically matched dimensions can successfully bridge defects.

The decision to pursue a custom design is obviously made preoperatively. In templating, the surgeon must be confident that an implant will achieve initial stability on host bone for any chance of durable fixation. Once fixed to host skeleton, metal can be relied on to take loads for decades. Given the importance of preoperative decision making, the quality of preoperative radiographs cannot be overemphasized. Poor radiographs often underestimate bone loss, creating unanticipated problems at the time of reconstruction. A complete set should include long-leg views of both extremities, standing anteroposterior (AP) views of both knees, scaled AP and lateral views of both knees, and sunrise views. Comparing the failed knee with the opposite side allows assessment of bone loss, alignment, and size. The long-leg views provide information about alignment, bone loss, malalignment above and below the joint, internal fixation, or prostheses above and/or below the failed knee. Occasionally, computed tomography (CT) can assist in assessing volume loss from lysis, estimating canal diameters, or more precisely gauging distorted anatomy. The long-leg view helps establish the location of the joint line, the first step toward understanding the needed augmentation. Assessing the amount of bone loss may be difficult where the implant obscures the bone. Areas of osteolysis are frequently subtle and may be underestimated. On the ipsilateral knee film, landmarks such as the femoral epicondyles, the fibular head, and the tibial tubercle can be used as references. A tracing of the more normal side can be used as an overlay on the failed side to help with joint line assessment, component sizing, and bone loss severity.

The major step in surgical planning is the matching of bone loss with reconstruction method. We have simplified the classification of lost bone in total knee replacement into 3 categories: bone defects amenable to reconstruction with the use of augment blocks and wedges (shims); defects significant enough to require metaphysis-fitting cones (sleeves); and extensive defects, usually involving loss of ligamentous attachments, requiring the use of structural metal analogs of the distal femur or proximal tibia (segments). The amount and location of bone loss determines which method—shim, sleeve, segment, or combination of these—will be necessary to achieve implant stability. While shims are commonly available with standard revision knee systems, standardized sleeves and segments are rare. The increasingly severe bone loss found in revision total knee arthroplasty, however, will determine the future off-the-shelf availability of these devices. Sleeves are currently found only with the S-ROM total knee system (DePuy Orthopaedics, Warsaw, IN), although the availability of sleeves and cones will likely be expanded to other systems. Segmental replacements are most commonly found as a portion of tumor devices.

On the femoral side, bone loss that extends only to the epicondyles can usually be managed successfully with modular, off-the-shelf shims, sized to restore the joint line while stem fixation into the diaphysis provides the necessary support for load-sharing. If the bone loss extends into the metaphyseal bone, then prostheses with sleeves may allow sufficient stability on host bone while restoring the joint line. Cone-shaped metallic augments such as sleeves fill the bony defect with metal, which although not restorative of bone stock, does allow the surgeon to bypass poor bone stock in favor of fixation in the metaphyseal flare, where the implant can be wedged for stability. Bone loss that exceeds the metaphysis and extends into diaphyseal bone requires segmental replacement that can only be achieved with either allograft composite implants or custom-designed components.

The revision surgeon should quantify tibial bone loss as well. Cavitary and segmental defects that leave a medial or lateral column of bone sufficient to share load with a diaphyseal stem are readily handled with revision components. Shims can be used to gain additional support on a deficient medial or lateral column. On the femoral side augments can be stacked to address condylar bone loss to a point; however, stacking wedges on the tibial side to catch up to host bone should be avoided. This technique cannot match the acute flare of the tibial metaphysis, leading to overstuffing of the soft tissue envelope. This can lead to collateral ligament irritation or even difficulty with closure. A custom module to match the tibial contour would be more suitable. If both columns are little more than a thin sclerotic rim, as is often the case with large cavitary loss, then achieving fixation on the best available bone requires loading the metaphysis with a sleeve and stem construct. This effectively bypasses the deficient rim. Segmental tibial bone loss that destroys the metaphysis or extends into the diaphysis requires proximal tibial replacement with either a metal segment or allograft.

In addition to bone loss, the surgeon must identify any deformity that will result in a *mismatch* in alignment between the diaphysis and the distal femur or proximal tibia. When using press-fit stems, the canal orientation dictates the coronal and sagittal component alignment at the joint. A standard stem position may prevent the component from achieving adequate stability on the only available host bone. Likewise, offset in the sagittal plane may be needed to balance the flexion space and the patellofemoral articulation. Most revision systems offer small amounts of stem offset, but options are limited. For instance, no system currently allows a surgeon to use metaphyseal sleeves with offset stems. Furthermore, the offset needs for select cases of fracture malunion are not available with standard revision stems.

After bone loss and deformity have been critically evaluated, the surgeon must decide how to handle the soft tissue. Ligament instability is usually corrected by precise component sizing, reestablishment of a normal joint line with proper soft tissue tension, and correct alignment of the implant rotationally and in the antero-posterior and lateral planes. Epicondylar loss or proximal tibial bone loss below the fibular head, however, will mean some degree of collateral incompetence. Unilateral ligament incompetence can usually be managed with constrained inserts. Medial and lateral incompetence, however, as would be the case in segmental replacement, necessitates more constraint to achieve stability. The accepted reconstructive option in these cases is a hinged knee, but higher loosening and infection rates make this method undesirable, especially in younger patients. Therefore, if the surgeon would anticipate finding

collateral ligaments for reattachment, a custom-designed segmental replacement that uses Trabecular Metal (porous tantalum) *buttons* (Implex Corporation, Cedar Knolls, NJ; Zimmer, Inc., Warsaw, IN) for ligament reattachment should be considered. Trabecular Metal is made from tantalum, an elemental metal that is highly biocompatible and corrosion resistant. Trabecular Metal is 80% porous and has a structural stiffness similar to dense cancellous bone, while solid metals are 10 to 50 times stiffer than bone. Because of this low stiffness, animal studies indicate that bone remodels more normally around and within porous tantalum.[2] Despite this high porosity and low stiffness, it is strong enough to withstand most physiological loads and has predictable mechanical strength properties and a stress-to-strain relationship similar to solid metal. Primary reconstruction after tumor excision or revision of unfixable supracondylar femoral or proximal tibial periprosthetic fractures are ideal for this type of biologic constraint. Other uses for porous tantalum include the extensor mechanism reattachment for cases of profound proximal tibial loss or patellar resurfacing in knees with deficient or absent patella.

MODULAR REVISION KNEE IMPLANTS

The revision surgeon must be familiar with the newer modular revision implants to appreciate their limitations. It is true that today's modular systems can accommodate the majority of revision cases. Custom implants that were manufactured as recently as 10 years ago are now easily *manufactured* intraoperatively with modular augments and stems (Figure 10-1). More than likely the industry will continue to evolve, making today's custom tomorrow's modular implant.

Most modular systems attempt to bypass or fill bone defects with a variety of shims. The most common problem with shims is the finite number of augment sizes. These augments can be *stacked* to address distal femoral bone loss up to a point, but because of the acute flare of the tibial metaphysis, stacking wedges to catch up to host bone overstuffs the soft tissue envelope and can lead to ligament irritation or even difficulty with closure.

Reconstructing large cavitary defects is difficult with modular revision systems. Osteolysis or mechanical loosing commonly creates large cavitary defects in the top of the tibia or the end of the femur. Frequently, the only bone that remains is a thin sclerotic shell. This bone is usually strongest at the site of ligament and tendon

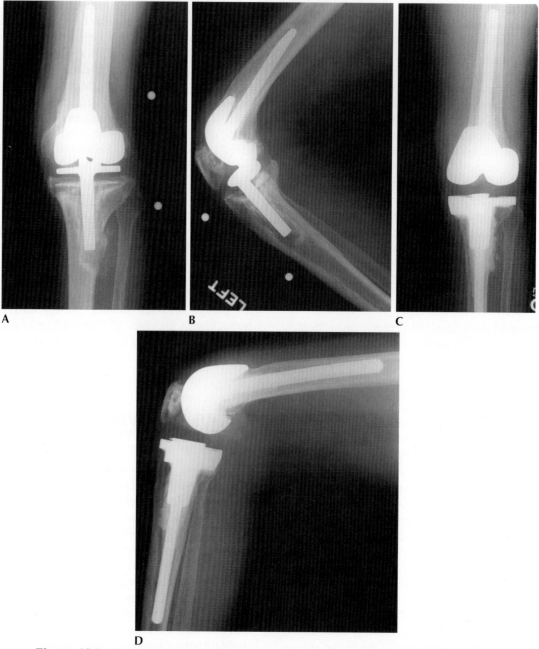

Figure 10-1. (A and B) Preoperative AP and lateral radiographs of a failed Kinematic (How-medica, Cheshire, CT) rotating hinge total knee arthroplasty with marked tibial bone loss and cortical perforation. The femoral component has subsided significantly. (C and D) Postoperative AP and lateral radiographs 9 years status post revision total knee arthroplasty with custom stemmed femoral and tibial components. These augments and stems are now available as standard devices in current modular revision knee systems.

attachments, because here the bone has been loaded even as the implant has failed. To achieve support and stability on host bone, the component would ideally be precisely matched to this thin margin.

Large femoral cavitary defects pose even greater reconstructive problems. The component must be precisely fit to the distal femur to balance the flexion and extension gaps. This makes it difficult to position the implants onto the remaining edge of bone. Current femoral augmentation wedges do not adequately address volumetric bone loss very well. Because augmentation wedges match the femoral component, there may be little contact with host bone at the margins of the femur. When a large femoral cavitary defect is present, the surgeon must rely on stems for added stability and any contact that can be achieved between the wedges and host bone.

Filling a bone defect with bone graft or cement is relying on a foundation not firmly anchored to host bone. One modular implant system, the S-ROM modular knee system (DePuy Orthopaedics, Warsaw, IN), addresses large volumetric defects by using modular stems and sleeves to fill the defects. While this system allows the filling of these large defects, there are significant problems and limitations. Symmetrical shapes do not fill asymmetrical volumes and accommodate the stem position dictated by the anatomy of the intramedullary canal. Furthermore, the current system must use a hinged articulation. As mentioned, the collateral insertions are often intact. Once proper tensioning has been achieved with a stable, well-positioned implant, there may be no need for a hinge.[3,4]

Segmental replacement is available from many companies as a tumor device. Until recently, press-fit stem options were not available. Once again, the articulation must be a hinge. In nontumor cases, such as failed allograft-prosthesis composites, or complex periprosthetic fractures, the collateral ligaments may very well be available for constraint. Custom prostheses, in which soft tissue can be secured to porous tantalum with a screw and washer, allow this possibility.

Recent modular knee designs include instrumentation that uses canal reamers to set the position of the tibial and femoral cutting blocks. These instruments guide preparation of the distal femur or proximal tibia to the orientation set by the stem of the component. Therefore, the surgeon must prepare the bone ends to the position dictated by the intramedullary guide or position of the instruments. On the tibial side this is commonly seen with extensive bone loss. Because the tibial base plate has no effect on the flexion and extension balance, there is great advantage in downsizing the tibial component to achieve stable contact with host bone. In these situations, a longer stem is required to achieve additional stability in the diaphysis, but the canal position relative to the remaining metaphysis commonly forces the base plate away from the center. A larger base plate should be avoided if it overhangs the medial side of the tibia. This tends to cause irritation and pain under the medial collateral ligament. Most systems include an offset stem as a standard option; however, the need for a higher offset custom stem should be determined preoperatively. Although modular implant systems are suboptimal in many complex revision procedures, clinical studies support the effectiveness of modular stems and augmentation wedges in revision cases with only minor bone loss.[5,6]

FOCUSED CUSTOMIZATION: MODULAR KNEE REVISION WITH CUSTOM MODULES

Many complex revision problems can be overcome by combining a modular knee system with custom modules directed at isolated deficiencies of a particular failed knee. In areas where the standard modules of the revision system are inadequate, a custom module is fabricated (Figure 10-2). Specialized modules can be designed to compensate for greater than normal or asymmetrical bone loss. When one side of the joint has significant bone loss, then the customization can be directed at designing an entire femoral or tibial component. In this case, the standard implant is used on the opposite side of the joint and the usual tibial inserts can be used. A custom component can even be designed to use the foundation system revision modules to compensate for unanticipated bone loss.

A custom module that is poorly designed or fits poorly creates a problem only marginally easier to solve than a poorly designed custom knee implant system. The surgeon's needs and the particular requirements of the custom module must be communicated to the design engineer, and the final design carefully reviewed. As with all custom designs, communication between the operating surgeon and the design engineer is paramount. While it is helpful to use a system with which the surgical team is familiar, it is critical to choose a manufacturer and engineer familiar with the process of custom design and fabrication. Implant design problems and delays in final production will be more common with a manufacturer who is unfamiliar with the process of custom design. An experienced custom engineer will be an asset throughout the design process. The experience gained from guiding previous surgeons through the process will be invaluable, as various design issues must be decided.

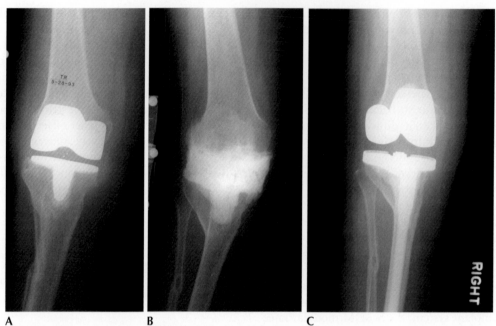

Figure 10-2. (A) Preoperative AP radiograph of an infected LCS Rotating Platform total knee arthroplasty (DePuy Orthopaedics, Warsaw, IN) with tibial canal distortion from a previous high tibial osteotomy. (B) Postoperative AP radiograph following resection of an infected total knee arthroplasty and placement of an antibiotic-loaded cement spacer. (C) Postoperative AP radiograph demonstrating medial offset of a long tibial stem on a custom tibial base plate (standard femoral component, tibial insert, and tibial stem used: CKS Modular knee system (Techmedica, Camarillo, CA); "focused" customization).

CUSTOM KNEE REVISIONS

Using custom-designed implants can best solve some of the problems caused by massive bone loss. Metal replaces the lost bone and provides stability on host bone. Designing the stem-implant intersection so as not to displace the articulating surfaces may salvage anatomic distortions. Designing the implant around the remaining bone can salvage knees with severe bone loss as long as the surgeon meets the basic requirements for successful revision.

Failed Allograft

An extreme example of bone loss is seen after a failed attempt at an allograft-prosthesis composite. The use of structural allograft has been discussed in a previous chapter (see Chapter 8). Several short-term analyses of its use in revision total knee arthroplasty have been reported.[7–9] Despite high union rates with rigid fixation and stems, graft resorption does occur with longer follow-up. As noted earlier, in a multicenter, midterm analyses, Clatworthy et al. reviewed 52 revision knee replacements in which 66 structural allografts were used to reconstruct major uncontained defects. Minimum follow-up was 60 months with a mean of 96.9 months. Survivor rate of the

allografts was 72% at 10 years. Five knees required revision for graft resorption and implant loosening at a mean of 92.8 months. An additional 3 knees had mild to moderate resorption, but were asymptomatic at latest follow-up.[1]

When structural allografts fail, reconstructive choices are limited. Resection arthroplasty or arthrodesis with an intercalary allograft are unattractive options from a functional standpoint. Revision surgery can be performed with another allograft; however, the biologic environment is unchanged and repeat failure is likely. Conversely, a custom device replaces the bone loss with metal, allowing accurate reestablishment of the joint line with a solid foundation on host bone (Figure 10-3).

Infection

Infection is another common cause of massive bone loss. Large segmental defects result from component removal and debridement. Some cases may not be amenable to reconstruction with current modular revision systems. Furthermore, allograft implantation in the setting of previous infection may not be optimal. Although success in a small number of patients has been reported, the risk of recurrent infection is a concern.[1,10] Nonvascularized allografts can serve as a nidus for the growth of organisms.[8]

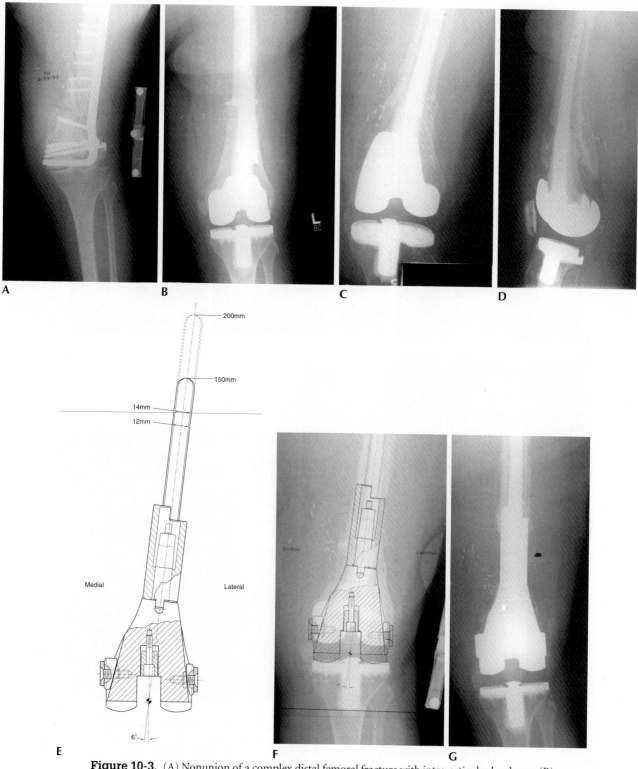

Figure 10-3. (A) Nonunion of a complex distal femoral fracture with intra-articular hardware. (B) Postoperative radiograph of distal femoral allograft/prosthesis composite with custom femoral stem. (C and D) At $2^{1}/_{2}$ years status post revision, radiographs demonstrate allograft failure. There is nonunion at the allograft-host junction, and there has been resorption and telescoping of the allograft. (E) Line drawing of proposed custom distal femoral replacement with modular implant. (F) Templated radiograph with overlay of custom proposal. (G) Postoperative radiograph at 4 years status post revision with a custom porous tantalum distal femoral segment.

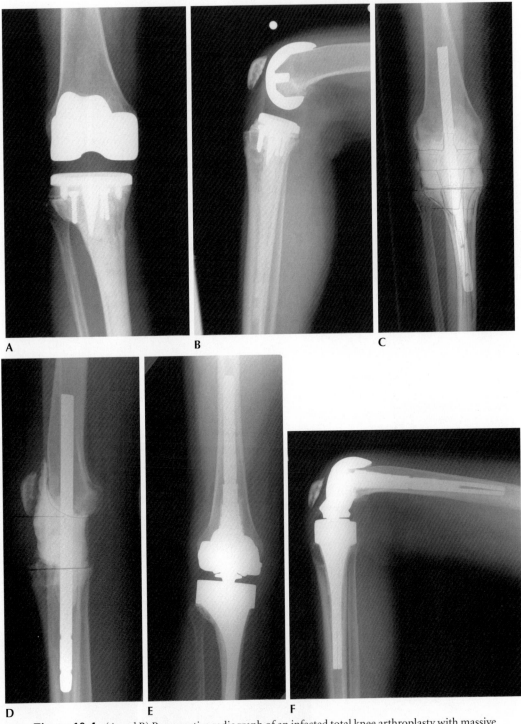

Figure 10-4. (A and B) Preoperative radiograph of an infected total knee arthroplasty with massive tibial bone loss. (C and D) Status post resection, the degree of tibial bone loss is even more impressive. (E and F) Postoperative radiograph showing revision with a custom tibial component and standard femoral component. Note the amount of tibial offset required by the anatomy.

When compared with revision knee arthroplasties without allograft, the infection rate in allograft procedures, on average, is almost double.[1,8,11–15] In this setting, a custom prosthesis can alleviate the need for grafting (Figure 10-4).

Total Femur

In the most extreme of cases, initial stability on host bone may be impossible to achieve even with long stems unless they are cemented. Cemented long stems in younger patients are undesirable. To achieve biologic fixation, the

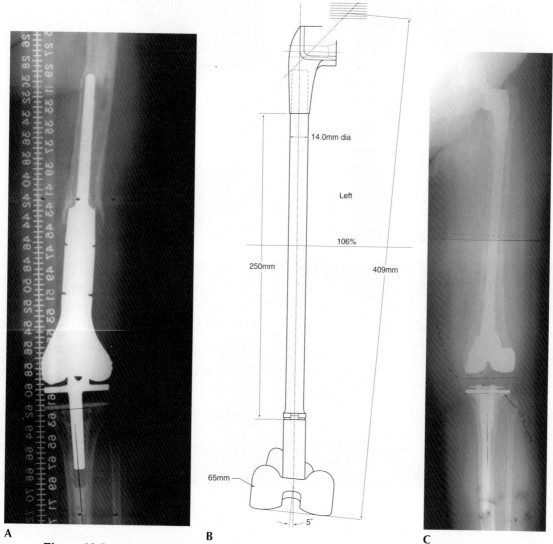

Figure 10-5. (A) Radiograph of failed cemented distal femoral tumor prosthesis with massive osteolysis and loosening. (B) Line drawing of proposed custom total femoral replacement. (C) Postoperative radiograph showing total femoral replacement with distal femoral allograft.

surgeon must *bypass* the deficiency and gain stability at the adjacent joint. Failed cemented segmental replacements of the distal femur are the most frequent cause of this type of femoral deficiency from a total knee standpoint. We have seen encouraging results with total femoral replacement in this circumstance (Figure 10-5). A modular total hip and knee system is linked together at a custom interface. Implant stability relies on the intact pelvis above and the tibia below.

Periprosthetic Fracture

The majority of clinical studies evaluating custom knee prostheses are found in the treatment of periprosthetic fractures.[16–19] Nondisplaced fractures have good outcomes with closed treatment; however, displaced fractures present a treatment dilemma. Closed treatment is doomed to failure.[20] Open reduction and internal fixation techniques have resulted in improved initial alignment, but the accompanying osteopenia and the presence of components makes this a technically challenging undertaking. Loss of reduction, malunion, and nonunion is not uncommon.[17,20,21] Custom components are an alternative for initial treatment when osteopenia or fracture position precludes rigid fixation, or when the component is loose. Alternatively, custom components can be reserved to salvage treatment failures.

Patellar Revision

At the time of revision knee arthroplasty, there may be substantial loss of patellar bone stock secondary to bone

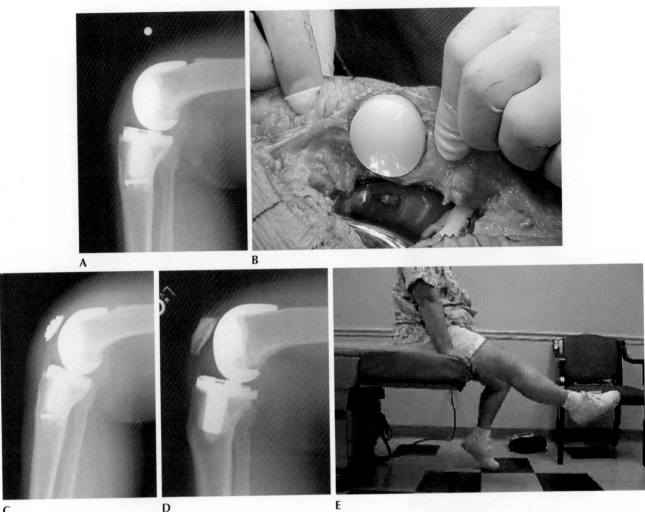

Figure 10-6. (A) Patellectomized patient status post primary total knee arthroplasty. (B) A Trabecular Metal custom patellar component in sutured into the soft tissue. (C) Postoperative radiograph showing good alignment of the component. (D) Postoperative radiograph of contralateral knee for comparison of patellar position. (E) The patient demonstrates active extension.

resection from prior resurfacing, osteolysis, or removal of a well-fixed patellar component. When possible, it is preferable to insert another patellar implant, but occasionally the amount of bone loss precludes adequate fixation of another prosthesis. Traditional treatment options in this setting have been either patellectomy or retention of the remaining patellar shell. Primary and revision total knee arthroplasty in patellectomized patients has consistently resulted in inferior outcomes.[22–24] Patellectomies in the revision setting have likewise yielded poor results, including difficulties with weakness and extensor mechanism disruption.[25,26] Retention of the osseous shell has also been associated with lower knee scores and persistent pain.[27,28]

We have used a custom patellar component made of porous tantalum (Trabecular Metal) for selected revision cases as a tool to replace or restore a patella with deficient bone stock. We have also used it successfully to reconstruct the biomechanics of the extensor mechanism in patellectomized patients with a poor outcome following primary total knee arthroplasty (Figure 10-6).

CONCLUSION

Custom-designed implants can solve some of the problems faced by revision surgeons. Custom revision arthroplasty, however, brings with it a host of unique problems that prevent it from becoming a panacea. Surgeons do not have familiar instrumentation to use with custom implants. Custom instruments can be designed but add expense and require additional foresight and planning from the surgeon and engineer. Little is required in the way of instruments, since the prosthesis is designed to fit the remaining bone. There are no trial implants available. These can be manufactured, but their cost is prohibitive in the current health care environment.

Custom implants require a great deal more planning and require 4 to 6 weeks to manufacture. Frequently, the added expense of a custom implant is a major issue, but several factors may compensate for the added cost. Using a custom implant may decrease or eliminate the need for structural allografts, the associated cost of the graft, and the operative time to prepare and shape it. Intraoperative problem solving is reduced because this has been done preoperatively during the design process. As the complexity of modular implants has increased, the cost gap compared with custom implants narrows.

Successful use of a custom implant for revision depends on the quality of preoperative planning. The consequences of inadequate planning may be severe. The implant may not fit if the implant is not sized correctly or if intraoperative problems with bone loss or soft tissues are not adequately anticipated. Time must be devoted to planning the reconstruction with the design engineer. It is important to design for greater bone loss than is expected from the radiographs. If the surgeon anticipates the potential pitfalls and plans accordingly, custom implants are a useful and effective method to salvage a failed knee replacement.

REFERENCES

1. Clatworthy MG, Ballance J, Brick GW, Chandler HP, Gross AE. The use of structural allograft for uncontained defects in revision total knee arthroplasty. A minimum five-year review. *J Bone Joint Surg Am.* 2001;83-A:404–411.
2. Bobyn JD, Stackpool GJ, Hacking SA, Tanzer M, Krygier JJ. Characteristics of bone ingrowth and interface mechanics of a new porous tantalum biomaterial. *J Bone Joint Surg Br.* 1999;81:907–914.
3. Rand JA, Chao EY, Stauffer RN. Kinematic rotating-hinge total knee arthroplasty. *J Bone Joint Surg Am.* 1987;69:489–497.
4. Springer BD, Hanssen AD, Sim FH, Lewallen DG. The kinematic rotating hinge prosthesis for complex knee arthroplasty. *Clin Orthop.* 2001;392:283–291.
5. Brand MG, Daley RJ, Ewald FC, Scott RD. Tibial tray augmentation with modular metal wedges for tibial bone stock deficiency. *Clin Orthop.* 1989;248:71–79.
6. Haas SB, Insall JN, Montgomery W III, Windsor RE. Revision total knee arthroplasty with use of modular compo-
7. Mnaymneh W, Emerson RH, Borja F, Head WC, Malinin TI. Massive allografts in salvage revisions of failed total knee arthroplasties. *Clin Orthop.* 1990;260:144–153.
8. Stockley I, McAuley JP, Gross AE. Allograft reconstruction in total knee arthroplasty. *J Bone Joint Surg Br.* 1992;74:393–397.
9. Harris AI, Poddar S, Gitelis S, Sheinkop MB, Rosenberg AG. Arthroplasty with a composite of an allograft and a prosthesis for knees with severe deficiency of bone. *J Bone Joint Surg Am.* 1995;77:373–386.
10. Tsahakis PJ, Beaver WB, Brick GW. Technique and results of allograft reconstruction in revision total knee arthroplasty. *Clin Orthop.* 1994;303:86–94.
11. Mow CS, Wiedel JD. Revision total knee arthroplasty using the porous-coated anatomic revision prosthesis: six- to twelve-year results. *J Arthroplasty.* 1998;13:681–686.
12. Friedman RJ, Hirst P, Poss R, Kelley K, Sledge CB. Results of revision total knee arthroplasty performed for aseptic loosening. *Clin Orthop.* 1990;255:235–241.
13. Goldberg VM, Figgie MP, Figgie HE III, Sobel M. The results of revision total knee arthroplasty. *Clin Orthop.* 1988;226:86–92.
14. Ghazavi MT, Stockley I, Yee G, Davis A, Gross AE. Reconstruction of massive bone defects with allograft in revision total knee arthroplasty. *J Bone Joint Surg Am.* 1997;79:17–25.
15. Lord CF, Gebhardt MC, Tomford WW, Mankin HJ. Infection in bone allografts. Incidence, nature, and treatment. *J Bone Joint Surg Am.* 1988;70:369–376.
16. Kress KJ, Scuderi GR, Windsor RE, Insall JN. Treatment of nonunions about the knee utilizing custom total knee arthroplasty with press-fit intramedullary stems. *J Arthroplasty.* 1993;8:49–55.
17. Figgie MP, Goldberg VM, Figgie HE III, Sobel M. The results of treatment of supracondylar fracture above total knee arthroplasty. *J Arthroplasty.* 1990;5:267–276.
18. Madsen F, Kjaersgaard-Andersen P, Juhl M, Sneppen O. A custom-made prosthesis for the treatment of supracondylar femoral fractures after total knee arthroplasty: report of four cases. *J Orthop Trauma.* 1989;3:332–337.
19. Keenan J, Chakrabarty G, Newman JH. Treatment of supracondylar femoral fracture above total knee replacement by custom made hinged prosthesis. *The Knee.* 2000;7(3):165–170.
20. Moran MC, Brick GW, Sledge CB, Dysart SH, Chien EP. Supracondylar femoral fracture following total knee arthroplasty. *Clin Orthop.* 1996;324:196–209.
21. Schatzker J, Lambert DC. Supracondylar fractures of the femur. *Clin Orthop.* 1979;138:77–83.

22. Kang JD, Papas SN, Rubash HE, McClain EJ Jr. Total knee arthroplasty in patellectomized patients. *J Arthroplasty.* 1993;8:489–501.

23. Larson KR, Cracchiolo A III, Dorey FJ, Finerman GA. Total knee arthroplasty in patients after patellectomy. *Clin Orthop.* 1991;264:243–254.

24. Martin SD, Haas SB, Insall JN. Primary total knee arthroplasty after patellectomy. *J Bone Joint Surg Am.* 1995; 77:1323–1330.

25. Dennis DA. Extensor mechanism problems in total knee arthroplasty. *Instr Course Lect.* 1997;46:171–180.

26. Laskin RS. Management of the patella during revision total knee replacement arthroplasty. *Orthop Clin North Am.* 1998;29:355–360.

27. Barrack RL, Matzkin E, Ingraham R, Engh G, Rorabeck C. Revision knee arthroplasty with patella replacement versus bony shell. *Clin Orthop.* 1998;356:139–143.

28. Pagnano MW, Scuderi GR, Insall JN. Patellar component resection in revision and reimplantation total knee arthroplasty. *Clin Orthop.* 1998;356:134–138.

CHAPTER 11

Femoral Alignment

James Huddleston, Reuben Gobezie, and Harry Rubash

The goal of total knee arthroplasty is to relieve pain and to improve function by creating a knee with adequate range of motion as well as osseous and ligamentous stability. Axial alignment is achieved with resections of the distal femur and proximal tibia. The tibial cut, with the aid of either intramedullary or extramedullary alignment guides, is generally made perpendicular to its long axis. A perpendicular cut is preferred because it is easier to reproduce and, when performed properly, helps to recreate the mechanical axis of the limb and thus improve the clinical outcome.[1-4] Axial alignment of the femur is generally made by resecting the distal femur in 5 to 7 degrees of valgus. Rotational alignment of the femur is achieved with the anterior and posterior distal femoral resections. The mechanics of the patellofemoral joint are heavily dependent on this rotational alignment. Improper rotational alignment may cause patellofemoral problems or gross changes in the foot progression angle during the gait cycle.

This chapter addresses the various methods used to achieve proper axial and rotational alignment of the femur in total knee arthroplasty. The influence of femoral alignment on patellofemoral mechanics and how it relates to achieving balanced flexion and extension gaps is also discussed. Particular attention is given to the current technique for achieving proper alignment in the revision setting.

ANATOMY

A tremendous amount of variation occurs in *normal* limb alignment. Static alignment is affected by height, weight, and bony morphology. Knee kinematics are influenced by the degenerative changes found in arthritic knees. The geometry of the human femur has been well described,[5] and several studies examine the specific sizes and shapes of the femur.[6,7]

In the coronal plane, the *anatomic axis* is defined as a line drawn down the centers of the femur and tibia (Figure 11-1). On average, this creates an angle of 5 to 7 degrees of valgus at the knee joint. The tibiofemoral angle results from a combination of the varus tilt of the tibial plateau (3 degrees) and the valgus alignment of the femoral condyles, on average 7 degrees.[8] The *mechanical axis* is defined as a line drawn from the center of the femoral head, through the center of the knee, and ending in the center of the ankle joint. In general, the mechanical axis lies 3 degrees off the *vertical axis*.

The flexion axis of rotation of the knee is thought to transect a line drawn between the medial and lateral epicondyles at the origins of the medial and collateral ligaments. This axis should lie transverse to the long axis of the tibia. At 90 degrees of flexion, the medial condyle extends 1–6 mm more posterior than the lateral condyle[9] (Figure 11-2). This axis undoubtedly has wide variation, and the amount of the condyles that fall below the transepicondylar axis varies as well.

BIOMECHANICS

The lower extremity goes through 2 stages during the gait cycle. It bears weight in the stance phase and is advanced in the swing phase. Stance phase can be divided into a period of double-limb support followed by a time of single-limb support. The single-limb support segment is further divided into multiple parts: heel strike, foot flat, heel off, and toe off. The contralateral foot enters heel strike shortly after the initial foot passes through heel rise. Stance phase comprises 62% of the gait cycle while swing phase accounts for 38%.[10]

In stance phase of the gait cycle, the medial compartment of the knee experiences approximately 60% to 70% of the weightbearing forces in a lower extremity with 7 degrees of anatomic valgus or a neutral mechanical axis. Any perturbation in the alignment will likely lead to changes in this distribution, and even small changes may predispose the joint to degenerative arthritis.[11–14] Establishing the correct axial and rotational alignment during total knee arthroplasty should serve to reproduce, as closely as possible, the normal distribution of forces seen across the knee joint during gait. This in turn should lead to an overall better clinical result and improve the survivorship of the components.[4] It has been shown that even a 5-degree axial malalignment can change the load seen across the knee joint by up to 40%.[15] This work was supported by the study of Ritter et al., who concluded that

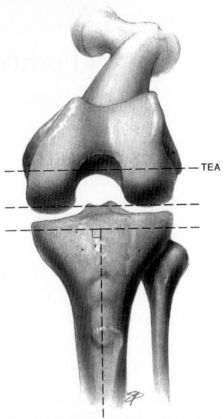

Figure 11-2. Transepicondylar axis. (From Pollice, Lotke, Lonner,[9] by permission of Lippincott Williams & Wilkins, 2003.)

Figure 11-1. The LE axes. (From Pollice, Lotke, Lonner,[9] by permission of Lippincott Williams & Wilkins, 2003.)

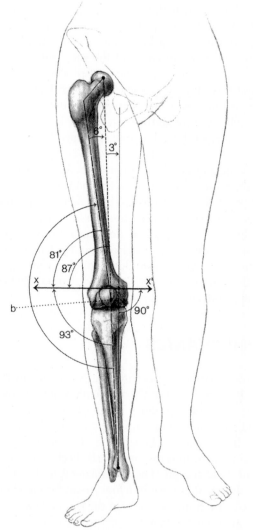

early failures in total knee arthroplasty were correlated with tibial varus of greater than 5 degrees.[16] Further, Berger and Rubash, in comparing 30 patients with isolated patellofemoral complications after total knee arthroplasty to 20 patients with well-functioning total knee arthoplasties, found that patellofemoral complications were directly correlated with combined internal rotation of the femur and tibia.[2] They noted that internal rotation of 1 to 4 degrees produced lateral tracking and patellar tilt. Patellar subluxation was seen with 3 to 8 degrees of internal rotation. As the internal rotation increased to 7 to 17 degrees, they reported patellar dislocation and early patellar component failure.

AXIAL ALIGNMENT

The mechanical axis of the lower extremity must be restored to neutral for a revision total knee arthroplasty to be successful. Most surgeons will perform the distal femoral resection by aligning it in 5 to 7 degrees of valgus.[17,18] It is commonly believed that the tibiofemoral angle should be restored to 6 degrees (+/−1 to 2 degrees) of valgus. Despite the average 3-degree varus angulation of the native tibial plateau, most surgeons prefer a tibial cut that is perpendicular to the long axis of the tibia. It is important to realize that these numbers may vary slightly depending on such variables as preoperative alignment, collateral ligament integrity, and obesity.

Historically, there are 2 methods for cutting the distal femur and proximal tibia. The tensioning or gap technique relies on an initial transverse tibial resection to assist in achieving rectangular flexion and extension gaps.[9] It cannot be overemphasized that a cut perpendicular to the long axis of the tibia is crucial for this technique to be successful. The dimensions of the flexion and extension gaps can only be assessed properly once all osteophytes are removed and all ligaments are balanced before tensioning (Figure 11-3).

In the measured resection technique, the surgeon attempts to restore proper alignment by replacing what has been removed by arthritis with exactly the same amount of prosthetic material. When using this method, the femoral resections (distal, anterior, and posterior)

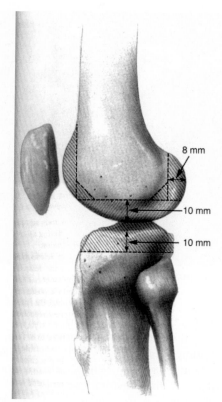

Figure 11-4. Measured resection technique. (From Pollice, Lotke, Lonner,[9] by permission of Lippincott Williams & Wilkins, 2003.)

Figure 11-3. (A and B) Tensioners. (From Insall, Scott,[23] by permission of Churchill Livingstone.)

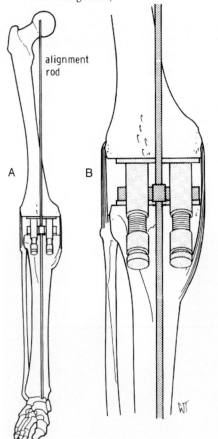

should reflect the thickness of the condylar surfaces of the prosthesis to be implanted. On the tibial side, if 12 mm of tibial plateau is resected, then the thickness of the tibial implant (tray and insert if using a modular tibia) should be equal to 12 mm (Figure 11-4).

Both extramedullary and intramedullary guides are available to assist the surgeon in cutting the distal femur in 5 to 7 degrees of valgus. It has been shown in multiple series that intramedullary (IM) guides improve the accuracy of the distal femur resection. In a review of 201 knee arthroplasties in which a standard IM guide was used, Teter et al. used radiographs to show that distal femoral alignment was considered to be accurate 92% of the time.[19] They identified femoral bowing and capacious femoral intramedullary canals as risk factors for inaccurate distal femoral alignment. The largest series comparing the 2 methods involved 200 consecutive total knee replacements, in which extramedullary guides were used in 75 cases and intramedullary guides were used in 125 cases. The postoperative distal femoral alignment was defined as "acceptable" if it fell between 4 and 10 degrees of valgus. They reported that 72% of the extramedullary group versus 86% of the intramedullary group had acceptable alignment. Further, they found that joint line

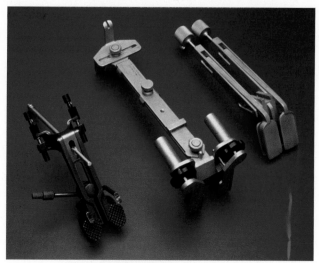

Figure 11-5. Tensioners in laboratory.

orientation was outside of the "normal" range twice as frequently in the extramedullary guide group.[20] Based on these findings, most surgeons elect to use an intramedullary femoral guide when performing total knee arthroplasty. In the revision setting, the use of intramedullary rods is particularly helpful to assist the surgeon in dealing with bone loss and distorted anatomy.

To use an intramedullary alignment guide, the surgeon begins by establishing an entry point located just anterior to the origin of the posterior cruciate ligament. Flexing the knee facilitates this process. It is advisable in the revision setting to obtain full-length anteroposterior and lateral weightbearing radiographs of the lower extremity. This allows the surgeon to determine the preoperative axial alignment and to assess the morphology of the femoral intramedullary canal. This is particularly

important in cases of posttraumatic arthritis after femur fracture. The drill hole starting point is usually slightly medial to the center of the intercondylar notch. Placement of the guide too medially or too laterally results in cuts that are in excessive varus or valgus, respectively. Most current knee systems offer cutting jigs that allow the distal femur to be cut in 4 to 7 degrees of valgus alignment.

Fat emboli syndrome is a concern with the use of intramedullary guides. Two techniques have helped to diminish its incidence. Overdrilling of the starting point allows for the release of the intramedullary contents, which diminish intramedullary pressures when the rod is inserted.[21] Further, overdrilling should allow for the rod to engage in diaphyseal bone. Flutes in the guide rod have also been shown to decrease intramedullary pressures and to reduce the incidence of fat embolism.[21,22]

The tensioning technique, as described originally by Insall, can also be used to perform the distal femoral resection.[23] This technique relies on a tibial cut that is perpendicular to the long axis of the tibial shaft. Before making any bony cuts, all osteophytes should be removed and soft tissues should be balanced. The extension space is then created under tension by cutting the distal femur parallel to the cut tibial plateau; this ensures a rectangular extension space. The knee is then flexed to 90 degrees, and the tensioners are re-inserted (Figure 11-5). The posterior femoral cut is then performed parallel to the tibial plateau. In the primary total knee arthroplasty of a varus knee, proper external rotation can usually be achieved by resecting more off the medial posterior condyle than the lateral posterior condyle. This may not always be the case with revision total knee arthroplasty, as the posterior femoral condyles, if present at all, are likely to be severely distorted (Figure 11-6).

Figure 11-6. (A and B) Intraoperative technique. (From Insall, Scott,[23] by permission of Churchill Livingstone.)

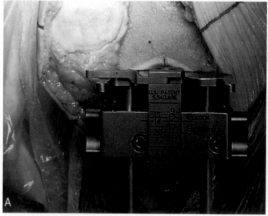 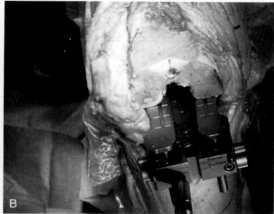

planning is crucial in estimating the size of the last reamer to be used.

The valgus angle of the distal femur is then checked by inserting a straight stem into the intramedullary canal. A standard revision cutting block is then attached to the stem. If this device sits flush on the distal femur, then, for most systems, 5 to 7 degrees of valgus alignment exists between the anatomic axis and the distal cut. If the device does not sit flush, then the distal femur must be recut. Before doing so, the surgeon should check that the proper side (right vs. left) has been selected.

Recutting of the femur begins by attaching a stem extension onto the distal femur revision cutting block. Once this has been impacted, a distal femoral cutting guide is attached to the extension (Figure 11-9). The distal femoral cutting guide is then stabilized with 2 headless pins. The intramedullary guide is then removed with an extractor. At this point, the position of the joint line can be adjusted by using the +2, −2, +4, and −4 holes that are found on most distal femur cutting guides. These markings correspond to millimeters of bone that will be removed with the resection. The final joint line should be approximately 2.0 to 2.5 cm distal to the epicondyles. An

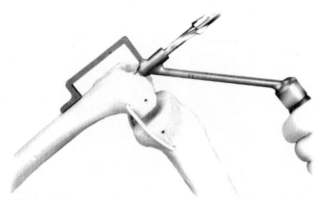

Figure 11-7. Finding the starting hole for the femoral reamer. (From Rubash H, et al. CCK Technique Guide. In NexGen LCCK Revision, 2001. Courtesy of Zimmer, Inc., Warsaw, IN.)

Revision systems with cutting slots provide a third alternative for achieving proper distal femoral alignment. The surgeon begins by locating the starting point for the femoral reamer. Some systems offer an IM hole locator to assist in finding this position. This device has an outrigger that lies flat on the anterior cortex of the femur and parallel to its anatomic axis (Figure 11-7). Once the starting point has been chosen, the starter reamer is then inserted into the medullary canal. Eccentric placement of the intramedullary guide can be avoided by reaming parallel to the shaft of the femur in both the anteroposterior and medial-lateral planes. Once the canal has been located, the starting hole is enlarged with a step drill. The canal is then reamed progressively larger, generally by hand, until cortical contact is made (Figure 11-8). We stop when cortical engagement occurs. Proper preoperative

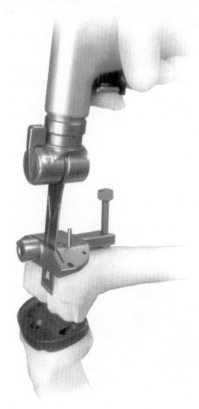

Figure 11-9. Distal femoral cut. (From Rubash H, et al. CCK Technique Guide. In NexGen LCCK Revision, 2001. Courtesy of Zimmer, Inc., Warsaw, IN.)

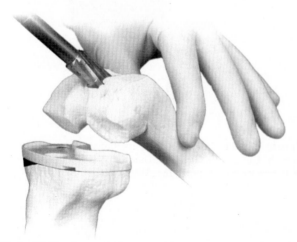

Figure 11-8. The medullary canal is then reamed larger until cortical contact is made. (From Rubash H, et al. CCK Technique Guide. In NexGen LCCK Revision, 2001. Courtesy of Zimmer, Inc., Warsaw, IN.)

oscillating saw is then used to make the distal femoral cut.

The femur must then be evaluated for the proper size. Again, preoperative templating will ensure an accurate estimate as to the final size of the femoral component to be used. Many systems come with sizing templates that can be attached to the intramedullary alignment guide. These should serve as an estimate only, as the final size will ultimately be selected when one balances the flexion and extension gaps.

The last step is to establish proper femoral rotation and component placement. To do so, the surgeon attaches a femoral base-guide flange to the cutting block. The proper right-left indication must be selected. The flange is then secured to the cutting block, and the device is reinserted over the intramedullary alignment guide. The cutting block should be flush with the distal femur, and the flange should rest on the anterior femoral cortex. An alignment guide is then attached to the posterior edge of the cutting block. We prefer to orient this guide parallel to the surgical epicondylar axis[24] (Figure 11-10). If the cutting block is not properly positioned on the distal femur, then an offset femoral stem can be used. This allows for adjustment of the cutting block several millimeters in both the anteroposterior and medial-lateral planes. Once the final position has been selected, 2 headless pins are used to secure the device to the distal femur. The intramedullary alignment guide is then removed, and the proper anterior and posterior femoral cuts can be made through the corresponding slots (Figure 11-11). Any bony defects that remain can be addressed with the use of augments. After the size and location of the augment to be used has been determined, the surgeon prepares the femur by cutting through the corresponding augment cutting slots on the femoral cutting guide (Figure 11-12).

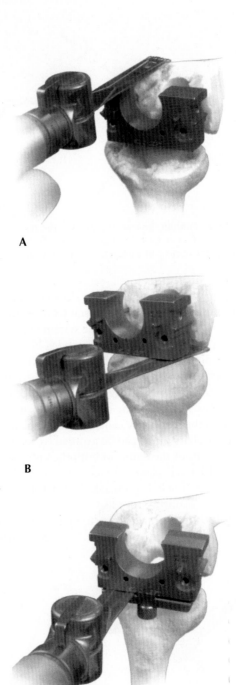

A

B

C

Figure 11-11. (A–C) Setting rotational alignment. (From Rubash H, et al. CCK Technique Guide. In NexGen LCCK Revision, 2001. Courtesy of Zimmer, Inc., Warsaw, IN.)

Figure 11-10. Rotational alignment guide. (From Rubash H, et al. CCK Technique Guide. In NexGen LCCK Revision, 2001. Courtesy of Zimmer, Inc., Warsaw, IN.)

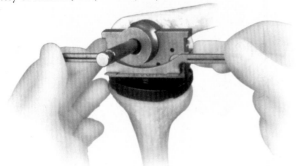

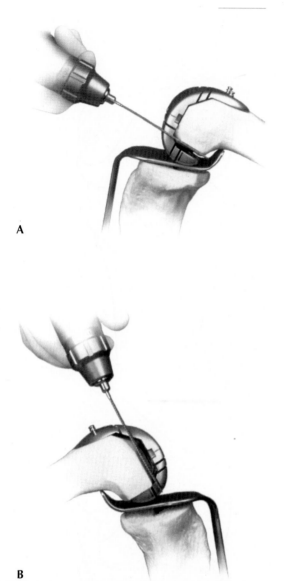

A

B

Figure 11-12. (A and B) The femur is prepared by cutting through the corresponding augment cutting slots on the femoral cutting guide. (From Rubash H, et al. CCK Technique Guide. In NexGen LCCK Revision, 2001. Courtesy of Zimmer, Inc., Warsaw, IN.)

ROTATIONAL ALIGNMENT

It has been shown that slight external rotation of the femoral component helps to optimize patellar tracking. Optimal patellofemoral kinematics help the surgeon to avoid the many pitfalls that may arise from the patellofemoral articulation.[3,25] The rotation of the femoral component is critical in determining the surgeon's ability to achieve a rectangular flexion space. Problems with the patellofemoral joint are among the most common postoperative complications encountered

in total knee arthroplasty today, affecting 4% to 41% of total knee arthroplasties in which the patella was resurfaced.[26,27] Up to 45% of all revision total knee arthroplasties and 30% to 41% of re-revisions are related to the patellofemoral joint.[1,28] These problems include poor tracking, subluxation, anterior knee pain, patellar clunk, and accelerated patellofemoral component wear.[2,3,24,29,30] Despite the technological advances afforded by the current generation of total knee prostheses, patellofemoral complications continue to plague surgeons.[2,31–34]

In general, 2 methods are used to achieve proper femoral rotational alignment. The first method involves the use of tensioners. The second method relies on bony landmarks. The literature is filled with numerous supporters and detractors of the various methods. The revision surgeon must be familiar with the different techniques, as the distortion of anatomy and the bone loss that often accompany revision arthroplasty may not allow the surgeon to use any one particular reference.

In the *classic* method, the knee is initially balanced in full extension. It is then flexed to 90 degrees, and a cut perpendicular to the long axis of the tibia is performed. The knee is then tensed in 90 degrees of flexion, and anteroposterior resections, parallel to the tibial plateau, are performed on the femur. This should produce a rectangular flexion space, thus assuring proper rotational orientation of the femur relative to the patella and the tibia.[35] It is important to realize that this technique may be difficult in cases of substantial preexisting ligamentous imbalance.

Hungerford and Krackow proposed in 1985 that equal amounts of bone must be resected from the medial and lateral posterior femoral condyles[36] (Figure 11-13). When unequal amounts of bone are resected off the tibial plateau (as is usually the case in varus osteoarthritis), the femoral component will be internally rotated, if equal amounts of bone are then taken from the medial and lateral posterior femoral condyles. The increased Q-angle likely causes patellar maltracking with subsequent eccentric polyethylene wear, subluxation, or even dislocation of the patellofemoral joint. To prevent this problem in the majority of knees, the surgeon must resect more posterior condyle from the medial side than from the lateral side. The damage to the posterior femoral condyles from osteolysis or during removal of the primary component will likely render this technique impractical in revision total knee arthroplasty.

The clinical epicondylar axis is one bony landmark that may be used to ensure proper femoral rotation. In 1987 Yoshioki et al. defined the *clinical* epicondylar axis as the line connecting the lateral epicondylar prominence and the most prominent aspect of the medial epicondyle.[37] Their group also described the condylar twist

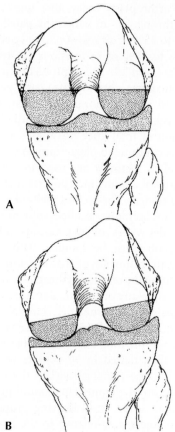

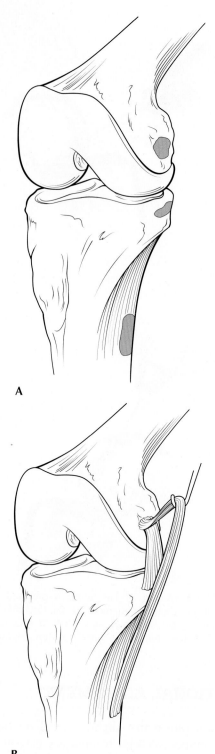

Figure 11-13. (A and B) Posterior condyle, equal resections and appropriate resections. (From Krackow KA. *The Technique of Total Knee Arthroplasty.* St. Louis: Mosby; 1990:131.)

angle as the angle subtended by the posterior condylar line and the clinical epicondylar axis (Figure 11-14). The medial prominent point can be palpated through the skin and soft tissues and is located on the crescent ridge that is the point of attachment for the superficial fibers of the medial collateral ligament (Figure 11-15). Many other current total knee systems use the posterior condylar line as their reference point for determining rotational alignment. The jigs are usually based on a pre-fixed 3 degrees of external rotation off the line drawn between the posterior condyles (posterior condylar line) (Figure 11-16).

Figure 11-14. Condylar twist angle. (From Berger, Rubash, Seel, et al.[24] by permission of *Clin Orthop.*)

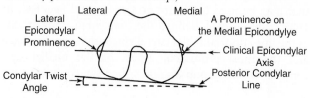

Figure 11-15. (A and B) MCL origin. (Adapted from Berger, Rubash, Seel, et al.[24] by permission of *Clin Orthop.*)

Again, this point of reference is not always available when revising a total knee arthroplasty. Further, this technique may be unreliable with the cartilage wear and bony defects that are present with arthritis.[38]

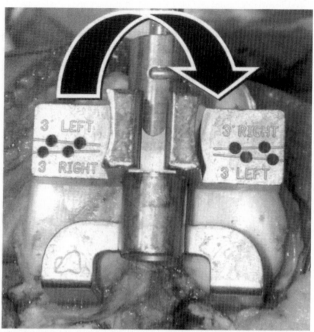

Figure 11-16. ER off posterior condylar line. (From Callaghan J, Rosenberg A, Rubash H, Simonian P, Wickiewicz T, eds. *The Adult Knee.* By permission of Lippincott Williams & Wilkins, 2003.)

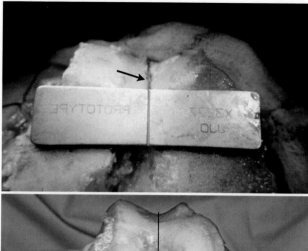

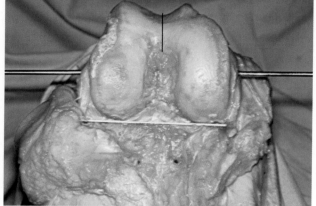

Figure 11-17. (A and B) Whiteside's line. (From Callaghan J, Rosenberg A, Rubash H, Simonian P, and Wickiewicz T, eds. *The Adult Knee.* By permission of Lippincott Williams & Wilkins, 2003.)

Whiteside's line is another bony landmark that may assist the surgeon in determining rotation of the femoral component. Described by Whiteside and Arima in 1995, this line runs in the deepest part of the trochlear groove and should be perpendicular to the epicondylar axis[39] (Figure 11-17). It is useful as an intraoperative check to ensure proper orientation of the femoral cutting block. Unfortunately, patellofemoral arthritis may obscure this reference. Further, the anterior and posterior femoral cuts from the index procedure may make it difficult to use this technique in revision arthroplasty.

It is our feeling that the *surgical* epicondylar axis provides both an important secondary anatomic reference in primary total knee arthroplasty as well as a useful primary anatomic landmark that can be used when the posterior condylar surfaces are not available to accurately gauge rotation of the femoral component. Berger, Rubash, et al. have defined the surgical epicondylar axis as a line drawn between the lateral epicondylar prominence and the medial sulcus of the medial epicondyle (Figures 11-18 and 11-19). The medial sulcus may be difficult to find intraoperatively. If this is the case, the authors advocate removing any superficial soft tissues and then using a surgical marker to define the entire medial epicondyle. The medial sulcus can be found as a depression in the center of the prominence. It is from the medial sulcus that the deep fibers of the medial collateral ligament take origin. The superficial medial collateral ligament is the fanlike

insertion that overlies the deep fibers. Once identified, the anterior and posterior femoral resections should be performed parallel to this axis.

The anterior trochlear groove is also a useful intraoperative reference to assist in determining the correct amount of external rotation of the femoral component. It has been well described that in a normal femur, the lateral side is more prominent than the medial side. When the surgeon performs the anterior femoral cut, more of the lateral side should be resected than the medial side. When the cut is performed correctly, more cancellous

Figure 11-18. Line drawing of the surgical epicondylar axis. (From Berger, Rubash, Seel, et al.[24] by permission of *Clin Orthop.*)

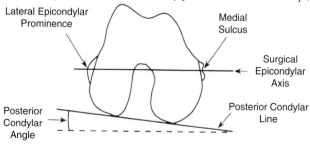

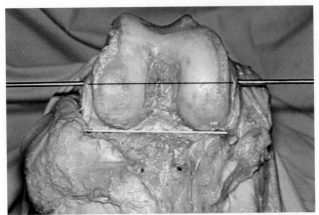

Figure 11-19. Photograph of the surgical epicondylar axis. (From Callaghan J, Rosenberg A, Rubash H, Simonian P, Wickiewicz T, eds. *The Adult Knee.* By permissions of Lippincott Williams & Wilkins, 2003.)

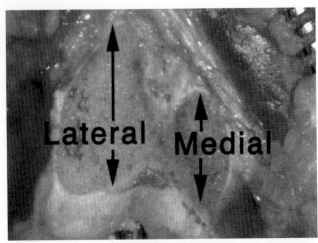

Figure 11-20. Insall boot. (From Callaghan J, Rosenberg A, Rubash H, Simonian P, Wickiewicz T, eds. *The Adult Knee.* By permissions of Lippincott Williams & Wilkins, 2003.)

bone should be visible laterally (Figure 11-20). This sign is commonly referred to as the *Insall boot*. If the resection is made in neutral or in internal rotation, one would see more cancellous bone on the medial side. If this is the case, we recommend reassessing and performing a cut parallel to the surgical epicondylar axis.

In 1999, Olcott and Scott compared the efficacy of these various reference axes.[40] They evaluated 100 consecutive primary total knee arthroplasties in 81 patients performed for both osteoarthritis (93 knees) and rheumatoid arthritis (7 knees) by one surgeon (R.D.S.). The femoral alignment necessary to create a balanced flexion gap was determined and compared with Whiteside's line, the transepicondylar axis, and a line in 3 degrees of external rotation off the posterior femoral condyles. They found that the transepicondylar axis most consistently recreated a balanced flexion space. The 3 degrees off the posterior condyles was least consistent, especially in valgus knees.

Katz et al. found that the tension technique, as described initially by Insall, was the most reliable in determining the correct femoral rotation.[41] Their group also reported that the transepicondylar axis (both clinical and surgical) had the greatest variation. Agaki et al. in 2001 reached conclusions similar to those reached by Olcott and Scott with regard to the posterior condylar line.[42] They used computed tomography to evaluate the posterior condylar line, the anteroposterior line, and the transepicondylar axes (surgical and clinical) in 111 symptomatic arthritic knees. The tibiofemoral and distal femoral valgus angles were then compared with the previously mentioned reference angles. Their group found that the posterior condylar angle became unreliable when the tibiofemoral valgus angle exceeded 9 degrees. They

were unable to locate the medial sulcus of the surgical epicondylar axis in 25% of the cases. The authors concluded that the anteroposterior axis was more reliable in valgus knees, and they advocated the use of computed tomography for knees with severe valgus deformity.

The medial/lateral placement of the femoral component should not be overlooked, as it may influence patellar tracking as well.[25] In most cases, the mediolateral width of the femoral component occupies most of the bony surface. However, if some cancellous bone remains visible, we recommend lateralizing the component. The femoral component should be adjusted until the lateral edge of the prosthesis bisects the cut lateral surface of the femur (Figure 11-21). This effectively lateralizes the trochlear groove and thus optimizes patellar tracking.

Figure 11-21. Mediolateral placement of the femoral component. The femoral component should be adjusted until the lateral edge of the prosthesis bisects the cut lateral surface of the femur.

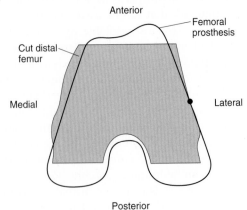

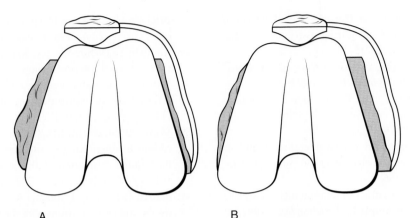

A   B

Figure 11-22. (A and B) Mediolateral placement of the femoral component. Medialization of the prosthesis causes lateralization of the patella relative to the trochlear groove, which should be avoided. (Adapted from Callaghan J, Rosenberg A, Rubash H, Simonian P, Wickiewicz T, eds. *The Adult Knee.* By permission of Lippincott Williams & Wilkins, 2003.)

Conversely, medialization of the prosthesis causes lateralization of the patella relative to the trochlear groove (Figure 11-22). This should be avoided, as it is likely to have a negative impact on patellar tracking.

SUMMARY

The alignment of the femoral component is vital to the success of any total knee arthroplasty. Alterations in the normal alignment likely lead to decreased component survivorship and poor clinical outcomes. Revision total knee arthroplasty poses particular challenges to the surgeon with regard to femoral alignment.[43,44] At the Massachusetts General Hospital, we believe that proper axial alignment can be achieved with the use of an intramedullary alignment guide. This should allow for the distal femur to be cut reliably in 5 to 7 degrees of valgus. Proper rotational alignment is achieved by making the anterior and posterior femoral resections parallel to the surgical epicondylar axis. It is our feeling that the surgical epicondylar axis is a reliable landmark that can be used in even the most difficult revision cases. Restoration of the native axial and rotational alignment of the femur improves the chances of achieving a successful and durable revision total knee arthroplasty.

REFERENCES

1. Elia EA, Lotke PA. Results of revision total knee arthroplasty associated with significant bone loss. *Clin Orthop.* 1991; 271:114–121.

2. Berger RA, Crossett LS, Jacobs JJ, Rubash HE. Malrotation causing patellofemoral complications after total knee arthroplasty. *Clin Orthop.* 1998;356:144–153.

3. Figgie HE, Goldberg VM, Heiple KG, et al. The influence of tibial-patellofemoral location on function of the knee in patients with the posterior stabilized condylar knee prosthesis. *J Bone Joint Surg.* 1986;68A:1035–1040.

4. Lotke PA, Ecker ML. Influence of positioning of prosthesis in total knee replacement. *J Bone Joint Surg.* 1977;59A: 77–79.

5. Kapandji A. *The Physiology of Joints.* 2nd ed. New York: Churchill Livingstone; 1970:232–233.

6. Burr D, Cook L, Cilento E, et al. A method for radiographically measuring true femoral rotation. *Clin Orthop.* 1982; 167:139.

7. Mensch J, Amstutz H. Knee morphology as a guide to knee replacement. *Clin Orthop.* 1975;112:231.

8. Johnson F, Leitl S, Waugh W. The distribution of load across the knee. *J Bone Joint Surg.* 1992;62B:346.

9. Pollice P, Lotke P, Lonner J. Principles of instrumentation and component alignment. In: Callaghan J, Rosenberg A, Rubash H, Simonian P, Wickiewicz T, eds. *The Adult Knee.* Philadelphia: Lippincott, Williams & Wilkins; 2003: 1085–1093.

10. Mann R, Coughlin M. *Surgery of the Foot and Ankle.* 6th ed. St. Louis: C.V. Mosby; 1993:15.

11. Harrington IJ. A biomechanical analysis of force actions at the knee in normal and pathologic gait. *Biomed Eng.* 1976; 11:167.

12. Harrington IJ. Static and dynamic loading patterns in knee joints with deformities. *J Bone Joint Surg.* 1983;65A: 247–259.

13. Hsu R, Himeno S, Coventry M. Normal axial alignment of the lower extremity and load-bearing distribution at the knee. *Clin Orthop.* 1990;255:215–217.

14. Morrison J. Bioengineering analysis of force actions transmitted by the knee joint. *Biomed Eng.* 1968;3:164.

15. Hsu H, Garg A, Walker P, et al. Effect of knee component alignment on tibial load distribution with clinical correlation. *Clin Orthop.* 1989;248:135.

16. Ritter M, Faris P, Keating E, et al. Post-operative alignment of total knee replacement: its effect on survival. *Clin Orthop.* 1994;299:153–156.

17. Reed SC, Gollish J. The accuracy of femoral intramedullary guides in total knee arthroplasty. *J Arthroplasty.* 1997;12:677–682.

18. Ries MD. Endosteal referencing in revision total knee arthroplasty. *J Arthroplasty.* 1998;13:85–91.

19. Teter K, Bregman D, Colwell C. The efficacy of intramedullary alignment in total knee replacement. *Clin Orthop.* 1995;321:117–121.

20. Cates H, Ritter M, Keating E, et al. Intramedullary versus extramedullary alignment systems in total knee replacement. *Clin Orthop.* 1993;286:32–39.

21. Fahmy N, Chandler H, Danylchuk K, et al. Blood-gas and circulatory changes during total knee replacement. role of the intramedullary alignment rod. *J Bone Joint Surg.* 1990;72A:19–26.

22. Gleitz M, Hopf T, Hess T. [Experimental studies on the role of intramedullary alignment rods in the etiology of fat embolisms in knee endoprosthesis]. *Z OrthopIhre Grenzgeb.* 1996;134:254–259.

23. Insall J, Scott WN. *Surgery of the Knee.* 3rd ed. Philadelphia: Churchill Livingstone; 2001:1560.

24. Berger RA, Rubash HE, Seel MJ, et al. Determining the rotational alignment of the femoral component in total knee arthroplasty using the epicondylar axis. *Clin Orthop.* 1993;286:40–47.

25. Rhoads D, Noble P, Reuben J, et al. The effect of femoral component position on patellar tracking after total knee arthroplasty. *Clin Orthop.* 1990;260:43.

26. Boyd A, Ewald F, Thomas W, Poss R, Sledge C. Long-term complications after total knee arthroplasty with or without resurfacing of the patella. *J Bone Joint Surg.* 1993;75A:674–681.

27. Stuart M, Larson J, Morrey B. Reoperation after condylar revision total knee arthroplasty. *Clin Orthop.* 1993;286:168–173.

28. Thornhill T, Hood R, Dalziel R, et al. Knee revision in failed non-infected total knee arthroplasty—the Robert B.

Brigham Hospital and Hospital for Special Surgery experience. *Orthop Trans.* 1982;6:368–369.

29. Anouchi YS, Whiteside LA, Kaiser AD, Milliano MT. The effects of axial rotational alignment of the femoral component on knee stability and patellar tracking in total knee arthroplasty demonstrated on autopsy specimens. *Clin Orthop.* 1993;287:170–177.

30. Mantas JP, Bloebaum RD, Skedros JG, Hofmann AA. Implications of reference axes used for rotational alignment of the femoral component in primary and revision total knee arthroplasty. *J Arthroplasty.* 1992;7:531–535.

31. Aglietti P, Buzzi R, Gaudenzi A. Patellofemoral functional results and complications with the posterior stabilized total condylar knee prosthesis. *J Arthroplasty.* 1988;3(1):17.

32. Brick G, Scott R. The patellofemoral component of total knee arthroplasty. *Clin Orthop.* 1988;231:163.

33. Insall JN, Binazzi R, Soudry M, et al. Total knee arthroplasty. *Clin Orthop.* 1985;192:13.

34. Bryan R, Rand J. Revision total knee arthroplasty. *Clin Orthop.* 1982;170:116.

35. Fehring T. Rotational malalignment of the femoral component in total knee arthroplasty. *Clin Orthop.* 2000;380:72–79.

36. Hungerford D, Krackow K. Total joint arthroplasty of the knee. *Clin Orthop.* 1985;192:23.

37. Yoshioka Y, Siu D, Cooke TD. The anatomy and functional axes of the femur. *J Bone Joint Surg.* 1987;69A:873–880.

38. Griffin F, Insall J, Scuderi G. The posterior condylar angle in osteoarthritic knees. *J Arthroplasty.* 1988;13:812.

39. Whiteside LA, Arima J. The anteroposterior axis for femoral rotational alignment in valgus total knee arthroplasty. *Clin Orthop.* 1995;321:168–172.

40. Olcott CW, Scott RD. The Ranawat Award. Femoral component rotation during total knee arthroplasty. *Clin Orthop.* 1999;367:39–42.

41. Katz M, Beck T, Silber J. Determining femoral rotational alignment in total knee arthroplasty: reliability of techniques. *J Arthroplasty.* 2001;16:301.

42. Agaki M, Yamashita E, Nakagawa T, et al. Relationship between frontal knee alignment and reference axes in the distal femur. *Clin Orthop.* 2001;388:147–156.

43. Hoeffel DP, Rubash HE. Revision total knee arthroplasty. Current rationale and techniques for femoral component revision. *Clin Orthop.* 2000;380:116–132.

44. Bertin K, Vince K, Booth R, Paprosky W, Rosenberg A, Rubash H. *Zimmer LCCK Revision Instrumentation Surgical Technique.* Warsaw, IN: Zimmer, Inc.; 2000.

CHAPTER 12

Tibial Alignment

James V. Bono

Precise component alignment in both the anteroposterior and lateral planes is essential for proper implant function and longevity in total knee arthroplasty (TKA). Inability to achieve proper alignment can generate eccentric implant loading resulting in early aseptic loosening and failure (Figure 12-1). In addition, correction of the mechanical axis of the lower extremity (Figure 12-2) to within 5 to 7 degrees of valgus has been shown to improve TKA implant longevity both biomechanically and clinically.[1–14]

Both intramedullary and extramedullary alignment guide systems are used to correct deformity in TKA. Both systems are dependent on the degree to which each guide rod approximates the anatomic axes of the femur and tibia. Intramedullary alignment of the femur in TKA has been generally accepted as superior to extramedullary alignment.[15–22] The femoral shaft is difficult to locate through a large, surrounding soft tissue envelope. Additionally, femoral extramedullary alignment systems require estimation of the center of the femoral head. Radiographic skin markers often can be used; however, bulky surgical drapes and obesity may present problems. Alternatively, intraoperative fluoroscopy or surgical navigation can be used to define the center of the femoral head.

On the tibial side, there is considerable debate as to whether intramedullary or extramedullary alignment is superior. Tibial intramedullary alignment devices are based on the assumption that the angle between the anatomical and the mechanical axis is not significantly different from zero in either the coronal or sagittal planes.[23–27] This chapter seeks to define the indications and emphasize the contraindications for intramedullary alignment of the tibia in revision total knee arthroplasty. Furthermore, specific case examples are reviewed that illustrate the pitfalls of and alternatives

to intramedullary alignment of the tibia in total knee arthroplasty.

In our previous report,[28] 44 adult cadaveric tibiae without obvious clinical deformity were harvested. Using a stepped drill bit, the proximal medullary canal was entered anterior to the tibial attachment of the anterior cruciate ligament. The starting hole was oversized with a rasp and a long 8-mm diameter solid intramedullary fluted guide rod was passed down the medullary canal until it was firmly engaged distally. The bone cut was made referencing off the intramedullary cutting jig. Anteroposterior and lateral radiographs were taken and the anatomical, mechanical, and guide rod axes were assessed on each radiograph. The accuracy of the guide rod was assessed by measuring how closely the guide rod axis approximated the anatomic and mechanical axis in both the anteroposterior and lateral planes. The difference between the anatomic axis and the guide rod axis was measured and defined as the axis angle.

Observations obtained from this cadaveric study revealed that certain deformities and clinical situations would preclude the use of intramedullary alignment of the tibia in total knee arthroplasty. The clinician needs to be aware of the contraindications and alternatives to intramedullary alignment of the tibia in total knee arthroplasty.

RESULTS OF ANATOMIC STUDIES

Anatomic requirements for successful intramedullary alignment require a patent intramedullary canal for complete seating of the guide rod. In the cadaveric tibiae examined, analysis of the anteroposterior radiographs of all 44 specimens revealed the guide rod to be on average in 0.56 degrees of valgus (range 1.4 degrees varus to 2.8

degrees extension) compared with the mechanical axis. Analysis of the lateral radiographs of all 44 specimens revealed the guide rod to be in 0.2 degrees of extension (range 3.3 degrees flexion to 2.5 degrees extension) compared with the mechanical axis.

The anteroposterior guide rod-mechanical axis angle was examined in 10% increments of guide rod insertion. There was a tendency for this angle to increase as the insertion amount decreased, from 0.75 degrees at 90% to 100% insertion to 1.90 degrees at 40% to 50% insertion. Maximum accuracy of the tibial intramedullary alignment guide rod required complete seating of the device to the level of the distal physeal scar ($p < 0.05$). The valgus tibiae, i.e., the tibia with a valgus bow, demonstrated an increased anteroposterior guide rod-mechanical axis angle as compared with the neutral or varus tibiae. Furthermore, the intramedullary guide was more accurate in reproducing the mechanical axis in the non-valgus tibiae ($p < 0.05$). This finding suggests that the valgus tibia may be a relative contraindication to relying exclusively on intramedullary alignment.

In addition to the findings described previously, other clinical situations can prohibit the use of intramedullary alignment in total knee arthroplasty. Any situation that blocks the passage of a straight guide rod would disallow the use of intramedullary alignment. Both anatomic abnormalities and retained implants can result in mechanical obstruction of the intramedullary canal (Figures 12-3A, B and 12-4A, B).

FIGURE 12-1. Massively obese 70-year-old woman with early mechanical failure following TKA. Varus alignment of the tibial component contributed to mechanical overloading of the medial compartment.

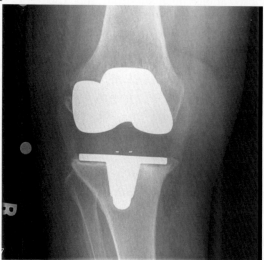

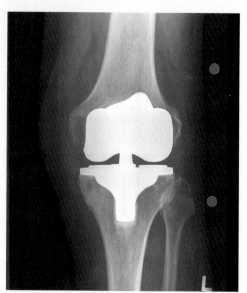

FIGURE 12-2. Proper alignment of the femoral and tibial component allows even distribution of stress over the medial and lateral compartment.

OBSERVATIONS IN REVISION TOTAL KNEE ARTHROPLASTY

The incidence of revision TKA is increasing, largely due to the increased number of primary procedures performed annually. The leading indications for revision TKA include reimplantation after infection and aseptic loosening. Bone stock loss is invariably encountered at revision resulting from mechanical collapse of bone, osteolysis, or a result of aggressive debridement in the setting of post-septic reimplantation. The use of intramedullary stems in this setting is advisable due to the compromised bony platform of the tibial plateau, as well as to offset the stresses transmitted to the bone, which accompany the use of constrained and semi-constrained revision components.

Intramedullary extension stems may be used both with and without cement and are discussed further in the following chapter. Cementless fixation is typically achieved by intimate contact of an uncoated, fluted extension stem within the intramedullary canal of the tibia and femur. The intramedullary canal is prepared with rigid axial reamers to match the diameter of the selected intramedullary extension stem. The intramedullary extension stem is assumed to replicate the intramedullary axis of the femur or tibia. As a result, component position is dictated by the use of an intramedullary extension stem. If a cementless extension stem is selected, greater stability of the intramedullary extension stem occurs with circumferential filling of the stem within the intramedullary canal.

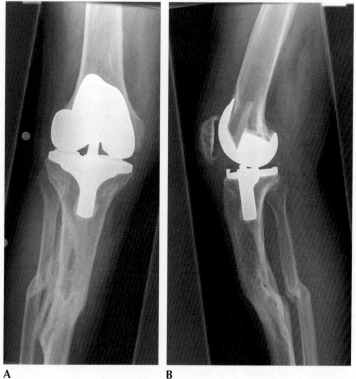

A   **B**

FIGURE 12-3. (A and B) AP and lateral views of the tibia depict a well-healed fracture of the tibial diaphysis, which would block the passage of an intramedullary guide rod into the tibia.

FIGURE 12-4. (A and B) Nonanatomic alignment of the tibial diaphysis precludes the use of intramedullary alignment.

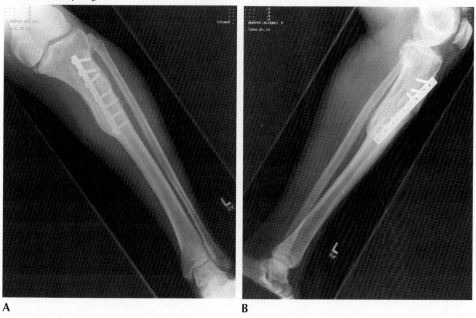

A   **B**

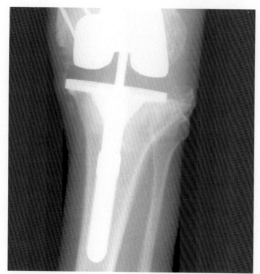

FIGURE 12-5. Following revision TKA using a press-fit intramedullary tibial stem, the tibial component is noted to overhang medially, leaving the lateral plateau uncovered. The position of the tibial component is dictated by the placement of the stem and does not always result in symmetric coverage of the tibial plateau.

Intramedullary extension stems may be used in two distinct manners, based on surgeon preference. First, if the surgeon elects to emphasize stability of the stem within the canal based on a line to line fit, the component position will by necessity be dictated by the intramedullary stem, and may not result in symmetric coverage by the underlying bone (Figure 12-5). If, however, the surgeon prefers symmetric positioning of the component, the diameter of the intramedullary extension stem may have to be compromised, to shift the component from the intramedullary axis of the tibia or femur (Figure 12-6A, B). If this is done, the stability of the cementless stem within the canal will suffer. Stability may be recovered by cementing the stem within the canal, acknowledging an asymmetric cement mantle.

If an intramedullary extension stem is used, component position will be dictated by the position of the intramedullary rod. In a previous study,[29] we sought to determine whether the use of a press-fit, canal-filling, cementless intramedullary extension stem in revision TKA resulted in asymmetric placement of the tibial component.

RESULTS OF RADIOGRAPHIC DATA

Radiographs of 24 patients undergoing revision total knee arthroplasty with a stemmed tibial component were reviewed. The same modular revision implant system was in each case. There were 14 male and 10 female subjects, with an average age of 66.7 years (range, 37 to 93).

FIGURE 12-6. (A) An attempt to place the tibial component symmetrically on the tibial plateau results in non-anatomic placement of the tibial stem, illustrating the conflict between the intramedullary axis of the tibia and the anatomy of the tibial plateau. (B) A custom-made tibial component with an offset tibial stem allows for axial alignment of the stem with anatomic coverage of the tibial plateau.

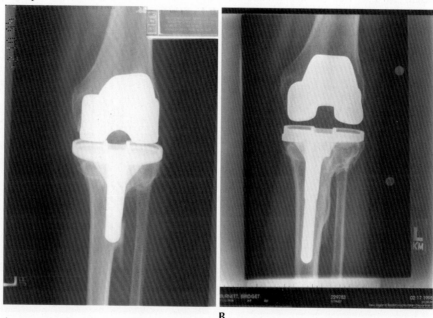

A   B

Intramedullary tibial stem extensions were used in each case, with an average diameter of 14.9 mm (range, 10 to 20 mm) and an average length of 68.5 mm (range, 30 to 115 mm). Augmentation wedges were required in 5 patients, with two 10 degree full medial wedges, one 15 degree full medial wedge, one 15 degree half-medial wedge, and one 10 degree half-lateral wedge. Measurements of tibial component medial, lateral, anterior, and posterior displacement were made and corrected for magnification.

The tibial component was noted to be eccentrically positioned on the tibial plateau in 24 of 24 patients, with medial placement noted in 20, lateral in 3, posterior in 17, and anterior in 3. Medial tibial component overhang was most common (46%), averaging 2.5 mm (range, 1.7 to 4.3 mm). Of the 11 patients with medial component overhang, the lateral aspect of the tibial plateau was noted to be uncovered by an average of 5.4 mm (range, 1.8 to 9.9 mm) in 8 patients.

IMPLICATIONS FOR REVISION TOTAL KNEE ARTHROPLASTY

Medial eccentricity of the tibial component was found to be the most common problem (20 of 24) encountered when intramedullary extension stems were used in revi-

FIGURE 12-7. A modular offset tibial stem is used to shift the tibial component laterally and posteriorly to allow symmetric coverage of the tibial plateau. The press-fit tibial stem is centered within the diaphysis and fills the canal.

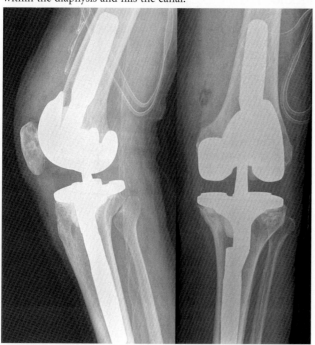

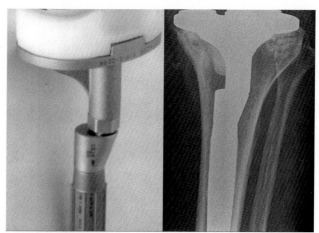

FIGURE 12-8. An offset adapter (Stryker, Allendale, NJ) is available in 4, 6, and 8 mm increments and is used to shift the tibial component (360 degrees) about the intramedullary axis, which is defined by the intramedullary extension stem.

sion TKA,[29] resulting in medial overhang in 11 of 24 cases despite downsizing of the tibial component. Posterior placement of the tibial component was similarly noted in 17 of 24 cases. This is the result of altered anatomy due to loss of proximal tibial bone stock and the restriction placed on tibial component positioning by the intramedullary stem. This finding suggests that an allowance for lateral and anterior offset be incorporated into tibial component design when used with an intramedullary stem extension (Figures 12-7 and 12-8).

Therefore, if an intramedullary extension stem is used, component position will be dictated by the position of the intramedullary rod. Asymmetric placement of the component typically results. A component, which would be of appropriate size, is found to overhang on one side and be uncovered on the other. This typically requires downsizing of the component to remedy the overhang, which accentuates the amount of bone uncovered by prosthetic component. The results of this study confirmed our belief that the use of a canal filling cementless, press-fit intramedullary extension stem creates asymmetric positioning of the tibial component.

DISCUSSION

Appropriate orientation of prosthetic components is crucial for arthroplasty survival. Postoperative alignment of the lower extremity has a direct effect on the durability of the implant. Significant varus or valgus malalignment may predispose the tibial component to early loosening.

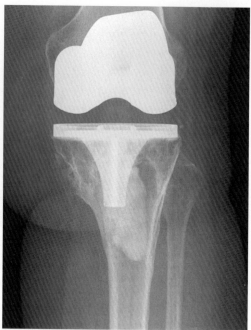

FIGURE 12-9. Previous fracture has distorted the tibial metaphysis, which must be recognized in order to achieve proper alignment and fixation.

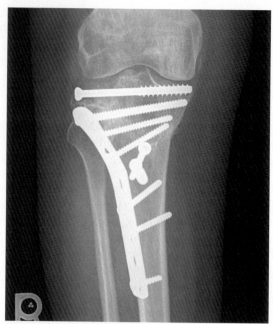

FIGURE 12-11. A lateral tibial plateau fracture with bone loss. Hardware is removed before TKA.

Anatomic deformity can result from previous fracture (Figure 12-9), sepsis, or metabolic bone disease (e.g., Paget's disease). Implant barriers to intramedullary alignment occur after fracture fixation (Figures 12-10 through

12-12), broken retained hardware, or below a femoral component in total hip arthroplasty.

Whether an intramedullary or extramedullary alignment guide is used, accurate reproduction of bony cuts is

FIGURE 12-10. Posttraumatic arthritis following ORIF of a tibial plateau fracture. The tibial metaphysis has been distorted. Hardware is removed before TKA.

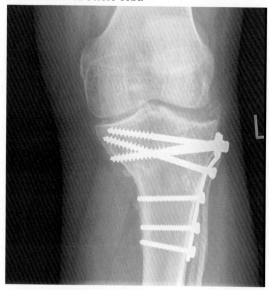

FIGURE 12-12. A 2-stage reconstruction is planned. The first stage consists of hardware removal with simultaneous creation of fasciocutaneous flaps, which tests the integrity of the soft tissues before implantation.

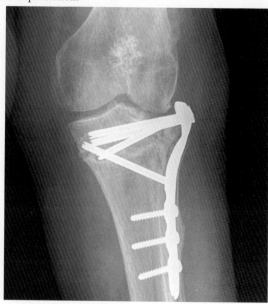

a prerequisite for successful arthroplasty. Either guide system relies on the similarity between the anatomic and mechanical axes. Our previously reported cadaveric tibiae data confirm this assumption; the anatomic axis approached the mechanical axis to within 1° on average in both the anteroposterior and lateral planes.[28]

For the tibia, many surgeons prefer extramedullary alignment, using bony landmarks about the ankle as reference points. Because the center of the talus is slightly medial to the midpoint between the malleoli, the surgeon must estimate the center of the talus based on these bony landmarks, which may be obscured by soft tissue excess, bony abnormalities, or bulky surgical drapes. Even if surgical navigation systems are employed, alignment is still based on where the surgeon estimates the center of the talus to be located.

Some authors have suggested that for the tibia, intramedullary alignment is more accurate and reproducible than extramedullary alignment and allows consistent and accurate long bone cuts. Our cadaveric tibiae data confirm the reliability of intramedullary alignment in assessing the anatomic axis in total knee arthroplasty. However, when passage of the intramedullary guide rod is prevented from complete seating to the distal tibial physeal scar, the reliability of this technique in assessing the anatomic axis of the tibia is impaired. Simmons et al. were unable to template a long tibial intramedullary guide rod from a central entry point in 42% of cases. In addition, they were able to achieve a 90 degree cut to the long axis of the tibia in 30 of 35 knees (85.7%) when complete seating of the guide rod was achieved and only in 2 of 25 knees (8%) when the long tibial intramedullary guide was incompletely seated.[24] Our data demonstrate that when penetration of the guide rod was incomplete, the resultant malalignment corresponded inversely with the depth of insertion. In cases in which penetration of the guide rod was complete (>80%), the accuracy of the intramedullary alignment system increased ($p < 0.05$) to within 1 degree in both the anteroposterior and lateral planes.

Angular deformities in the tibia can interfere with the use of intramedullary devices and prevent passage of the guide rod. Simmons et al. suggested that intramedullary alignment is less predictable in the valgus knee and may lead to malalignment. Our data support the decreased accuracy of tibial intramedullary alignment in valgus versus neutral and varus tibiae ($p < 0.05$). Therefore, valgus deformity of the tibia may be a contraindication to absolute reliance on intramedullary alignment.

In addition to a valgus bow of the tibia, anatomic bony deformity may be a contraindication to the use of intramedullary alignment when performing total knee arthroplasty. Previous fracture, osteotomy, sepsis, or metabolic bone disease, such as osteopetrosis or Paget's disease, can result in a long bone deformity of the tibia that precludes the use of intramedullary alignment guides. Furthermore, retained hardware after fracture fixation or intramedullary cement/hardware after total knee arthroplasty act as barriers to intramedullary alignment. Careful preoperative planning with standing long leg radiographs will identify the patient at risk for incomplete passage of an intramedullary alignment guide rod and should be obtained in all TKA candidates in whom an intramedullary alignment system is considered.

CONCLUSION

There is considerable debate whether intramedullary or extramedullary tibial alignment provides a more accurate reproduction of the mechanical axis of the affected limb.[2,17,18,23,28] In the absence of severe bowing of the tibia, which precludes complete seating of the guide rod, intramedullary tibial alignment is reproducibly accurate and consistent to within 1 degree in the varus-valgus and flexion-extension planes. Maximum accuracy of tibial intramedullary alignment requires complete seating of the device to the distal tibial physeal scar ($p < 0.05$) and is best suited for the nonvalgus tibiae ($p < 0.05$).

Theoretical disadvantages of intramedullary alignment in TKA include the increased risk of fat embolization and medullary bone loss with guide rod passage to the tibia. A reduction in guide rod diameter from 8 to 6mm, in conjunction with lavage and suction of the intramedullary canal, can help decrease the potential for fat embolization during insertion of intramedullary alignment devices. Anatomic angular deformity resulting from previous fracture, osteotomy, sepsis, or metabolic bone disease may represent additional contraindications to intramedullary alignment use. Furthermore, mechanical obstruction resulting from retained hardware after fracture fixation, osteotomy, or intramedullary cement/hardware after total knee arthroplasty may preclude the use of an intramedullary guide rod. Careful preoperative planning identifies the patient at risk for incomplete intramedullary guide rod passage. In these patients, the use of extramedullary alignment and intraoperative radiographs maximizes accuracy of tibial component position and improves implant longevity.

In revision TKA, alignment is equally critical. Our data have shown that the intramedullary axis of the tibia does not bisect the tibial plateau.[29] Therefore, if a cementless intramedullary extension stem is used, tibial component position will be dictated by the position of the stem. In the majority of cases, this results in asymmetric position of the tibial component with respect to the tibial plateau. This creates the potential for component overhang and diminished support. The use of offset cementless intramedullary extension stems is recommended to address these shortcomings. An asymmetric stem reduces the potential for component overhang while reclaiming areas of uncovered bone for component coverage. In most cases, the need to downsize components is eliminated, allowing a larger component to be used; this allows for an increase in surface area for component support and fixation. The results of this study support the use of an offset stem, which allows for both anteroposterior and mediolateral translation to maximize bony contact between the tibial component and host bone.

REFERENCES

1. Insall JN, Binazzi R, Soudry M, Mestriner LA. Total knee arthroplasty. *Clin Orthop.* 1985;192:13–22.

2. Laskin RS. Alignment of total knee components. *Orthopaedics.* 1984;7:62.

3. Lotke PA, Ecker ML. Influence of positioning of prosthesis in total knee replacement. *J Bone Joint Surg.* 1977;59A: 77–79.

4. Moreland JR. Mechanisms of failure in total knee arthroplasty. *Clin Orthop.* 1988;226:49–64.

5. Townley CO. The anatomic total knee resurfacing arthroplasty. *Clin Orthop.* 1985;192:82–96.

6. Smith JL, Tullos HS, Davidson JP. Alignment of total knee arthroplasty. *J Arthroplasty.* 1989;4:55.

7. Tew M, Waugh W. Tibiofemoral alignment and the results of knee replacement. *J Bone Joint Surg.* 1985;67B:551–556.

8. Bargren JH, Blaha JD, Freeman MAR. Alignment in total knee arthroplasty: correlated biomechanical and clinical observations. *Clin Orthop.* 1983;173:178–183.

9. Hsu RW, Himeno S, Coventry MB, Chao EYS. Normal axial alignment of the lower extremity and load-bearing distribution at the knee. *Clin Orthop.* 1990;255:215–227.

10. Hvid I, Nielsen S. Total condylar knee arthroplasty: prosthetic component positioning and radiolucent lines. *Acta Orthop Scand.* 1984;55:160–165.

11. Uematsu O, Hsu HP, Kelley KM, Ewald FC, Walker PS. Radiographic study of kinematic total knee arthroplasty. *J Arthroplasty.* 1987;2(4):317–326.

12. Petersen TL, Engh GA. Radiographic assessment of knee alignment after total knee arthroplasty. *J Arthroplasty.* 1988; 3:67–72.

13. Engh GA, Petersen TL. Comparative experience with intramedullary and extramedullary alignment in total knee arthroplasty. *J Arthroplasty.* 1990;5:1–8.

14. Moreland JR, Bassett LW, Hanker GJ. Radiographic analysis of the axial alignment of the lower extremity. *J Bone Joint Surg.* 1987;69A:745–749.

15. Tillett ED, Engh GA, Peterson T. A comparative study of extramedullary and intramedullary alignment systems in total knee arthroplasty. *Clin Orthop.* 1988;230:176–181.

16. Ishii Y, Ohmori G, Bechtold JE, Gustillo RB. Extramedullary versus intramedullary alignment guides in total knee arthroplasty. *Clin Orthop.* 1995;318:167–175.

17. Brys DA, Lombardi AV, Mallory, TH, Vaughn, BK. A Comparison of intramedullary and extramedullary alignment systems for tibial component placement in total knee arthroplasty. *Clin Orthop.* 1991;263:175–179.

18. Dennis DA, Channer M, Susman MH, Stringer EA. Intramedullary versus extramedullary tibial alignment systems in total knee arthroplasty. *J Arthroplasty.* 1993;8: 43–47.

19. Moreland JR, Hungerford DS, Insall JN, Scott RD, Whiteside LA. Symposium: total knee instrumentation. *Contemp Orthop.* 1988;17(5):93–126

20. Cates HE, Ritter MA, Keating EM, Faris PM. Intramedullary versus extramedullary femoral alignment systems in total knee replacement. *Clin Orthop.* 1993;286:32–39.

21. Giang C, Insall JN. Effect of rotation on the axial alignment of the femur: pitfalls in the use of femoral intramedullary guides in total knee arthroplasty. *Clin Orthop.* 1989;248: 50–56.

22. Siegel JL, Shall LM. Femoral instrumentation using the anterosuperior iliac spine as a landmark in total knee arthroplasty. an anatomic study. *J Arthroplasty.* 1991;6: 317–320.

23. Laskin RS, Turtel A. The use of intramedullary tibial alignment guide in total knee replacement arthroplasty. *Am J Knee Surg.* 1989;2:123.

24. Simmons ED, Sullivan JA, Rackenmann S, Scott RD. The accuracy of tibial intramedullary alignment devices in total knee arthroplasty. *J Arthroplasty.* 1991;6:5.

25. Whiteside LA. Intramedullary alignment of total knee replacement. *Orthop Rev.* 1989;18:89–112.

26. Whiteside LA, McCarthy DS. Laboratory evaluation of alignment and kinematics in a unicompartmental knee arthroplasty inserted with intramedullary instrumentation. *Clin Orthop.* 1992;274:238–247.

27. Oswald MD, Jakob RP, Schneider E, Hoogweoud H. Radiological analysis of normal axial alignment of femur and tibia in view of TKA. *J Arthroplasty.* 1993;8:419–426.

28. Bono JV, Roger DJ, Laskin RS, Peterson MGE, Paulsen CA. Tibial intramedullary alignment in total knee arthroplasty. *Am J Knee Surg.* 1995;8(1):7–12.

29. Jamison J, Bono JV, McCarthy MC, Turner RH. Tibial component asymmetry in revision total knee arthroplasty: a case for tibial component offset. *J Arthroplasty.* 1998;13(2):241.

CHAPTER 13

Use of Stems in Revision Total Knee Arthroplasty

Thomas K. Fehring

Revision total knee arthroplasty is becoming an increasingly common reconstructive procedure. As the number of primary total knee arthroplasties continues to increase on a yearly basis, the need for revision surgery will likewise increase exponentially. Therefore, it is important to determine the best surgical techniques to manage revision problems as they are encountered.

Most major manufacturers of total knee replacement offer modular revision knee systems. They use modular augmentations to deal with tibial and femoral bone loss. Most also feature intramedullary jig systems to make accurate revision bone cuts. In addition, manufacturers provide a variety of stems to enhance fixation in revision situations. Variable length stems designed to engage in the metaphysis or diaphysis are commonly offered options. Offset stems are also available to deal with altered anatomy. This variety of stems can be implanted in a press-fit or cemented fashion.

Despite this wide array of options available, little comparative information exists to guide the revision knee surgeon in making a proper prosthetic selection for his patient. This chapter reviews the salient biomechanical literature available regarding stem fixation as well as reviews the effect of canal filling stem fixation on limb alignment and implant position. A comparative study concerning methods of stem fixation is also presented, along with current recommendations for stem use in revision TKA.

BIOMECHANICAL ISSUES

Important biomechanical issues that have been studied in the laboratory include the length of stem necessary for fixation, the potential for juxta-articular stress shielding, and the type of stem fixation.

While stable fixation is an integral part of revision total knee surgery, how to achieve such stability in a revision situation with compromised periarticular bone remains controversial. To enhance stability, implants with extended stems have been used during revision knee surgery. The use of such stems transfers stress from the deficient plateau to the shaft.[1]

There were early concerns that the use of such stems might cause significant periarticular stress shielding with subsequent failure. Bourne and Finlay[2] in a strain gauge study noted that the use of intramedullary stems was accompanied by marked stress shielding of the proximal tibial cortex over the length of the stem. They therefore discouraged the use of long intramedullary stems in revision total knee arthroplasty.

In contrast, the successful use of extended stems in revision knee surgery without significant stress shielding was predicted by a number of authors through biomechanical testing. Brooks et al.[3] noted that a 70mm tibial stem carried approximately 30% of the axial load and relieved the deficient proximal bone to that extent. They concluded that it was unlikely that serious juxta-articular osteoporosis would result through the use of such stems. Reilly et al.[4] noted that if a 60mm tibial stem was used with incomplete coverage, decreased proximal strains would be noted. However, if the tibial plateau was completely covered, no load bypass would occur. Jazrawi et al.[5] concurred with this assessment, noting no significant decrease in proximal tibial strain with the use of either cemented or cementless stems. The proximal tibia was substantially loaded in each stem construct tested by these authors.

Therefore, it seems that the use of extended stems is not harmful to juxtaarticular bone in the form of stress shielding following long stem revision surgery. In our revision knee practice encompassing over 500 revision

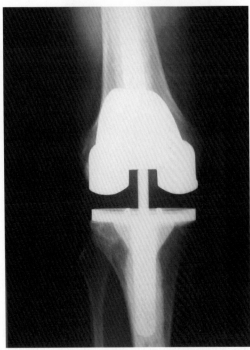

FIGURE 13-1. Revision implant with metaphyseal engaging stems.

knees, metaphyseal engaging stems are used in the vast majority of instances (>90%) (Figure 13-1). The use of diaphyseal engaging stems in our revision practice is rare (<10%). Such stems are reserved for use with large juxtaarticular allografts or periarticular osteotomes or bridging existing cortical defects (Figure 13-2). The ideal method of fixation for such stems remains controversial. While the use of extended stems has become a routine part of revision knee surgery, the ideal method of fixation for such stems remains controversial.

Since little comparative clinical information is available when comparing cemented versus cementless stems in revision total knee surgery, biomechanical studies may help the operating surgeon determine which method of stem fixation is optimal.

Stern et al.[1] in a cadaveric study of tibial stems compared cemented and cementless implants. Configurations were subjected to axial as well as eccentric loads. Micromotion and magnitude of migration were quantified. These authors found that cemented implants were associated with significantly less micromotion compared with uncemented components for all configurations tested. They also noted a decreased magnitude of migration with the use of cement. It should be recognized that in this study when cementless stems were used, the tibial tray was not cemented. This is in contrast to the usual clinical use

of cementless stems in which the tray is cemented and the stem remains cementless.

Bert et al.[6] in a biomechanical study that more closely mirrors clinical use of these stems compared fully cemented constructs with one in which only the tibial tray was cemented and the stem was press-fit. They found that a tibial tray implanted with a press-fit cementless stem had significantly increased micromotion compared with a fully cemented construct. They concluded that the tibial component should be completely cemented under the base plate and around the tibial stem. It should be recognized that this was a study of primary implants without extended length stems.

In another study, Jazrawi et al.[5] looked closely at the mode of fixation on tibial component stability in a revision setting. In evaluating cemented and cementless tibial stems in the laboratory, they noted that longer diaphyseal engaging cementless stems had similar micromotion when compared with shorter cemented metaphyseal engaging tibial stems. They did, however, note that cemented metaphyseal engaging stems had significantly less tray motion than a cementless construct of the same length. These laboratory predictions from different centers consistently found less micromotion with the use of cement stem fixation (Figure 13-3).

FIGURE 13-2. Diaphyseal engaging stem used to fix tibial osteotomy.

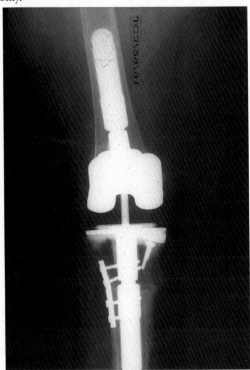

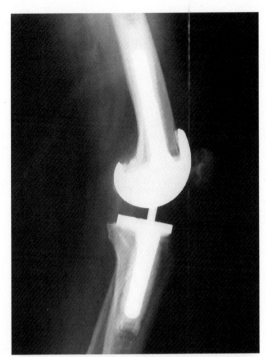

FIGURE 13-3. Well-fixed cemented revision implant.

STEM FIXATION AND ALIGNMENT

Another controversial aspect in revision total knee surgery deals with the type of fixation and ability to maintain normal axial and sagittal limb alignment with canal-filling stems. The revision knee surgeon must be aware of the potential malignment issues that can occur with canal filling cementless stems. On the tibial side, valgus bowing of the tibial diaphysis is not uncommon. Thus, when a canal filling diaphyseal engaging stem is used, axial malalignment can ensue (Figure 13-4).

In addition to the potential for axial malalignment, anteromedial overhang of the tibial tray may occur with the potential for postoperative anteromedial knee pain.

Hicks et al.[7] noted significant variability in the location of the tibial canal to the tibial plateaus. In their cadaveric review, they found that the intramedullary canal center was usually anterior and medial to the tibial plateau. This study highlighted the need for offset stems in revision total knee arthroplasty, especially if engaging the diaphysis of the tibia (Figures 13-5 and 13-6)

Canal filling stems can also have an effect on alignment on the femoral side. A canal filling femoral stem can lead to anterior displacement of the femoral component. Such displacement increases the height of the patellofemoral space with the potential for limiting motion. In addition, such anterior displacement by defi-

nition increases the flexion gap, which can lead to flexion instability (Figure 13-7).

Strategies to prevent such translation include offset stems or stem bolts, which can move the stem anteriorly or posteriorly as necessary to prevent sagittal malignment. Alternatively, a narrow cemented stem can be placed posteriorly in the canal limiting this effect (Figure 13-8).

Another potential problem is that canal filling femoral stems can affect implant position at the joint line. Since most femurs have an anterior bow, a canal filling stem that engages this bow will lead to flexion of the femoral component.

A final alignment issue that can affect implant position occurs when the shaft of the femur is slightly lateral to the condylar bone. If one uses a canal filling stem in this situation, lateral shift of the implant occurs. This helps patellar tracking. However, the eccentric lateral box position can compromise distal femoral bone stock (Figure 13-9).

Many of the described axial and sagittal malalignment issues can be handled in one of 2 ways. A narrow cemented stem can be used in most situations to prevent the previously mentioned malalignment issues. The stem

FIGURE 13-4. Diaphyseal engaging stem causing malalignment in a tibia with valgus bowing.

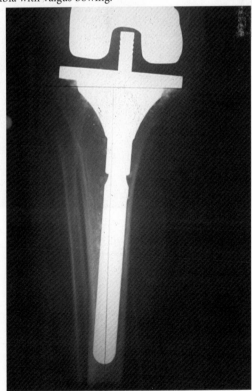

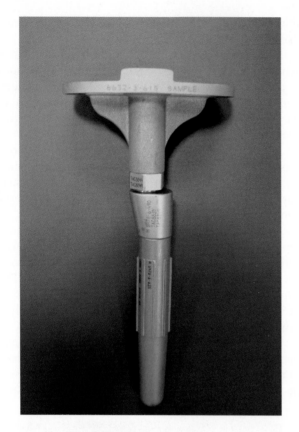

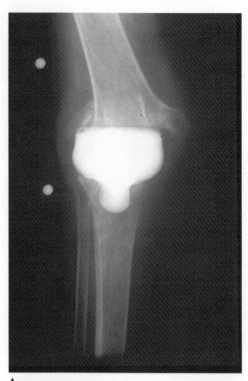

A

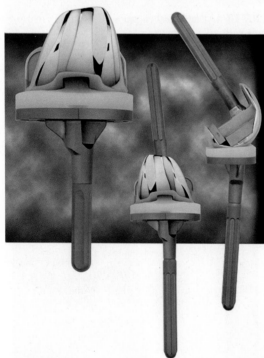

FIGURE 13-5. Various offset modular stems.

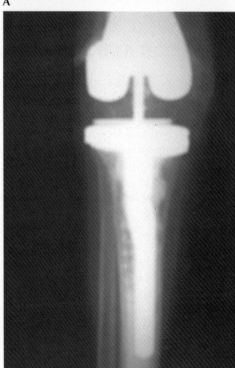

B

FIGURE 13-6. (A) Status post-resection arthroplasty for sepsis. Standard tibial stem would lead to anteromedial overhang. (B) Postoperative view with offset stem and centered tibial base plate.

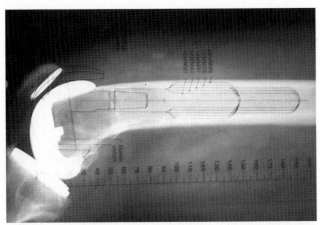

FIGURE 13-7. Canal filling stem template illustrating anterior displacement of the femoral component with corresponding increase in flexion gap.

FIGURE 13-9. Canal filling stem shifting the femoral component laterally.

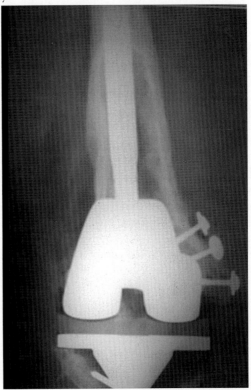

is simply placed eccentrically in the canal to prevent malalignment. Care must be taken to ensure an adequate cement mantle. Alternatively, most manufacturers now offer adjustable offset stems that can compensate for limb malalignment and implant malposition that can occur when using straight canal filling stems.

The revision surgeon must, however, recognize the potential problems noted previously to have the necessary equipment available at the time of revision.

STEM FIXATION

From the previous discussion, one can surmise that cemented fixation has certain advantages over its cement-

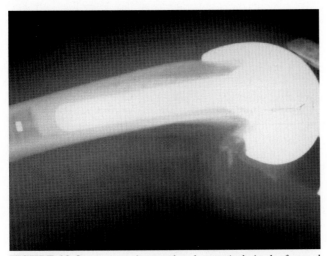

FIGURE 13-8. Cemented stem placed posteriorly in the femoral canal.

less stem counterpart. In the laboratory less micromotion has been reported. In addition, the limb alignment and implant position problems noted previously rarely occur with cemented constructs. To determine what type of stem fixation is best for the revision knee patient, it is also important to review the literature to date on this subject.

Although no prospective study comparing cemented versus cementless stems in revision total knee arthroplasty is available, proponents of each method have reported their results.[8–11] Murray et al.[9] reported the clinical and radiographic results of 40 patients who underwent cemented long stem revision total knee arthroplasty at an average follow-up of nearly 5 years. Only one patient had asymptomatic radiographic loosening of the femoral component, while no tibial component was categorized as loose. They concluded that it was necessary to compare the durability of revisions performed with press-fit cementless stems to the excellent results they reported with fully cemented constructs.

Bertin et al.[11] first described the use of juxta-articular cementing with the use of long uncemented stems in their analysis of 53 revision total knees. At a follow-up of only 18 months, 18% had complete radiolucent lines at the femoral bone cement interface, while 21% of the tibial implants had a complete radiolucent line at the tibial bone cement interface. The widths of the radiolucent zones were not thought to be progressive by the authors. Thin white lines were frequently seen around the cementless stems in Bertin's study. Of the 73 stems with radiopaque lines next to the stems, 18 were tightly approximated to the stem, 40 were parallel within a few millimeters of the implant, while six had divergent sclerotic lines. The authors believed that these lines did not imply loosening but needed to be followed longer to establish their significance as the follow-up in this study was extremely short.

Peters et al.[10] reviewed 57 revision total knee arthroplasties performed for aseptic failures. Eighteen tibial stems and 34 femoral stems were used in this group of revisions. Thirty-two of these stems were cemented and 20 were cementless. Adequate radiographs were available for only 39 of these 52 implants (75%). Unfortunately, while the Knee Society's Radiographic Scoring System was used to determine the location and size of radiolucent lines, implants were not categorized according to the Knee Society guidelines as stable, possibly loose requiring close follow-up, or loose. In Peters' series, radiolucent lines were more prevalent adjacent to press-fit femoral stems compared with cemented constructs (p < 0.02). There was no significant difference in the total number of radiolucent lines around cemented and cementless tibial stems in their series (p = 0.73).

Haas et al.[8] reviewed 65 patients who underwent revision total knee surgery for aseptic loosening. Each patient had cement used on the cut surfaces in the metaphyseal region of the femur and tibia along with a cementless fluted stem. Once again, while the Knee Society Radiographic Scoring System was used to determine location of radiolucent lines, implants were not categorized according to Knee Society guidelines as stable, possibly loose requiring close follow-up, or loose. Radiolucent lines at the bone cement interface were noted in 33% of the femoral implants and 64% of the tibial implants. Most were 1–2 mm and nonprogressive. Complete radiolucent lines at the bone cement interface were noted in 7% of the tibial components and 1% of the femoral components.

In the study by Haas et al., radiopaque lines about the stems were common, being seen in 67% of the femoral stems and 69% of the tibial stems. Complete radiopaque lines were seen about 34% of the femoral stems and 27% of the tibial stems. The average follow-up for this group of patients was only 3.5 years. The authors stated that there was no association between radiopaque lines and clinical knee scores at this time. They also stated that they did not understand the importance of these frequently occurring radiopaque lines but did not note an association with outcome at this time.

We have become concerned regarding the significance of these radio-opaque lines observed around cementless stems in our own revision practice. After revising a number of patients with cementless stem fixation (Figure 13-10), we sought to determine which type of stem fixation was superior in a large series of revision total knee arthroplasties.

We have reviewed our experience with metaphyseal engaging stems in revision total knee arthroplasty. Fortunately, we used a similar number of cemented and cementless stems, allowing a comparative measure of stem fixation.

Between 1986 and 2000, 475 revision total knee arthroplasties were performed in 419 patients. Of the 475 TKAs, 393 full-component revisions in 279 patients were performed using 484 stems. The remaining 82 revisions were performed without the use of stems. Of these 279 patients, 85 patients with 131 stems were deceased, re-revised within 2 years, or revised with diaphyseal engaging stems. Eighty-seven patients with 151 stems had less than 2-year follow-up. The final data set is 113 patients with 202 metaphyseal engaging stems implanted at the time of full component revision. Radiographic analysis was performed using the Knee Society Radiographic Scoring System. According to this system, implants were categorized as stable with insignificant radiolucencies, possibly loose needing close follow-up, or loose. Implants with cemented stems were compared with cementless stem fixation.

Of the 202 metaphyseal only engaging stems, 107 were cemented and 95 were cementless. The average follow-up was 57 months. Of the 107 implants with cemented stems, 100 (93%) were categorized as stable, 7 (7%) require close follow-up, and none were loose (Figure 13-11). Of the 95

FIGURE 13-10. Loose revision implant with cementless stem.

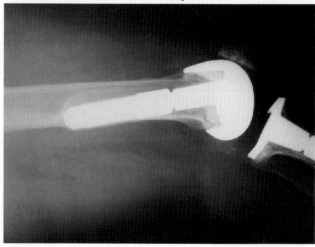

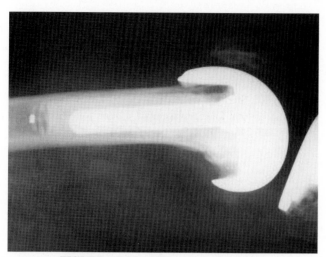

FIGURE 13-11. Stable cemented fixation.

implants placed with cementless stems, only 67 (71%) were categorized as stable, 18 (19%) required close follow-up, and 10 (10%) were loose (2 tibial and 8 femoral implants) (Figure 13-12). Components with cemented stems and components implanted with cementless stems were compared using a 3 by 2 χ^2 at the 0.05 level. Implants placed with cemented stems were significantly more radiographically stable than those

implanted with cementless stems, χ^2 (2) = 19.92. This difference was significant at the p = 0.0001 level.

We have shown that cemented metaphyseal engaging stems work well in the majority of revision total knees at midterm follow-up. We are also concerned about the radiographic appearance of implants placed with cementless stems at similar follow-up.

CONCLUSION

At this time, we would urge caution in using cementless metaphyseal engaging stems in revision knee arthroplasty. The biomechanical data favoring cemented constructs as well as the alignment problems that can ensue when using a cementless canal filling stem argue against the routine use of cementless stems. In addition, the midterm radiographic findings present here concerning cementless stems are disturbing. Although we have only re-revised four implants to date for aseptic loosening of a revision implant, we are concerned that each of these implants was initially revised with a cementless stem. This fact coupled with the radiographic findings described in our study prevents us from considering the use of cementless stems at this time. Until we determine if the early radiographic results presented here will lead to premature clinical failure, we cement all of our metaphyseal engaging stems when they are used in revision total knee surgery.

REFERENCES

1. Stern SH, Wills D, Gilbert JL. The effect of tibial stem design on component micromotion in knee arthroplasty. *Clin Orthop.* 1997;345:44–52.
2. Bourne RB, Finlay JB. The influence of tibial component intramedullary stems and implant-cortex contact on the strain distribution of the proximal tibia following total knee arthroplasty. *Clin Orthop.* 1986;208:95–99.
3. Brooks PJ, Walker PS, Scott RD. Tibial component fixation in deficient tibial bone stock. Clin Orthop. 1984;184:302–308.
4. Reilly D, Walker PS, Ben-Dov M, Ewald FC. Effects of tibial components on load transfer in the upper tibia. Clin Orthop. 1982;165:273–282.
5. Jazrawi LM, Bai B, Kummer FJ, Hiebert R, Stuchin SA. The effect of stem modularity and mode of fixation on tibial component stability in revision total knee arthroplasty. *J Arthroplasty.* 2001;16:759–767.
6. Bert JM, McShane M. Is it necessary to cement the tibial stem in cemented total knee arthroplasty? *Clin Orthop.* 1998;356:73–78.

FIGURE 13-12. Unstable cementless fixation.

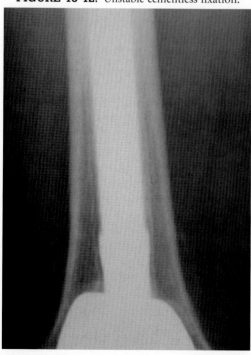

7. Hicks CA, Noble P, Tullos H. The anatomy of the tibial intramedullary canal. *Clin Orthop.* 1995;321:111–116.

8. Haas SB, Insall NJ, Montgomery W, Windsor RE. Revision total knee arthroplasty with use of modular components with stems inserted without cement. *J Bone Joint Surg.* 1995; 77A:1700–1707.

9. Murray PB, Rand JA, Hanssen AD. Cemented long-stem revision total knee arthroplasty. *Clin Orthop.* 1994;309: 116–123.

10. Peters CL, Hennessey R, Bade RM, Galante JO, Rosenberg AG. Revision total knee arthroplasty with a cemented posterior-stabilized or constrained condylar prosthesis. *J Arthroplasty.* 1997;12:895–903.

11. Bertin KC, Freeman MAR, Samuelson KM, Ratcliffe SS, Todd RC. Stemmed revision arthroplasty for aseptic loosening of total knee replacement. J Bone Joint Surg. 1985; 67B:242–248.

CHAPTER 14

Restoration of Stability, Maintaining Joint Line, Gap Balancing, and Constraint Selection

Brian McDermott

The most common aseptic cause of revision total knee arthroplasty is instability. The source of the instability can be straightforward or multifactorial. Instability can result from improper balancing of the flexion and extension spaces, malpositioning of the joint line, or imbalance of the soft tissue sleeve surrounding the knee. The reason for the instability must be identified for the revision to be successful.[1,2] The goals of revision total knee arthroplasty are the same as those of primary surgery, to restore the original anatomy of the knee, regain function, and provide stability.[3–7]

MAINTAINING THE JOINT LINE

A major goal of revision total knee arthroplasty is to restore *normal* knee kinematics. This can be accomplished by balancing soft tissues and the remaining bony anatomy of the knee. Reestablishing a correct joint line position is recognized as one of the most important factors in achieving normal ligament balance and normal knee kinematics.[8,9]

Joint line malposition can lead to various problems. In primary knee arthroplasty, using a posterior stabilized implant, elevating the joint line more than 8 mm was associated with an inferior clinical outcome.[10] Similarly, lowering the joint line has also been associated with poor results. Joint line elevation after revision total knee arthroplasty is a more frequent occurrence. Excessive elevation has been associated with worse clinical and functional outcomes. Every attempt should be undertaken to place the joint line in the correct anatomical position.

What Causes an Elevated Joint Line?

An elevated joint line occurs when bone is lost from the distal femur. The most common causes of distal femoral bone loss are aseptic loosening, osteolysis, and migration of the femoral component.[10] Other causes of distal femoral bone loss include excessive resection during primary knee arthroplasty or damage to bone during removal of components in revision surgery.

Historically, this loss of femoral bone would cause the prosthesis to be placed superiorly on the remaining good bone to achieve stability of the component. This would result in large polyethylene inserts being used, and an elevated joint line. Contemporary revision knee arthroplasty systems have addressed this issue by using augments. By using distal femoral augments, the joint line can be lowered, resulting in improved knee kinematics. Hoping to avoid the otherwise certain joint line elevation, some authors have actually advocated the use of distal femoral augments in all revision arthroplasties. Most revision surgeons also favor substitution of the posterior cruciate ligament (PCL) during revisions. If the ligament is maintained, there is less forgiveness for an elevated joint line. In PCL-retained knees the joint line needs to be within 3 mm of normal to restore proper knee kinematics. However, in PCL-sacrificed knees the joint line can be elevated up to 8 mm and not grossly affect kinematics.

Unfortunately, an elevated joint line cannot always be avoided. Some patients may have excessive scarring, bone loss, or flexion contractures. These problems can be difficult to handle and occasionally cannot be corrected by soft tissue release alone. If a choice has to be made between achieving full extension or an elevated joint line, full extension should prevail. Inability to achieve full extension would lead to quadriceps fatigue and gait abnormality.

How To Assess Proper Joint Line Position

Identifying the *anatomic* joint line in a revision situation is difficult. Multiple authors have reported on bony landmarks and their relationship to the joint line.[11] These include the medial femoral epicondyle, lateral femoral epicondyle, fibular head, and inferior pole of the patella. A properly placed joint line should be approximately 30 mm distal to the medial femoral epicondyle, 25 mm distal to the lateral epicondyle, and 10 to 15 mm proximal to the fibular head. These landmarks are easily palpable in revision knee replacements. In patients in whom there is scarring over the medial epicondylar sulcus, a metal ruler may be passed under the medial collateral ligament until it abuts onto the origin of the ligament. In the revision knee situation, referencing off of the patella (Insall-Salvati ratio) is not as accurate.[12] This may be secondary to lengthening of the patellar tendon. Contralateral knee radiographs can always obtained for additional confirmation of a patient's normal joint line location.

Complications from Malposition of the Joint Line

Joint line malposition after revision surgery is not uncommon. The more common error is joint line elevation. An elevated joint line has been associated with anterior knee pain, patella baja, and midflexion laxity. Although not as common, a lowered joint line can be equally disabling.

Anterior knee pain is a common consequence of joint line elevation. In an attempt to achieve stability of the revision knee, multiple soft tissue releases may be performed. While adequate soft tissue balance and limb alignment may be achieved, this may come at the cost of joint line elevation. As the patellar tendon is fixed in length, such a change in the axial position of the joint line of the prosthesis would change the function of the extensor mechanism. The increased tension in the extensor mechanism can lead to pain and loss of range of motion. A study by Figgie et al. showed that knees with a joint line elevation of less than 8 mm after knee replacement had better range of motion and no patellofemoral symptoms compared with those of more than 8 mm.[10]

Patella baja is a common complication of joint line elevation. A distalized patella can impinge against the lip of a tibial insert or post of a posterior-stabilized insert. Although a patient with patella baja is frequently asymptomatic, impingement can lead to increased wear, anterior knee pain, or patellar tendon attrition. Contemporary polyethylene inserts have an anterior *scalloping* to try to lessen the incidence of impingement.

Midflexion laxity is often the most disabling complication of an elevated joint line. As the name implies, the knee in a patient with midflexion laxity is stable in both full extension and 90 degrees of flexion. However, during early flexion the knee becomes unstable. This phenomenon is related to an imbalance between location of the

joint line and collateral ligament tension. Most commonly, it is a result of femoral bone loss either distally or posteriorly leading to a misplaced joint line. A tight posterior capsule causes overresection of the distal femur to allow full extension. This overresection elevates the joint line. The knee is stable in extension secondary to a tight posterior capsule; as the knee is flexed it becomes unstable due to relaxing of the posterior capsule and laxity in the collateral ligaments. The clinical significance of midrange laxity is relatively obvious when of sufficient magnitude, but when the malpositioning error is of a lesser degree, the clinical significance may not be clear until later. It is conceivable that midrange laxity leads to progressive stretching of secondary restraints and increased instability over time.[13] Midflexion laxity is avoided by releasing the posterior capsule if contracted, minimizing resection of the distal femur, and reapproximating the anatomic joint line.

FLEXION-EXTENSION GAP BALANCING

After component removal, the goal of revision total knee surgery is to create equal flexion and extension gaps. This usually is achieved with soft tissue releases to correct fixed angular deformities and assessment of the residual femoral and tibial bone, which will be the foundation for the subsequent reconstruction. Freeman,[14] Insall, and Ranawat were the first to recommend balancing the knee ligaments by restoring the flexion and extension gaps. They, along with others, designed condylar prosthetic components that relied on passive soft tissue tension, together with tibiofemoral congruency, to provide stability in both flexion and extension.[15]

Proper balancing of the flexion-extension gaps correlates with proper tensioning of the soft tissue sleeve surrounding the knee and maintenance of correct mechanical alignment. Unequal resection or loss of bone versus implant thickness leads to altered tension of the collateral ligaments and posterior capsular structures, if present. As the flexion-extension gaps will be affected by tension in the medial and lateral soft tissue constraints, ideally medial and lateral balance should be obtained with appropriate releases of contracted soft tissues, and then the flexion-extension gap sizes should be determined. Once the medial and lateral balance is obtained and the components are removed, spacer blocks are used to analyze the flexion-extension gaps. The use of spacer blocks allows assessment of medial-lateral symmetry of both gaps as well as the overall size of each gap. If there is excessive bone loss or irregularity of the bony surfaces, use of the spacer block may not be feasible. It is also important to decide if the bone loss will require augmentation to preserve equal flexion and extension gap dimensions.[16] Symmetric medial and lateral collateral ligament tension in both flexion and extension should be sought. Soft tissue balance in flexion and extension and medial-lateral are important components of a successful revision TKA.[17,18] If these balances cannot be achieved, a more constrained condylar prosthesis must be used.

There are some general rules that may be considered when balancing the flexion and extension gaps. First, the changes to the tibial platform affect both the flexion and extension gaps. Second, isolated extension gap problems can be addressed on the distal femur. For a tight extension gap, further resection of the distal femur can be performed. If the extension gap is loose, augmentation of the distal femur helps. Third, isolated flexion gap problems are handled with shifting the femoral component in the anterior or posterior direction or increasing the overall AP dimension of the component. Posterior augmentation on the condyles can also be performed.

Assessing the Flexion Gap

The flexion gap is often enlarged compared with the extension space during a revision TKA. The enlargement of the flexion space may be caused by malrotation of the primary femoral component, collateral ligament insufficiency, excessive bone loss, or an improperly sized femoral component. Excessive internal rotation of the primary femoral component leads to overresection of the posterior lateral femoral condyle. This causes a larger flexion gap laterally. Care must be taken to restore proper rotational alignment of the femoral component. This often requires the augmentation of the lateral posterior femoral condyle. The transepicondylar axis, if present, is the best landmark to help restore correct alignment. The new rotational axis should be parallel to the transepicondylar axis.

Collateral ligament insufficiency can cause flexion gap imbalance. The collateral ligaments are the primary check rein of the flexion gap. If these ligaments are insufficient, the flexion gap will be enlarged, since the posterior structures are loose in flexion. It is important to displace the extensor mechanism laterally when assessing the flexion gap. In a reduced position a contracture of the extensor mechanism will narrow the flexion gap even if collateral ligaments are lax. While this may provide medial-lateral stability in full flexion, early and midflexion laxity would be present.

Excessive bone loss and improperly sized femoral component are intertwined. Bone loss can result from removal of the components, a loose component on osteopenic bone, osteolysis, or bone resection during the primary surgery. This bone loss can result in inappropri-

ate undersizing of the femoral component. An undersized component results in a decreased anteroposterior dimension and an enlarged flexion space. This may result in the use of an oversized polyethylene component requiring excessive distal femoral resection to achieve full extension. Undue resection of distal femur results in an unacceptable proximal migration of the joint line.

When choosing the size of the femoral component that stabilizes the knee in flexion, ignore the residual bone. Try to visualize what the original anatomy of the distal femur would have been before surgery. This can be accomplished by using the size of the removed component or contralateral knee x-rays. If the original component was sized appropriately, a comparably sized femoral component should be reimplanted. On revision of knees that were unstable in flexion, use of a larger femoral component may be indicated. When revisions are performed for the knee that flexes poorly, a smaller femoral component may be helpful to decrease the tension in flexion and enhance motion. In those cases on extensive bone loss, liberal use of either metal or bone graft augmentation should be performed to restore the correct flexion gap.

Assessing the Extension Gap

Balancing the extension gap is often more straightforward. Once the femoral component position has been established to stabilize the flexion gap, the knee is brought to full extension. If the knee achieves full extension and is stable, the extension gap is balanced. If the knee achieves recurvatum, distal femoral augmentation should be considered. Caution should be taken not to make the joint line too far distally because this may adversely affect patellar tracking.

Failure to reach full extension may have many causes. In knees with a preoperative flexion contracture, inability to fully extend the knee is usually because of a contracted posterior capsule. Knees with good preoperative extension should not have a contracted posterior capsule, and further distal femoral resection may be required. Care must be taken not to resect too much bone and elevate the joint line inappropriately. Patients who have a large polyethylene insert used to stabilize the flexion gap and subsequent inability to achieve full extension may benefit from a femoral component change. A decision to increase the anteroposterior dimension of the femoral component and decrease the size of the tibial insert may stabilize the knee in flexion, allow the knee into extension, and maintain the joint line. With the use of an offset stem it is also possible to seat the femoral component more posteriorly, resulting in the need for less polyethylene. By downsizing the polyethylene size, distal femoral augmentation is more easily achieved. The result will be a better positioned

TABLE 14.1. Treatment of Gap Imbalance Possibilities.

	Extension Normal	*Extension Tight*	*Extension Loose*
Flexion Normal	Nothing	Resect distal femur Release posterior capsule	Distal femoral augmentaion
Flexion Tight	Resect posterior femur Shift femoral component anterior Downsize femoral component	Downsize polyethylene insert Resect proximal tibia	Downsize femoral component, augment distally Shift femoral component ant, and augment distally
Flexion Loose	Shift femoral component posterior Posterior augmentation	Resect distal femur Larger femoral component	Larger polyethylene insert

joint line, since most revision total knee arthroplasties result in distal femoral bone loss.

There are multiple gap imbalance possibilities. Each of these imbalances requires its own unique approach and protocol to correct the situation. These approaches have been described by many authors and are listed in Table 14.1.

Gap Mismatch

One situation that may arise while balancing the flexion and extension gaps is gap mismatch. This condition results when there is irreconcilable mismatch between a capacious flexion gap and a less accommodating extension gap. The enlargement of the flexion gap is secondary to soft tissue failure. Gap mismatch is important to identify in any revision. If unidentified, it is unlikely that the flexion and extension gaps could be balanced by conventional releases or component selection and positioning. The imbalance would lead to flexion instability and recurrent failure of the knee arthroplasty. When mismatch is identified appropriately, a constrained component is necessary to avoid instability. It is the surgeon's preference to use either a linked component or nonlinked constrained device with concurrent soft tissue repair.

CONSTRAINT SELECTION

Revision total knee arthroplasty is a complex undertaking that requires attention to detail to restore a functional joint. As stated earlier, the goals of revision surgery are the same as those of primary knee arthroplasty. As for the goal of stability, it is preferable to implant the prosthesis

with the least degree of constraint that offers a stable construct.[19–22]

The revision prosthesis selected by the surgeon should provide the degree of stability necessary to solve the anticipated stability challenges. A thorough preoperative clinical and radiological examination should be performed to help elicit any signs of instability to be encountered. This should be supplemented with an examination under anesthesia just before surgery to uncover any signs of instability masked in the office. The majority of revision total knees can be performed with a posterior stabilized implant. Posterior cruciate retaining knees are rarely useful in a revision setting and will not be discussed further. In those cases where stability is not achieved with a posterior stabilized implant, more constrained devices such as nonlinked constrained or rotating hinged designs must be used.

PROSTHETIC DESIGNS

Revision total knee prosthetic design is a balance between conformity and constraint, which relies on the simultaneous interaction of the supporting soft tissues and the contoured prosthetic surface. The prostheses have evolved from fully constrained to semiconstrained to contemporary constrained designs. The prosthetic features that contribute to stability include femoral-tibial congruence, posterior stabilized cam, extended and thickened post of non-inked constrained designs, and linking of the prosthesis. Newer modular revision knee systems also are equipped with augmentation and stem options. The more constrained the knee becomes, the higher the stress load on the bone-cement interface. Femoral and tibial stems should be added for stability as the components become more constrained or there are significant bony defects of the condyles. As the construct becomes more constrained, stems have been shown to function as oad-sharing devices.[23] Stems can be either press-fitted or cemented in place depending on the quality of the bone and the size of the stem used.

Posterior Stabilized

Posterior-stabilized implants, with their conforming articulation and spine and cam mechanism, provide adequate stability when the collateral ligaments are functional. The spine and cam mechanism offers enhancement of component stability in flexion. This is achieved by resisting posterior subluxation of the tibial component in flexion. Flexion and extension gaps need to be balanced appropriately for posterior-stabilized implants. Excessively large flexion gaps can allow posterior dislocation of the spine. Inability to balance the flexion and extension gaps requires the use of a constrained condylar prosthesis. Although the spine and cam mechanism acts as a mechanical posterior cruciate ligament, it provides no varus or valgus restraint. When using a posterior stabilized implant, the host soft tissues and any soft tissue repairs or reconstructions must be able to provide sufficient stability to the knee. Therefore, if there is insufficiency of either collateral ligament, a more constrained prosthesis should be used. As a rule, slight lateral ligamentous insufficiency is better tolerated than medial collateral ligament insufficiency. The benefit of modular revision implant systems is the ability to exchange posterior-stabilized and constrained condylar polyethylene inserts on the same tibial base plate. Multiple studies have shown good results of revision total knee arthroplasty with a posterior-stabilized implant.[24–28]

Constrained Designs

The following sections address prosthetic options when posterior stabilized components are not sufficient to provide a stable construct. These situations typically include settings of deficient collateral ligament support and result in intrinsic varus-valgus instability or flexion gap laxity that is too large to be accommodated by a posterior-stabilized prosthesis. Inappropriate use of constrained prostheses includes failure to perform necessary soft tissue releases to correct deformity that was left uncorrected at the time of the original arthroplasty that failed. In addition, it is inappropriate to select constrained devices when the instability results from pseudolaxity of collateral ligaments caused by deficient bone. In many revision knees, stability is restored when the soft tissues are balanced and the bone stock has been restored, thus

allowing use of a less constrained prosthesis. Once the decision has been made that a posterior-stabilized prosthesis is not sufficient to stabilize the knee, the surgeon must choose between a nonlinked constrained and a rotation hinge design. There are advantages and disadvantages to both designs.

Nonlinked Constrained Nonlinked constrained prostheses are selected in cases of collateral ligament insufficiency or flexion-extension gap mismatch. These prostheses have a taller and thicker polyethylene intercondylar post. This post imparts stability by limiting rotation, medial-lateral translation, and varus-valgus angulation of the knee articulation. As a result of the increased constraint, stems should be used for supplemental fixation due to increased forces across the bone-cement interface. Advantages of this design over rotating hinge designs include a changing center of rotation during flexion, thereby theoretically imparting less tangential anterior-posterior stress across the prosthetic interface.[29] In addition, because they are not linked they allow the soft tissue sleeve, rather than prosthetic interfaces, to absorb hyperextension forces. In cases of insufficient soft tissues to prevent hyperextension, such as muscular weakness, deficient posterior capsule, massive bone loss, or segmental resection, a hinged device with a hyperextension stop should be used. A disadvantage of nonlinked constrained designs compared with rotating hinge designs is they are more rotationally constrained and theoretically impart greater rotational stress to the bone-cement interface.

Keys to achieving good long-term results with nonlinked constrained knees include proper alignment and maintaining a sufficient soft tissue sleeve. In regard to alignment, both rotational and coronal alignment need to be critically evaluated before final implantation. A valgus mechanical axis in a patient with residual medial collateral ligament insufficiency or a varus mechanical axis in a patient with lateral collateral ligament insufficiency can be problematic. Also, because there is a limited amount of rotation allowed in the design, proper rotational alignment must be achieved.

In those patients with soft tissue instability so extreme that a nonlinked constrained design is insufficient to provide stability, the surgeon can either perform a soft tissue reconstruction with a nonlinked constrained design or use a rotating hinge design. If a soft tissue repair is to be performed, a constrained design should be used to protect the repair. However, failure of the nonlinked constrained design has been observed when there is total deficiency of the medial collateral ligament or when severe malalignment of the limb exists.[30,31] These failures have included breakage of the enlarged post.

TABLE 14.2. Results of Nonlinked Constrained Prosthesis in Revision Total Knee Arthroplasty.

Author	No. of Knees	Follow-up (yrs)	Rate of Excellent/Good (%)
Kim[32]	14	6.3	93
Rand[33]	21	4	50
Rosenberg et al.[34]	36	3.8	69

Results of the nonlinked constrained design have been encouraging. To date there have been no prospective randomized studies comparing nonlinked constrained with rotating hinge designs. However, there are multiple studies reporting the short- to midterm results of the use of nonlinked constrained prosthesis. The results of their use in revision-only situations are listed in Table 14.2. Most patients at mean follow-up of at least 4 years show excellent or good outcomes. There is concern that with the increased constraint there will be an increased rate of failure long term. Studies by Font-Rodrigues[35] and Trousdale[36] have revealed the opposite. Trousdale showed an 80% survivorship at 15 years, while Font-Rodriguez at 7 years reports a 98% cumulative survivorship.

Rotating Hinge Constrained Rotating hinge constrained designs are used in extreme cases to obtain stability. The reason for their use in revision knee arthroplasty can include absence of the medial collateral ligament, global instability, periprosthetic fracture, or severe bone loss. As with all revision knee arthroplasties, in order to achieve the best results, appropriate release of soft tissue contractures and assessment of the remaining bone stock must be performed. With the appropriate soft tissue and bone preparation, as well as the continuing improvement of modular revision knee systems, the use of rotating hinge prostheses has become rare.

Historically the use of hinged prostheses was associated with suboptimal outcomes. Early designs, such as the Shiers, Walldius, and Guepar were used routinely, even for primary arthroplasty.[37,38] These designs were easy to implant, since at the time of surgery all the ligaments were resected and the stems dictated the alignment. Unfortunately, long-term results were not as enticing as their ease of use. The early hinged prosthesis did not allow any axial rotation, thereby resulting in high rates of aseptic loosening. Other pitfalls were poor extension mechanism stability, high infection rates, and large amounts of bone loss due to the bulky size of the prosthesis.[39–42]

The development of the rotating hinge design corrected a lot of the early flaws. In addition to allowing rotational movement, these newer generation implants also improved extensor mechanism articulation, modular augments and stems, and tibial base plates. These design improvements have resulted in better short-term results.[43,44] However, there have been few studies reporting long-term success with these implants. Also, failure of a rotating hinged prosthesis leaves few reconstructive options. The large amount of bone resection necessary for implantation makes arthrodesis extremely difficult as a salvage operation. Reimplantation of a modular tumor prosthesis, allograft-prosthesis composite, and above-the-knee amputation become the remaining options. The unknown long-term results and poor salvage options are the reasons these prostheses should be used only in the elderly low-demand patient with a limited life expectancy or in the indications listed previously.

In summary, the prosthesis options for revision knee arthroplasty are vast. The final decision by the surgeon cannot be made until full evaluation of the remaining soft tissues and bone stock is performed intraoperatively. While improvements in constrained designs have been made, the least constrained design that offers adequate stability should be chosen. The development of modular revision knee systems has made this goal more easily attainable.

REFERENCES

1. Callaghan JJ, O'rourke MR, Saleh KJ. Why knees fail: lessons learned. *J Arthroplasty.* 2004;19(4 Suppl 1):31–34.
2. Windsor RE, Scuderi GR, Moran MC, et al. Mechanisms of failure of the femoral and tibial components in total knee arthroplasty. *Clin Orthop.* 1989;248:15–20.
3. Engh GA, Rorabeck CH. *Revision Total Knee Arthroplasty.* Philadelphia: Williams & Wilkins; 1997.
4. Bourne RB, Crawford HA. Principles of revision total knee arthroplasty. *Orthop Clin North Am.* 1998;29(2):331–337.
5. Dennis DA. Revision knee arthroplasty: how I do it. In: Insall JN, Scott WN, eds. *Surgery of the Knee.* Vol 2. 3rd ed. New York: Churchill Livingstone; 2001:1934–1941.
6. Dorr LD. Revision knee arthroplasty: how I do it. In: Insall JN, Scott WN, eds. *Surgery of the Knee.* Vol 2. 3rd ed. New York: Churchill Livingstone; 2001:1925–1933.
7. Sanchez F, Engh GA. Revision knee arthroplasty: how I do it. In: Insall JN, Scott WN, eds. *Surgery of the Knee.* Vol 2. 3rd ed. New York: Churchill Livingstone; 2001:1942–1967.
8. Yoshii I, Whiteside LA, White SE, Milliano MT. Influence of prosthetic joint line position on knee kinematics and patellar position. *J Arthroplasty.* 1991;6(2):171–177.

9. Lotke PA, Echer ML. Influence of positioning of prosthesis in total knee replacement. *J Bone Joint Surg Am.* 1977; 59A:77.

10. Figgie HE, Goldberg VM, Heiple KG, et al. The influence of tibial-patellofemoral location on function of the knee in patients with the posterior stabilized condylar knee prosthesis. *J Bone Joint Surg Am.* 1986;68A(7):1035–1040.

11. Stiehl JB, Abbott BD. Morphology of the transepicondylar axis and its application in primary and revision total knee arthroplasty. *J Arthroplasty.* 1995;10:785.

12. Laskin RS. Joint line position restoration during revision total knee replacement. *Clin Orthop.* 2002;404:169–171.

13. Martin JW, Whiteside LA. The influence of joint line position on knee stability after condylar knee arthroplasty. *Clin Orthop.* 1990;259:146–156.

14. Freeman MAR, Insall J, Besser W, et al. Excision of the cruciate ligaments in total knee replacement. *Clin Orthop.* 1977;126:209.

15. Krackow KA, Mihalko WM. The effects of severe femoral bone loss on the flexion extension joint space in revision total knee arthroplasty: a cadaveric analysis and clinical consequences. *Orthopedics.* 2001;24(2):121–126.

16. Stulberg SD. Revision total knee arthroplasty: Managing bone loss with augmentation. *Orthopedics.* 1997;20(9): 845–848.

17. Whiteside LA. Soft tissue balancing. the knee. *J Arthroplasty* 2002;17(4):23–27.

18. Ries MD, Haas SB, Windsor RE. Soft-tissue balance in revision total knee arthroplasty. *J Bone Joint Surg.* 2003; 85-A(Suppl 1):38–42.

19. Scuderi GR. Revision total knee arthroplasty. how much constraint is enough? Clin Orthop. 2001;392:300–305.

20. Bugbee WD, Ammeen DJ, Engh GA. Does implant selection affect outcome of revision knee arthroplasty? *J Arthroplasty.* 2001;16(5):581–585.

21. Hartford JM, Goodman SB, Schurman DJ, Knoblick G. Complex primary and revision total knee arthroplasty using the condylar constrained prosthesis. *J Arthroplasty.* 1998;13(4):380–387.

22. Cuckler JM. Revision total knee arthroplasty: how much constraint is necessary? *Orthopedics.* 1995;18(9):932–936.

23. Brooks PJ, Walker PS, Scott RD. Tibial component fixation in deficient tibial bone stock. *Clin Orthop.* 1984;184: 302.

24. Takahashi Y, Gustilo RB. Nonconstrained implants in revision total knee arthroplasty. *Clin Orthop.* 1994;309: 156–162.

25. Rand JA, Bryan RS. Results of revision total knee arthroplasties using condylar prosthesis. a review of 50 cases. *J Bone Joint Surg.* 1988;70A:738–745.

26. Rosenberg AG, Verner JJ, Galante JO. Clinical results of total condylar III prosthesis. *Clin Orthop.* 1991;273:83–90.

27. Haas SB, Insall JN, Montgomery W, Windsor RE. Revision total knee arthroplasty with use of modular components with stems inserted without cement. *J Bone Joint Surg.* 1995; 77A:1700–1707.

28. Murray PB, Rand JA, Hanssen AD. Cemented long-stem revision total knee arthroplasty. *Clin Orthop.* 1994;309: 116–123.

29. Nelson CL, Gioe TJ, Cheng EY, Thompson RC. Implant selection in revision total knee arthroplasty. *J Bone Joint Surg.* 2003;85A(Suppl 1):43–51.

30. McPherson EJ, Vince KG. Breakage of a total condylar III knee prosthesis. a case report. *J Arthroplasty.* 1993;8: 561–563.

31. Hohl WM, Crawford E, Zelicof SB, et al. The Total Condylar III prosthesis in complex reconstruction. *Clin Orthop.* 1991;273:91–97.

32. Kim YH. Salvage of a failed hinge knee arthroplasty with a Total Condylar III type prosthesis. *Clin Orthop.* 1987;221: 272–277.

33. Rand JA. Revision total knee arthroplasty using the Total Condylar III prosthesis. *J Arthoplasty.* 1991;6:279–284.

34. Rosenberg AG, Verner JJ, Galante JO. Clinical results of total knee revision using the Total Condylar III prosthesis. *Clin Orthop.* 1991;273:83–90.

35. Font-Rodriquez DE, Scuderi GR, Insall JN. Survivorship of cemented total knee arthroplasty. *Clin Orthop.* 1997;345: 79–86.

36. Trousdale RT, Beckenbaugh JP, Pagnano MW. 15-year results of the Total Condylar III implant in revision total knee arthroplasty. Proceedings of the 68th Annual Meeting of the American Academy of Orthopaedic Surgeons. San Francisco, 2001; 585.

37. Shiers LP. Arthroplasty of the knee. *J Bone Joint Surg Br.* 1954;36:553–560.

38. Walldius B. Arthroplasty of the knee using an endoprosthesis. 8 years' experience. *Acta Orthop Scand.* 1960;30: 137–148.

39. Hui FC, Fitzgerald Jr RH. Hinged knee arthroplasty. *J Bone Joint Surg.* 1980;62A:513–519.

40. Jones EC, Insall JN, Inglis AE, et al. GUEPAR knee arthroplasty results and late complications. *Clin Orthop.* 1979;140: 145–152.

41. Jones GB. Arthroplasty of the knee by the Walldius prosthesis. *J Bone Joint Surg.* 1968;50B:505–510.

42. Bain AM. Replacement of the knee joint with the Walldius prosthesis using cement fixation. *Clin Orthop.* 1973;94: 65–71.

43. Jones RE, Barrack RL, Skedros J. Modular, mobile-bearing hinge total knee arthroplasty. *Clin Orthop.* 2001;392:306–314.

44. Westrich GH, Mollano AV, Sculco TP, Buly RL, Laskin RS, Windsor R. Rotating hinge total knee arthroplasty in severely affected knees. *Clin Orthop.* 2000;379:195–208.

CHAPTER 15

Management of the Extensor Mechanism During Revision Total Knee Arthroplasty

Richard S. Laskin and Burak Beksaç

Management of the extensor mechanism is one of the most difficult aspects of performing a good revision knee replacement. Problems with exposure, patellar tracking, removal of prior implants, avascular necrosis, fracture, and soft tissue deficits all can complicate the surgery. Even in the best of situations, extensor mechanism problems can jeopardize the outcome of the revision. Socrates, over 2300 years ago, believed that one of the best instructional methods was a series of questions that would then provoke thoughtful answers. This chapter is organized as a series of the questions that arise for the revision surgery and attempts to provide some answers and an algorithm for management of the extensor mechanism.

HOW CAN ONE EXPOSE THE KNEE EASILY WITHOUT DAMAGING THE EXTENSOR MECHANISM?

Nowhere is there a revision knee surgeon who at least once in his or her career has not wished that developmental anatomy had progressed in a different manner so that there was not a patella and quadriceps and patellar tendons "obstructing the view" during surgery. Having said that, however, the extensor mechanism does exist and does often obstruct the view of the revision. There should be, therefore, a stepwise method of managing the extensor mechanism so as not to damage it, but yet allow adequate exposure of the femur and tibia. What follows is the authors' personal algorithm.

The capsular exposure must be adequate. For almost all knees this means a median parapatellar arthrotomy extending for at least 4 to 5 cm proximal to the patella. Although there are clear indications and devotees of other incisions in primary knee replacement, such as the sub-

vastus, the midvastus, and the lateral parapatellar incision, these exposures are usually markedly inadequate in the revision setting.

After performing the medial parapatellar arthrotomy, the knee should be flexed maximally. At that point the surgeon should elevate the soft tissues from the medial tibial plateau and medial tibial metaphysis. On the medial side, this elevation progresses to beyond the widest extent of the tibial plateau and then slightly posterior to it. Initially it is easiest to begin the elevation with a diathermy scalpel and then continue medially and posteromedially using a curved periosteal elevator. While these soft tissues are being elevated, the surgical assistant should progressively externally rotate the knee. External rotation displaces the tibial tubercle laterally and decreases the tension that will be placed on it when the patella is eventually displaced laterally or everted.

Next, a Hohmann's retractor is placed around the lateral femoral condyle and the patella is gently displaced laterally. This places any scarring and adhesions in the lateral gutter on stretch, and at this point these adhesions can be released with a diathermy scalpel. These adhesions are intra-articular and therefore releasing them is not equivalent to performing a lateral parapatellar capsular release.

With the Hohmann's retractor still exerting lateral pressure on the patella, the surgeon should release any scarring from behind the patellar ligament and the lateral tibial plateau. Since direct visualization is often difficult in this area, a curved periosteal elevator is a safer tool to use than is a diathermy scalpel. If the tibial component is modular, exposure can be facilitated by removing the polyethylene insert at this point.

The patellar tendon should then be stabilized. Normally, the authors place a smooth Steinman pin through the center of the patellar ligament into the tibial tubercle.

152

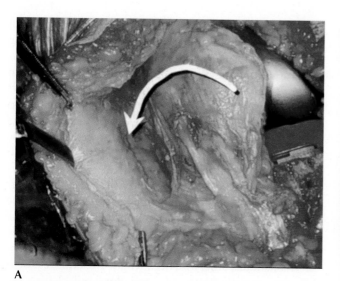

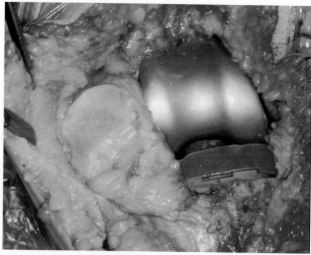

A   B

FIGURE 15-1. In obese patients a fascial pouch can be created (A) into which the patella is everted (B).

Should the patellar ligament begin to avulse when the patella is everted, the pin will act as a stress reliever and prevent complete avulsion. Other choices for stabilization include a surgical staple or a towel clip.

An erroneous idea is that the patella has to be completely everted to adequately visualize the femur and tibia. Actually, at times all that is necessary is lateral displacement of the bone, and indeed that technique is currently used when performing both revisions and minimally invasive primary knee replacements. Eversion places further stress on the patellar tendon, although it does increase the visualization somewhat as compared with displacement laterally.

At this stage the knee should be brought to a position of 45 degrees of flexion, and, with the knee in external rotation, the patella should be displaced laterally, or an attempt made to evert it.

In the obese patients with a thick subcutaneous adipose layer adjacent to the patella, it may be difficult, despite these surgical techniques, to displace or evert the patella. Whiteside[1] has suggested the creation of a subcutaneous pouch in these obese patients, into which the patella can be everted (Figure 15-1A, B). The pouch is developed by sharply dissecting in the subfascial layer under the adipose tissue. This layer is easily visible as a white glistening membrane and is easily discernible from the overlying yellow fatty layer. Dissecting in this tissue plane preserves the blood supply to the adipose layer and helps avoid potential vascular compromise to the overlying fat and skin. Eversion or displacement of the patella into the pouch causes less tension on the patellar ligament than would similar eversion over the thick skin and fat layer.

If the patella still cannot be displaced laterally or everted without undue tension on the patellar ligament, there are several possible solutions. Procedures may be performed either proximally or distally.

Proximal Releases

Coonse and Adams,[2] in 1943, described release of the quadriceps mechanism. In their technique, a V-incision is made in the extensor mechanism with its base at the level of the joint line and its apex at the junction of the tendinous and muscular junction of the rectus femoris (Figure 15-2). The distal portions of the rectus femoris tendon and patella are then *turned down* distally. Both the medial and lateral superior genicular arteries are sacrificed with this approach, and vascular compromise of the flap is a potential risk. Rarely is this type of release required for patellar exposure in the revision knee; however, in the knee that has undergone multiple operations, this release can give wide exposure, especially of the femur and patella.

Trousdale et al.[3] and Scott and Siliski[4] have described the results of using a modification of the Coonse-Adams approach. In this approach, often referred to as the V-Y incision, the lateral arm extends only for a short distance distally, preserving the lateral superior genicular artery (Figure 15-3). This allows mobilization of the patella in almost all cases and has the added advantage of permitting medial displacement of the patella and distal extensor mechanism at the time of closure to enhance patellar tracking. Postoperatively, aggressive motion exercises must be delayed to prevent disruption of the lengthened quadriceps apparatus from occurring.

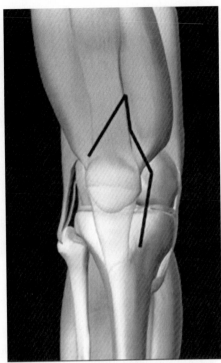

FIGURE 15-2. Coonse and Adams described an approach consisting of an inverted V incision in the quadriceps. The distal portion of the rectus and the patella are then turned down distally.

FIGURE 15-3. In the modified Coonse-Adams approach, the lateral limb does not come down to the joint line. This preserves the lateral superior genicular artery and aids in the viability of the flap.

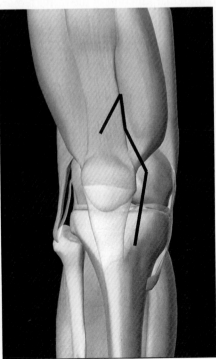

Insall[5,6] described the rectus snip procedure in which a short proximal lateral oblique incision is made, joining the medial capsular incision at the level of the musculotendinous junction of the rectus femoris (Figure 15-4). In this manner the rectus femoris tendon is severed, and this decompresses the extensor mechanism sufficiently to allow the patella to be everted without tension on the patellar ligament. If necessary, this procedure may be combined with a lateral release distally if necessary to enhance patellar tracking.

At the close of the procedure, the medial capsular incision is closed with interrupted sutures and the knee flexed to see the tension (if any) on the rectus snip. The rectus snip is then closed with several nonabsorbable interrupted mattress sutures. Unless the quadriceps mechanism has otherwise been lengthened, this release is for exposure purposes only, and does not change the normal postoperative physical therapy protocol as related to motion exercises or walking.

Distal Releases

Osteotomy of the proximal tibia decompresses the extensor mechanism and allows lateral patellar displacement. Although there have been descriptions of osteotomizing only a small fragment of the tibial tubercle,[7] this procedure is not recommended because of the potential of avulsion of the small bone fragment occurring in the postoperative period.

FIGURE 15-4. In the rectus snip approach, there is an upper lateral extension of the median parapatellar capsular incision.

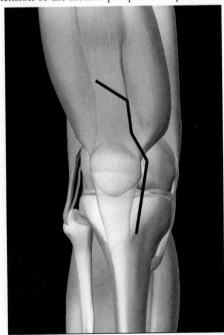

Whiteside[8] and Barrack et al.[9] have described an osteotomy of the crest of the tibia in which the crest is cut medially and then hinged laterally so as to retain the attachment of the lateral crural musculature to the fragment (Figure 15-5). With further soft tissue release in the anterolateral area of the tibia at the joint level, the extensor mechanism can easily be displaced laterally, giving extensive exposure of the knee joint.

At the completion of the surgery the fragment is reattached using either 3 wires or several screws (Figure 15-6). The authors prefer the wire technique with the individual wires inserted from proximal laterally to medial distally in the manner described by Whiteside and Rorabeck. With wire fixation, the patients are allowed to begin early motion of the knee in a manner analogous to that used for primary total knee replacement.

Ries[10] has described a modification of this osteotomy in which the fragment is tapered or thinned distally to avoid the potential stress riser distally. He prefers to reattach the fragment using screws that are aimed so as to avoid contacting any intramedullary stem on the tibial component. He likewise feels that this fixation will enable rapid early motion of the knee.

It has been suggested that a routine lateral retinacular release be performed in all total knee revisions so as to allow easy displacement and eversion of the patella. A routine lateral retinacular release in the face of a medial arthrotomy can cause severe impairment of blood flow to the remaining patellar remnant, already often somewhat avascular from the prior knee replacement.[11] Furthermore, the result of such an extensive lateral release is that the extensor mechanism is a large flap with a good soft

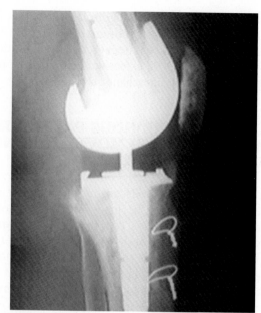

FIGURE 15-6. The tibial crest osteotomy is fixed back in position using stainless steel wires.

tissue attachment proximally, and a somewhat tenuous patellar tendon attachment distally (Figure 15-7).

The quadriceps snip and the tibial tubercle osteotomy are not mutually exclusive. If, after performing a quadri-

FIGURE 15-7. An extensive lateral release when combined with a median parapatellar approach results in a large bipedicle flap of tissue with a tenuous blood supply.

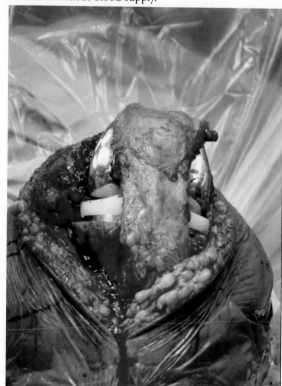

FIGURE 15-5. In the tibial crest osteotomy a fragment of bone that is laterally based and encompasses the tibial tubercle and the patellar tendon attachment is removed from the tibia. The fragment should be approximately 8 cm long and tapered distally. A small ledge is left proximally to help with stability after surgery.

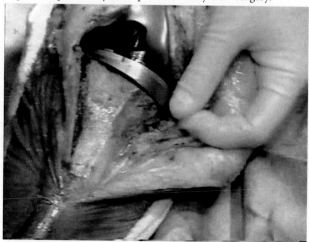

ceps snip, the authors still cannot displace the patella they will then progress on to a tibial tubercle osteotomy. This double exposure method has been used in several patients with severe infection with extensive scarring at the time of the second stage of an exchange revision.

SHOULD THE PREVIOUS PATELLAR COMPONENT BE REMOVED DURING REVISION SURGERY?

Once the patella has been adequately exposed and everted, a decision must be made whether or not to remove the previous implant. Twenty years ago, this question would have been moot. It was thought at that time that during a revision all the components had to be revised to prevent "further complications." At present, this is the regimen for septic cases; however, it is not so in the nonseptic situation. Greenwald[12] has shown that since the forces normally generated at the prosthetic patellofemoral joint are greater than the yield strength of polyethylene, there is always some wear or deformation of all patellar implants. Does that mean that all patellar implants should be revised?

Rosenberg et al.[13] have described 5 radiographic features associated with a loose patellar component. These include bone cement radiolucency, increased bone density in the patella, trabecular collapse of the bone, patellar fracture and/or fragmentation, and lateral subluxation of the residual patellar bone. Interestingly enough, all these findings were increased in patients who had undergone a prior lateral release.

In nonseptic situations in which the indication for revision was femoral or tibial component (loosening or wear) or the soft tissues (instability or contracture), the authors specifically evaluate the patellar component as to wear and fixation. To do this one must first remove the patellar meniscus.

Cameron and Cameron[14] and Laskin[15] have reported on the almost universal development of a patellar meniscus of fibrous tissue that surrounds the patellar implant within several months of the index surgery. This meniscus is avascular and aneural. At the time of revision only a small central portion of the patellar polyethylene may be visible. For this reason the entire meniscus must be removed out to and including the patellar rim to properly evaluate the implant and the underlying bone.

Most patellar components presently in use are symmetrical domes, and as such are compatible with the trochlear flange of many femoral components, both primary and revision. If this is the case, and if there are no large erosions or gouges in the polyethylene surface, the surgeon may elect to retain the patellar implant at the time of revision, *if* it is not loose from the patella. To ascertain this, one should grip the periphery of the implant with a small towel clip and gently attempt to move the implant. If there is no pistoning, the implant can be considered not to be loose.

Many metal-backed patellar components have been shown to have a high rate of failure. Bailey and Scott[16] and Lombardi et al.[17] reported a high incidence of wear-through of the polyethylene, especially in those metal-backed components in which there was a metallic endoskeleton and thin overlying polyethylene. Laskin and Bucknell[18] reported that the Tricon-M metal-backed patellar implant with a thick polyethylene and without a metallic endoskeleton demonstrated good function at 5 to 7 years after surgery; however, by 8 to 10 years these results have deteriorated as well. It is for these reasons that the authors believe that if there is a metal-backed patellar implant *in situ*, it should be removed at the time of revision, even in the absence of gross wear or loosening.

In the worst case scenario, the polyethylene is worn down to the metal base plate, with metal-on-metal abrasion between the base plate and the femoral component. The resultant metal debris stains the synovium adjacent to the prosthesis. Extreme metal wear may result in metal deposits in the suprapatellar bursa and posteriorly in the popliteal bursa. An attempt should be made to remove as completely as possible the metal-encrusted synovium. This must usually be performed by sharp dissection with avoidance of use of cutting cautery.

If the implant used in the index surgery was anatomical in shape, it will not normally fit the revision femoral flange. In such cases the prior implant should be removed even in the absence of gross wear or loosening.

WHAT IS THE SAFEST WAY TO REMOVE THE PATELLA COMPONENT?

The primary indications for removal of an all polyethylene patellar component are loosening and gross wear. A relative indication is the presence of a metal-backed patellar component, whether or not it is loose. The patella should be initially stabilized with 2 towel clips. In most cases, removal of an all-polyethylene implant requires separating it from its cement base and fixation pegs with a short oscillating saw or osteotome. The pegs may then be drilled out using a high-speed bur, and the remaining cement then removed with a rongeur. It is important to attempt to preserve as much residual patellar bone as possible for the revision. As an alternative, the surgeon can cut the implant into pie-shaped sections with a high-speed bur, such as the Midas Rex, and extract each section individually. When the polyethylene is sectioned, it is important to cover the remainder of the knee so that the debris from the bur (which is considerable) is not transplanted throughout the knee joint. If an osteotome is used, the instrument should be directed from a proximal and lateral position. Inserting and impacting it from the distal portion of the patella may cause sudden tension on the patellar ligament and lead to its avulsion.

Removal of a metal-backed, porous ingrowth type of implant is somewhat more difficult. Initially, the surgeon should remove the polyethylene first as described previously, and then use a metal cutting bur on the Midas Rex to section the base plate. A system of stacking osteotomes under the base plate axially extracts it from the bone.

HOW CAN ONE ASSURE THAT THE PATELLA IS PROPERLY PLACED IN RELATIONSHIP TO THE JOINT LINE SO AS TO AVOID A PATELLA BAJA?

Proper joint placement during revision surgery is important not only in balancing the capsular sleeve, but also in allowing the patella to track without inferior impinge-

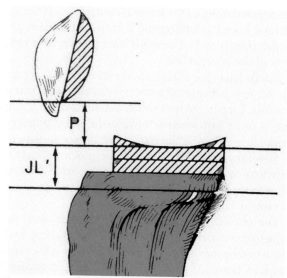

FIGURE 15-9. The patellar height (P) (as described by Figgie) is measured from the inferior pole of the patella to the superior surface of the tibial polyethylene. It should be more than 10 mm lest patellar impingement occur. *JL = joint line.*

FIGURE 15-8. Patella baja with impingement of the patella with the tibial polyethylene occurred due to a raising of the joint line.

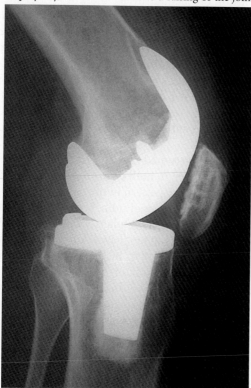

ment or proximal subluxation. A raised joint line can lead to patella baja with impingement of the patella and/or its implant on the tibial polyethylene (Figure 15-8). The clinical outcome can be anterior knee pain, diminished flexion, and polyethylene wear.[19–22]

It has been shown that when radiographs of revision knee replacements are evaluated, a patella baja was demonstrated in 80% of patients, and in cases in which this was more than 8 mm, there was a decrease in the Knee Society Scores.[23] Figgie and his coworkers[24] have demonstrated similar findings and described a patellar height, which they measured from the inferior portion of the patellar implant to the top of the tibial polyethylene. Optimally it should be no lower than 10 mm and more in the range of 10 to 30 mm (Figure 15-9). This measurement should be made with the knee in partial flexion to tense the extensor mechanism.

In primary total knee replacement, the surgical technique to properly place the patella height is fairly simple: An amount of femoral distal bone equal in thickness to that of the femoral component being used is removed. This replaces the femoral component, and by necessity the tibial component, in proper position. In the revision situation it is rarely so easy, since the level of the *normal* distal femur may be obscured by femoral component subsidence or osteolysis. One solution is to use the contralateral knee for guidance. The preoperative radiographic distance between the medial epicondyle and the transfemoral line can be measured, corrected for magnification, and then used at surgery to determine the proper positioning of the femoral component. If the contralateral knee has undergone a knee replacement, then this determination can be made on a preoperative radiograph of the affected knee.

Patella baja (See Figure 15-8) can occur during revision surgery because of uncompensated distal femoral bone loss. Even in the best situations, some distal femoral bone is often lost when removing the prior prosthesis. Often, after trimming the remaining surface to flatten it, the femoral component comes to lie much more proximally than is normal; with filling of the extension space with a thick enough polyethylene to achieve stability, the joint line is raised.

The obvious solution is to add distal femoral augments to the underside of the femoral component to *distalize* it and restore joint line position. Where is the proper joint line, however? A rough guide is that it should be 25 mm distal to the medial epicondyle. When the patellar implant is inserted, its inferior pole of the bone should lay at least one fingerbreadth proximal to the tibial polyethylene surface.

In some revision situations a patella baja already exists. This can occur if there was an erroneous raising of the joint line during the index surgery, or from scarring behind the patellar ligament after primary TKR or previous high tibial osteotomy. Possible remedies at surgery include those described previously, as well as placing the patellar implant somewhat proximal on the patellar bone, resecting the distal pole, or nose, of the patella, and finally *proximalizing* the tibial tubercle. Whiteside has described this last procedure with the possibility of obtaining approximately 10 mm of proximal displacement of the extensor mechanism. The problem of fixation of the tibial tubercle fragment in its proximal position and the risk of its avulsion during the postoperative period do exist, however.

HOW SHOULD THE PATELLAR REMNANT BE ADDRESSED AFTER REMOVAL OF THE PRIOR PATELLAR COMPONENT?

After removal of the previous patellar implant one is often left with a thin avascular patellar remnant, one or more holes from which the previous implant pegs resided, and possibly areas of osteolysis. As for defects found in the femur and tibia during revision surgery, there are several possible surgical techniques that can be used during reimplantation.

If there is a rim with a central defect—as is usually the case—the authors have used a biconvex implant for the reconstruction. The patella is grasped with a reaming clamp, which provides peripheral stability for the bone.

The center of the bone is then gently reamed using a biconvex reamer to remove any remaining fibrous tissues and a 1 to 2 mm layer of underlying bone. A biconvex inlay implant is then used to fill the cavity.

The obvious major concern is the potential for fracture of the patella, and whether the preparation of the patellar bone, especially in the revision situation, affects the strength of the bone and the potential for fracture?

Gomes et al.[25] studied patellar strength using both conventional onset and inset techniques of implant insertion. For their studies they used 10 cadavers, studying both patellae from each cadaver.

In one patella from each cadaver they used a planer reamer to obtain a flat surface. In the other patella they used a convex reamer. In both cases the thickness of the patella remaining was such that the combined thickness of the resultant bone and implant would equal that of the patella before preparation. The cemented implants used were the Genesis Biconvex and the Genesis Three-Pegged Flat prostheses (Smith & Nephew, Memphis, TN). Ten cadavers were examined. Each patellar sample was tested in a 3-point bending mode, the end point being fracture of the bone.

Their testing demonstrated that the 3-point bending strength (as measured in Newton-centimeters) of those patellae that were reamed flat (as for preparation of an onset patellar implant) was statistically equal to the contralateral intact control patella. Subsequent cementing of a flat button on the flat surface did not further increase, nor decrease, the bending strength over the intact patella.

The 3-point bending strength of those patellae that were reamed (as for preparation of an inlay patellar implant) was statistically diminished as compared with the contralateral intact control patella. However, when they then cemented an inlay biconvex patellar implant in the bone, there was a statistically significant increase in the bending strength by more than 50% over that of the intact patella.

It was likewise noted that the fracture patterns that were eventually seen in both types of patellar preparation differed. The fracture pattern in the patellae with an inlay biconvex implant was longitudinal, while that in the flat cut patella with an onlay implant was transverse. Theoretically, one might argue that a longitudinal fracture would cause less disruption of the extensor mechanism than would a transverse fracture and might have less deleterious sequellae. Because of the small numbers of patellar fractures that do occur, an appropriate power value for this type of study would require several thousand knee replacements, and at this point, that study has not been performed.

During a primary total knee replacement, one can easily measure the thickness of the patella and use this as a guide in judging the amount of patellar resection

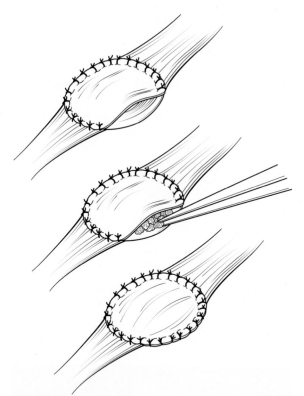

FIGURE 15-10. Hanssen has described forming a pouch from the soft tissues underlying the patellar tendon and filling it with cancellous bone to "reconstitute" a patella in situations in which the native patella is absent or extremely atrophic at the time of revision.

required. This is inapplicable, however, in the revision situation. Scott[26] has reported that the average thickness of the male patella is 25 mm and that of the female 22 mm. These can be used as rough approximations in judging how much further bone to resect and how thick an implant to use. In the revision situation the surgeon should attempt to make the combined thickness of the implant and the remaining bone slightly less than Scott's normal value, especially when a proximal or distal release has been employed, so as to avoid undue tension on the extensor mechanism.

Reuben[27] has described a minimum thickness of the patellar bone that should remain. He has noted that, for a transverse resection, if you leave less than 15 mm of bone, there is an increased risk of fracture.

If the patellar remnant is extremely thin, then the surgeon should consider not resurfacing the patella and performing a patelloplasty, as described in the subsequent sections.

Cameron (personal communication) has suggested inserting a large polyethylene patellar implant into the extensor retinaculum, drilling holes in its periphery, and securing it to the quadriceps tendon proximally and

to the patellar ligament distally with nonabsorbable sutures. In 4 cases the implant functioned well for over 3 years.

Nelson and his coworkers[28] have reported on bone grafting to the remnant of patellar bone and then inserting a porous coated tantalum cone into the remaining bone. A polyethylene button is then cemented on top of the cone.

Hanssen[29] has reported on creating a pouch from some of the tissues on the underside of the quadriceps tendon (Figure 15-10). The pouch is then filled with cancellous bone and the neck of the pouch secured. In this manner he has restored anterior bulk and recreated some of the lever arm normally afforded by the patella.

Ikezawa and Gustillo[30] reported on their technique in which they implanted a 5 mm thin biconvex polyethylene implant into a small patellar bony remnant. At 2 years' follow-up in their series, they had only an 8% rate of radiolucencies and no fractures.

WHAT SHOULD ONE DO IF THE PATELLA FRACTURED BEFORE THE REVISION OR IT FRACTURES DURING REMOVAL OF THE PATELLAR IMPLANT?

Most patellar fractures that occur in patients with total knee replacements are avascular in nature, with some degree of superimposed minor or major traumatic episode either preoperatively or during revision. Goldberg[31] has proposed a classification of patellar fractures in patients with total knee patients. Type I fractures usually involve the upper or lower aspects of the patella without involvement of the implant or its cement. These are avulsion-type injuries and are fairly easy to treat. Type II fractures result in either a loosening of the patellar component as a result of fracture through the body of the bone, or of disruption of the quadriceps mechanism. Type III fractures are those of the inferior pole with (type IIIA) or without (type IIIB) concomitant patellar ligament disruption. Finally, type IV is the most severe and represents a combination of a fracture of the patella with a dislocation of the bone and implant from the trochlear groove.

Because in many cases the patellar fragments are avascular, making secure internal fixation difficult, the surgeon may elect to attempt nonoperative treatment. This may be effective only in those fractures that are minimally displaced, without loosening of the patellar component. The largest reported series on nonoperatively treated fractures was by Hozack[32] in which he used 6 to 8 weeks of cast immobilization with weightbearing being allowed. He defined *nondisplacement* as 2 mm or less of displacement. His results were generally satisfactory in the nondisplaced fractures and poor in situations in which the fracture fragments were displaced. Goldberg as well found good results in 14 relatively nondisplaced fractures that were treated nonoperatively with cast immobilization. The authors have treated 4 nondisplaced fractures in this manner, 3 of which appeared to heal with fibrous union but were asymptomatic. The final fracture displaced while the patient was in the cast.

Comminuted fractures in which there is no disruption of the extensor mechanism should be treated nonoperatively. Windsor et al.[33] described using a long-leg cast in extension for about 2 months in these patients. If there is disruption of the extensor mechanism or loosening of the implant, he suggested performing a patellectomy.

As an alternative to patellectomy, the senior author has performed a patelloplasty in 14 patients with a comminuted patella fracture encountered during total knee revision. When evaluated 2 years after surgery, the incidence of anterior knee pain was 24%, as compared with 3.5% in those revision cases in which the patellar bone was retained and an implant used. In the former group only one patient could ascend or descend stairs in a reciprocal manner, while in the remainder of the revision cases this was possible in 40% of the patients. The average extensor lag in the patelloplasty group was 12 degrees (0 to 30 degrees range) while it was less than 5 degrees in the remainder of the revision cases. Interestingly, the mean flexion in the patelloplasty group was 123 degrees, while it was 105 in the remainder of the revision cases.

On occasion, one may encounter a displaced fracture of the patella that does not require fixation. Figure 15-11A demonstrates a fracture through a patellar remnant. The patient had previously undergone a revision knee replacement for a longitudinal fracture with a loose metal-backed component as well as loose femoral and tibial components. At the time of tibiofemoral revision, the loose lateral fragment was removed, as was the patellar implant. A patelloplasty was performed and no new implant inserted. Approximately 2 months later, when the patient was already flexing 120 degrees, she suffered an acute fracture of the remaining patellar remnant. Despite the radiographic appearance, the patient could actively straighten her knee against resistance with less than a 5-degree extensor lag (Figure 15-11B). It was thought that the retinaculum medially and laterally was intact, and it was elected to treat this patient nonoperatively with gradual restoration of function and elimination of her pain.

It is tempting to attempt an internal fixation using a tension band method in patients in whom there are 2

large patellar fragments. Again, the problem is that the bone is avascular, and this may preclude adequate healing (Figure 15-12). Likewise there must be no loosening of the component or the cement. For these reasons it is only a very occasional fracture that will be treated in this manner.

If there is a displaced fracture of the inferior or superior poles, Nelson et al.[28] have suggested fixation with a nonabsorbable Krackow suture passed through drill holes in the remaining patellar bone. He then allows some passive motion after surgery up to the level of the stability of the fragment at surgery.

FIGURE 15-11. (A and B) After removal of a patellar implant at the time of revision, there was insufficient bone remaining for reimplantation and a patelloplasty was performed. The patient subsequently fractured the remaining fragment of patella. Despite the radiographic appearance, the patient could actively extend the knee against resistance with less than a 5-degree extensor lag.

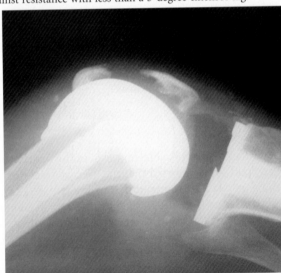

A

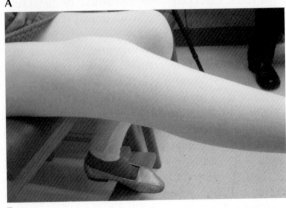

B

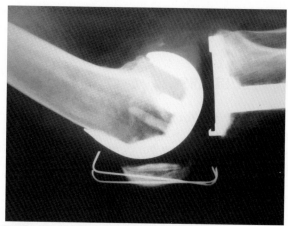

FIGURE 15-12. An attempt at internal fixation of a fractured patella after knee arthroplasty. The bone did not heal and a patelloplasty had to be subsequently performed.

WHAT IS THE BEST MANAGEMENT FOR A RUPTURE OF THE PATELLAR TENDON?

As with most other complications, the best treatment is avoidance, if possible. The patient at risk is one who has been on systemic corticosteroids, has marked limitation of flexion, a prior tibial osteotomy, or patella baja. The prevalence of such rupture varies from 1.4% to 3.2%.[34] Intraoperative rupture of the tendon during revision knee replacement or its avulsion from the tibial tubercle can be avoided using the methods described previously for exposure of the knee during revision. Again, it should be stressed that either a proximal or distal release should be considered in those knees with marked preoperative stiffness.

The results of primary repair of a patellar tendon or tibial tubercle avulsion during knee replacement have been horrible. Rand[35] reported a failure rate of over 90% using a variety of fixation materials. Nonabsorbable sutures, staples, screws, and screws with washers all were ineffective.

The repair for a ruptured patellar ligament is therefore more of a reconstruction rather than a repair. The tendon usually used for the repair is the semitendinosus, as described both by Cadambi and Engh[36] and Ecker.[37] The graft remains attached distally; the proximal portion of the graft is passed through a transverse tunnel in the patella above the implant and then rerouted distally though a transverse hole in the tibia just below the tubercle. The knee is kept immobile for approximately 6 weeks, although isometric exercises are encouraged during this period of time.

If the rupture of the patellar tendon is accompanied by comminution of the patellar fragment or insufficient bone for implantation of another implant, the surgeon should consider an extensor mechanism allograft as described by Emerson.[38] The allograft consists of a segment of quadriceps tendon, patella, patellar tendon, and an attached distal bony block. The block is placed and affixed with several screws slightly medial to the previous tibial tubercle. The proximal quadriceps is attached to the native quadriceps with nonabsorbable sutures. Proper tensioning of the mechanism is often difficult, and the most common complication is insufficient tension and a marked extensor lag. The anastomosis should be made with the knee fully extended but should allow at least 50 to 60 degrees of passive flexion at the time of surgery. The native tissues are then closed over the allograft in an attempt to encourage vascularization. The entire construct has to be carefully sculpted, and even when it is, the bulk makes skin closure at times difficult. Postoperatively the knee is kept in extension for 6 to 8 weeks and then started on gradual mobilization exercises.

WHAT SHOULD THE SURGEON DO IN A TOTAL KNEE REVISION WHEN THE PATELLA IS SUBLUXING LATERALLY?

Lateral subluxation of the patella after a knee replacement has a multiplicity of etiologies including internal rotation of the femoral component, internal rotation of the tibial component, an overthickened patella, lateral positioning of the patellar component on the patella, asymmetric patellar resection, excessive tibiofemoral alignment in valgus, and tightness of the lateral extensor retinaculum. All but the last represent surgical problems during the index knee replacement.

In the authors' experience internal rotation of the femoral component is the most common etiology for patients that they will see in conjunction with a subluxing patella after knee replacement. Again, prevention is the best treatment. Proper rotatory orientation of the femoral component at the time of index procedure through correct use of many references[30] including the transepicondylar line,[40] the midtrochlear line,[41,42] or the posterior condyles[43] can prevent this complication.

Internal rotation of the tibial component can likewise cause patellar subluxation. The author has shown that in over 90% of all primary and revision cases, proper tibial component rotation can be ensured if the front of the component is aligned with the medial third of the tibial tubercle.

Overthickening of the patella and patellar component can be avoided by measuring the thickness of the patella before implantation and attempting to reconstruct this thickness (or 1 or 2 mm thinner than this) during surgery.

Lateralization of the patellar component on the bone can cause patellar subluxation. Medialization or centralization of the implant is more optimal. If the implant is medialized, the surgeon should take care not to place it on the odd facet of the patella. Whether or not to resect the remaining lateral nonresurfaced area on the bone of a medially placed patellar implant remains controversial. The authors are presently performing a prospective trial of knees both with and about resection of the remaining lateral facet to evaluate the relationship, if any, to anterior knee pain, and stair climbing ability.

If the cause of the lateral subluxation is lateral retinacular tightness, and the components themselves are in proper position, the surgeon may elect to perform a lateral retinacular release. This may be performed arthroscopically or as an open procedure. The authors perform the procedure through an open approach in cases of marked patellar subluxation or dislocation. The retinaculum is released from the outside inward, attempting to keep the synovium intact. For those cases in which there is a remaining large Q-angle, a distal partial tendon

transposition, in a manner analogous to that described by Roux and Goldthwait, can be performed (Figure 15-13).

CONCLUSIONS

Avoidance remains the best treatment for potential extensor mechanism complications. Even though the patella is the smallest of the three bones involved in the arthroplasty, its failure almost assuredly leads to failure of the entire operation. Proper management is key to success of surgery.

REFERENCES

1. Whiteside L. Increasing exposure during knee replacement. In: Laskin RS, ed. *Controversies in Total Knee Replacement.* Oxford: Oxford University Press; 2001:339–350.
2. Coonse J, Adams JD. A new operative approach to the knee joint. *Surg Gynecol Obstet.* 1943;77:334–340.
3. Trousdale RT, Hanssen AD, Rand J, Calahan TD. V-Y quadricepsplasty in total knee arthroplasty. *Clin Orthop.* 1993;286:48–55.
4. Scott RD, Siliski JM. The use of a modified V-Y quadricepsplasty during total knee replacement to gain exposure and improve flexion in the ankylosed knee. *Orthopedics.* 1985; 8:45–48.
5. Insall JN. Surgical techniques and instrumentation in total knee arthroplasty. In: Insall JN, Windsor RE, Scott WN, Kelly MA, Aglietti P, eds. *Surgery of the Knee.* New York, Churchill Livingstone; 1993.
6. Garvin KL, Scuderi G, Insall JN. Evolution of the quadriceps snip. *Clin Orthop.* 1995;321:131–137.
7. Dolin MG. Tibial tubercle osteotomy in total knee replacement. *J Bone Joint Surg.* 1983;65A:704–706.
8. Whiteside LA. Exposure in difficult total knee arthroplasty using tibial tubercle osteotomy. *Clin Orthop.* 1997;321: 32–35.
9. Barrack RL, Smith P, Munn B, Engh G, Rorabeck C. Comparison of surgical approaches in total knee arthroplasty. *Clin Orthop.* 1998;356:16–21.
10. Ries MD, Richman J. Extended tibial tubercle osteotomy in total knee arthroplasty. *J Arthroplasty.* 1996;11:964–967.
11. Scuderi G, Scharf SC, Meltzer LP, Scott WN. The relationship of lateral release to patellar viability in total knee arthroplasty. *J Arthroplasty.* 1987;2:209–214.
12. Greenwald AS. In: Hamelynck KJ, Stiehl JB, eds. *LCS Mobile Bearing Knee Arthroplasty: 25 years of Worldwide Experience.* Berlin-Heidelberg: Springer Verlag; 2002:53–56.
13. Rosenberg AG, Jacobs JJ, Saleh KJ, et al. The patella in revision total knee arthroplasty. *J Bone Joint Surg Am.* 2003;85A:(Suppl 1):63–70.

FIGURE 15-13. A patellar tendon transfer for subluxation of the patella in situations in which the femoral and tibial components are well fixed and in proper alignment and orientation. (From Rosenberg, Jacobs, Saleh,[13] by permission of *J Bone Joint Surg.*)

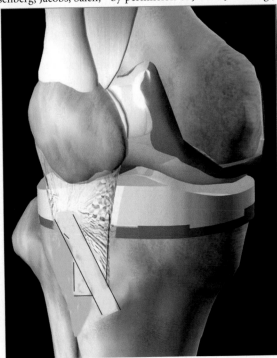

14. Cameron HU, Cameron GM. The patellar meniscus in total knee replacement. *Orthop Rev.* 1987;16:75–77.

15. Laskin RS. The use of an inset patella in total knee arthroplasty. In: Scuderi G, ed. *The Patella.* New York: Springer Verlag; 1997.

16. Bailey JC, Scott RD. Further observations on metal-backed patellar component failure. *Clin Orthop.* 1988;236:82–87.

17. Lombardi AV Jr, Engh GA, Volz R, Albrigo JL, Brainard BJ. Fracture/dislocation of the polyethylene in metal-backed patellar components in total knee arthroplasty. *J Bone Joint Surg.* 1988;70:675–679.

18. Laskin RS, Bucknell A. The use of a metal-backed patellar prosthesis in total knee arthroplasty. *Clin Orthop.* 1990;260: 52–55.

19. Paulos LE, Pinkowski JL. Patella infera. In: Fox JM, DelPizzo W, eds. *Patellofemoral Joint.* New York: McGraw-Hill; 1993: 205–214.

20. Laskin RS. Management of the patella during revision total knee replacement arthroplasty. *Orthop Clin North Am.* 1998;29:355–360.

21. Bryan RS. Patella infera and fat pad hypertrophy after total knee replacement. *Tech Orthop.* 1988;3:29–33.

22. Engh GA, McAuley JP. Joint line restoration and flexion-extension balance during revision total knee arthroplasty. In: Engh GA, Rorabeck CH, eds. *Revision Total Knee Arthroplasty: Techniques in Revision Surgery.* Baltimore: Williams and Wilkins; 1997:234–251.

23. Partington PF, Sawhney J, Rorabeck CH, Barrack RL, Moore J. Joint line restoration after revision total knee arthroplasty. *Clin Orthop.* 1999;345:165–171.

24. Figgie H, Goldberg V, Figgie M, Inglis AE. Kelly M, Sobel M. The effect of alignment of the implant on fractures of the patella after condylar total knee arthroplasty. *J Bone Joint Surg.* 1989;71A:1031–1039.

25. Gomes LSM, Bechtold JE, Gustilo RB. Patellar prosthesis positioning in total knee arthroplasty. *Clin Orthop.* 1988; 236:72–81.

26. Chmell MJ, McManus J, Scott RD. Thickness of the patella in men and women with osteoarthritis. *Knee.* 1996;2: 239–241.

27. Reuben JD. Effect of patellar thickness on patellar strain after total knee arthroplasty. *J Arthroplasty.* 1991;6:251–258.

28. Nelson C, Lahiji A, Lonner J, Kim J, Lotke P. The use of a porous metal shell for marked patellar bone loss during revision total knee arthroplasty. *J Arthroplasty.* 2003;18: 238–243.

29. Hanssen A. Bone grafting for severe patellar bone loss during revision knee arthroplasty. *J Bone Joint Surg.* 2001; 83A:171–176.

30. Ikezawa Y, Gustillo RB. Clinical outcome of revision of the patellar component in total knee arthroplasty. a 2- to 7-year follow up study. *J Orthop Sci.* 1999;4:83–88.

31. Goldberg VM, Figgie HE III, Inglis AE, et al. Patellar fracture type and prognosis in condylar total knee arthroplasty. *Clin Orthop.* 1988;236:115–122.

32. Hozack WJ, Golld SR, Lotke PA, et al. The treatment of patellar fractures after total knee arthroplasty. *Clin Orthop.* 1988;236:123–127.

33. Windsor RE, Scuderi DR, Insall JN. Patellar fractures in total knee arthroplasty. *J Arthroplasty.* 1989;4:S63–S67.

34. Kelly MA. Patellofemoral complications following total knee arthroplasty. *Instr Course Lect Am Acad Orthop Surg.* 2001;50:402–407.

35. Rand JA, Morrey BJ, Bryan RS. Patellar tendon rupture after total knee arthroplasty. *Clin Orthop.* 1989;244:233–239.

36. Cadambi A, Engh GA. Use of a semitendinosus tendon autogenous graft for rupture of the patellar ligament after total knee arthroplasty. *J Bone Joint Surg.* 1992;74A: 974–979.

37. Ecker ML, Lotke PA, Glazer RM. Late reconstruction of the patellar tendon. *J Bone Joint Surg.* 1989;61A:884–886.

38. Emerson RH, Head WC, Malini TI. Reconstruction of the patellar tendon rupture after total knee arthroplasty with an extensor mechanism allograft. *Clin Orthop.* 1990;260: 154–161.

39. Poilvache PL, Insall JN, Scuderi G, Font-Rodriguez D. Rotational landmarks and sizing of the distal femur in total knee arthroplasty. *Clin Orthop.* 1996;331:35–47.

40. Churchill DL, Incavo SJ, Johnson CC, et al. The transepicondylar axis approximates the optimal flexion axis of the knee. *Clin Orthop.* 1998;356:111–118.

41. Arima JA, Whiteside LA, McCarthy DS, White SE. Femoral rotational alignment, based on the anteroposterior axis, in total knee arthroplasty in the valgus knee. *J Bone Joint Surg.* 1995;77A:1331–1334.

42. Laskin RS. Lateral release rates after total knee arthroplasty. *Clin Orthop.* 2001;392:88–93.

43. Griffin FM, Insall JN, Scuderi GR. The posterior condylar angle in osteoarthritic knee. *J Arthroplasty.* 1998;14:812–815.

PART III

Special Considerations

CHAPTER 16

Infection in Total Knee Arthroplasty

Carl Deirmengian, Samir Mehta, and Jess H. Lonner

The specter of deep infection continues to temper the optimism regarding total knee arthroplasty (TKA), despite an incidence of less than 1% to 2%.[1-3] Infection after TKA is a topic of interest because of its diagnostic challenges, requisite intensity of care, and compromised outcomes. Efforts at reducing the rate of infection have allowed the identification of significant risk factors and the establishment of protocols for prevention.[4,5] Substantial progress has been made in the approach toward the diagnosis and treatment of the infected TKA.[6]

The primary goal of treatment in most patients with an infected TKA is the eradication of the infecting pathogen. Efforts aimed at achieving this goal should ideally result in a painless and functional extremity; however, function is occasionally sacrificed to clear the infection.

The cost of treating the infected TKA can be a burden for the patient, surgeon, hospital, and society. Hebert et al.[7] reported on the cost of caring for infected TKA in New Orleans between 1990 and 1993. Infected TKAs required 3 to 4 times the hospital resources when compared with primary TKAs, and double the resources when compared with aseptic revision TKAs. The net financial loss to the hospital was $15000 per patient, with an average loss of $30000 for Medicare patients. Sculco estimated the average annual cost of managing infected joint arthroplasties in the United States is $150 to $200 million.[8] This chapter reviews the currently available options for the diagnosis and management of infected TKAs.

ARTICLE I. RISK FACTORS FOR INFECTION

TKA infections are primarily the result of bacterial infections, which gain access to the knee intraoperatively or hematogenously, but fungal and viral infections have also been reported.[9] Host factors play a critical role in the establishment of infection. The immunocompromised state refers to a gradient of immune dysfunction, ranging from severe leukopenia to the more subtle effects of malnutrition. Leukocytes are instrumental in warding off infection, and any disease process affecting leukocyte count or function potentially increases the susceptibility of a TKA to infection.[10,11] Relatively recent evidence also suggests that the local synovial environment provides protection from infection by producing defensins, a family of antimicrobial peptides.[12,13] Although the role of local defense has not been completely elucidated, further research may prove that its dysfunction is also a form of immunocompromise.

During a TKA, possible sources of contamination include the operating room environment as well as the patient's own skin. Sterile techniques, iodophor drapes, laminar flow, and self-contained exhaust suits, among other things, attempt to minimize infection by addressing these sources of bacterial contamination, but the most important element is 24 to 48 hours of antibiotics, with the first dose given approximately 30 minutes before TKA. Bacteremia from any invasive procedure or chronic infection may also gain hematogenous access to the site of TKA. Dental, urologic, gynecologic, gastrointestinal, and podiatric procedures may all cause a transient bacteremia. Distant infection, such as chronic ulcers, dental abscesses, cellulitis, and urinary tract infections may also provide a source of organisms for the infection of TKAs. In the absence of obvious sources, one must be concerned of occult sources of bacteremia, such as endocarditis, that have systemic implications.

Overall, *Staphylococcus aureus* and *S. epidermidis* are the most commonly implicated organisms infecting TKA. In a review of 590 infected TKAs[14] comparing debridement versus direct exchange for the treatment of infected TKA, the most commonly infecting organisms were *Staphylococcus aureus* (48.7%), *Staphylococcus epidermidis* (16.3%), polymicrobial (5.4%), *Pseudomonas* (5.1%), *Streptococcus* (4.8%), *Enterococcus* (4.5%), and others (15.2%). However, specific clinical scenarios are often associated with particular types of organisms.[6] For example, early superficial infections tend to involve a high proportion of *Staphylococcus epidermidis*, while hematogenous infections often involve streptococcal organisms. Fungi have rarely been found to infect a TKA. Unlike native joints, infected more commonly by *Coccidioides immitis*, *Blastomyces dermatitidis*, and *Sporothrix schenckii*, TKA infections more commonly involve candidal infections.[15]

The ability of bacteria to form *biofilms* has been implicated as a factor that impedes our ability to treat periprosthetic infections. A biofilm is a bacterial aggregate that is protected by a slimy layer of polysaccharide and protein matrix.[16] Intercellular signaling molecules have been shown to provide a form of primitive communication that enables the formation of these bacterial communities.[17] Bacterial survival is enhanced within a biofilm, which not only serves as a barrier to the human immune system, but also protects against the diffusion and activity of antibiotics.[18] When inhabiting a biofilm, organisms are shielded from the immune system and may survive without causing symptoms, although they may serve as a nidus for future infection. The exact conditions[19] that promote biofilm formation, and methods of overcoming them have not been completely described.

Bacteria may also develop resistance by undergoing genetic changes that ultimately inactivate or block antibiotic action. Resistance in this form is usually specific to a certain type of antibiotic, as is demonstrated by vancomycin resistance and methicillin resistance. Resistant organisms are more difficult to eradicate because the anti-biotics available for their treatment are fewer in number, often more difficult to administer, and sometimes not tolerated by patients. Antibiotic resistance is a concerning trend that has been associated with a higher rate of treatment failure. Kilgus et al.[20] found that resistant organisms were eradicated from only 18% of 35 infected TKAs, while sensitive strains were eradicated in 89%. It is hoped that the development of improved treatment strategies and novel antibiotics will improve our ability to treat TKAs infected with resistant organisms.

SECTION 1.01 HOST RISK FACTORS AND HOST CLASSIFICATION

The host immune status has a tremendous influence on susceptibility to infection and the eventual response to treatment. Immune compromise may consist of an obvious deficiency to the immune system, such as neutropenia or hematologic malignancy. Alternatively, the more subtle effects on the immune system caused by conditions such as malnutrition, tobacco use, and advancing age may also result in states of immunocompromise. The identification and optimization of host factors are important for planning appropriate treatment. Furthermore, host factors should be considered when discussing the expectations and risks of TKA with the patient.

The maintenance of proper homeostasis in the local anatomic environment is critical to provide adequate defense against infection. At a microscopic level, tissue blood flow, oxygen tension, and cellularity are all factors that support local defense. Macroscopically, sufficient soft tissue coverage of the prosthesis is necessary to prevent skin breakdown and contamination. A vast number of local changes may compromise the ability to ward off infection. Areas of reduced blood flow and oxygen tension may result from skin bridges between multiple incisions, arterial disease, and venous stasis. Previous soft tissue injuries, fractures, and irradiation cause changes to the local tissue composition. Abscesses, sinuses, and active infections compromise local tissue coverage and may provide a nidus for reinfection.

Systemic illness is also associated with an increased susceptibility to infection. In addition to affecting local tissues surrounding a TKA, these diseases compromise the cellular and molecular responses that are critical for defense and the eradication of organisms. Systemic immune compromise is known to result from major organ insufficiency and diseases such as diabetes, immunodeficiencies, and malignancy. Environmental influences such as tobacco use, malnutrition, excessive alcohol consumption, and certain medications (e.g., steroids, chemotherapy agents, and some disease-modifying agents of rheumatoid disease, such as methotrexate and Enbrel) are also known to compromise the immune system.

Recognizing the importance of host factors, staging systems have been created to classify patients into host groups. McPherson et al.[21] reviewed 70 patients with an infected TKA and evaluated their outcomes as a function of one such staging system (Table 16.1). The staging system separately classified the infection type, the systemic host grade, and the local extremity grade in an effort to correlate stages with outcomes. They found that type III infections (late chronic) were associated with lower Knee Society scores and more pain after reimplantation, in addition to more complications, when compared with type I or II infections. Poor lower extremity status correlated with a higher complication rate and amputation, while worsening systemic host grade correlated with persistent or recurrent infection and permanent resections. Cierney and DiPasquale[10] also studied the usefulness of a staging system to prospectively compare the outcomes after treatment for infected TKA. Using the

TABLE 16.1. Prosthetic Joint Infection Staging System.*

Category	Grading	Description
Infection type	I	Early postoperative infection (<4 weeks postoperative)
	II	Acute hematogenous infection (<4 weeks duration)
	III	Late chronic infection (>4 weeks duration)
Systemic host grade	A	No compromise
	B	Compromised (2 or fewer factors)
	C	Significant compromise (>2 factors); or one of following:
		Absolute neutrophil count <1000
		CD4T cell count <100
		Intravenous drug abuse
		Chronic active infection (other location)
		Dysplasia/neoplasm of immune system
Lower extremity grade	1	No compromise
	2	Compromised (2 or less factors)
	3	Significant compromise (>2 factors)

From McPherson, Tontz, Patzakis, et al. (21), by permission of *Am J Orthop.*

*Note: The infection type describes the acuteness of the infection and data are adapted from Tsukayama DT, Estrada R, Gustilo RB. Infection after total hip arthroplasty: A study of the treatment of one hundred and six infections. *J Bone Joint Surg Am.* 1996;78:512–523.

osteomyelitis classification system, they classified patients based on local and systemic factors: Type A hosts are healthy and without healing deficiency, type B hosts are compromised by one or more systemic and/or local factors, and type C hosts are not able to withstand curative intervention due to concurrent illness. Of 43 patients in their study, 37 patients had wound healing deficiencies, and all were in patients with 3 or more comorbidities. All treatment failures, amputations, and mortalities were prospectively observed to involve high-risk patients.

Although host staging systems have not yet become standard practice, they raise an extremely critical concept that relates the patients' local and systemic health to the eventual treatment and outcome. The host-pathogen relationship defines the ability of an organism to establish a persistent infection. The identification of local and systemic host factors assists the surgeon in choosing an appropriate therapeutic intervention. For example, high-risk patients are not appropriate candidates for many of the same interventions that a healthy patient may receive. Additionally, the appreciation of host factors can help establish more realistic expectations after treatment of infected TKA, or in the most extreme cases, provide a basis for withholding TKA from certain at-risk patients.[10]

SECTION 1.01 DIAGNOSIS

The timely diagnosis of infection is absolutely critical; a delay can negatively affect the ultimate outcome and impede the ability to eradicate the infection. A detailed history of the nature of the presenting symptoms can often offer clues to the possibility of infection. In the acute postoperative setting, the treating physician should be concerned about the patient who presents with delayed wound healing, ongoing discomfort, limited motion, and failure to progress; this patient may be infected. Hematogenous infections, however, often present with a less insidious course and with the acute onset of pain, swelling, and perhaps cellulitis. The presence of risk factors such as remote infections or dental, urological, or other invasive procedures should raise the suspicion for infection, although often there are no clear, identifiable associated risk factors. The presence of fevers, chills, or malaise, while uncommon in a deep knee infection, are symptoms that should raise the suspicion of infection.

Unfortunately, the most glaring signs of infection— fevers, chills, sinus tracts, and purulent drainage—are uncommon in most infected TKAs (Figure 16-1). The more common presenting signs and symptoms—pain, swelling, warmth, and synovitis—are notoriously difficult to distinguish from aseptic failure. Nonetheless, patients who present with ongoing pain in the early postoperative period without clear reason, or those patients who present with the acute onset of pain should be evaluated for the possibility of infection. As a general tenet, patients who present with acute knee pain should be assumed to be infected until proven otherwise. The majority of patients with an infected knee arthroplasty, whether acute or chronic, will have pain, although occasionally a patient presents with malaise and fatigue, in the absence of pain. The latter is a relatively infrequent presentation, but one that should trigger suspicion regarding the possibility of a septic knee arthroplasty and septicemia. Cellulitis is an infrequent clinical sign, particularly in hematogenous infections, and it is often a challenge determining if the cellulitis is superficial or whether there is deep extension. As a general rule of thumb, cellulitis that is not accompanied by pain during knee motion is generally superficial and likely does not involve the deeper tissues, but aspiration of the knee joint through a noncellulitic area should be performed in these situations.

Weightbearing radiographs should be obtained on all patients presenting with a painful total knee arthroplasty. Radiographic signs of loosening are unlikely in the acute postoperative period or in late hematogenous infections that present acutely. TKAs with chronic long-standing infections may have evidence of loosening of the implants, but they are usually indistinguishable from those failures that occur for noninfectious reasons. Subtle findings, however, may be present with chronic infection, particularly when there is osteomyelitis, namely endosteal erosion, reactive periosteal bone, and occasionally heterotopic ossification (Figure 16-2).

While there are a variety of diagnostic tests that have been advocated and used to evaluate the painful TKA, the frustrating reality is that many are inaccurate and cannot be relied on in isolation to clearly establish whether or not

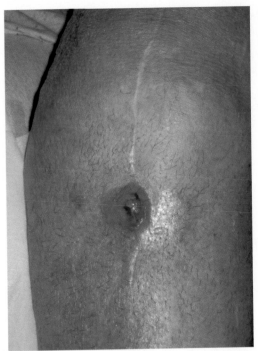

FIGURE 16-1. A small sinus present around the incision several years after TKA should raise the concern regarding the likelihood of a substantial chronic late infection.

FIGURE 16-2. (A–C) Anteroposterior radiograph of a knee after removal of an infected revision TKA and implantation of antibiotic-impregnated spacer blocks. Note periosteal reaction of the medial and lateral metaphyseal flares of the distal femur. Intraoperative biopsies of these bony sites showed chronic osteomyelitis. Distal femoral resection was necessary to eradicate the extensive osteomyelitis of the distal femur and eventually a hinged knee arthroplasty with distal femoral modular augments was necessary. (By permission of Lotke PA, Lonner JH, eds. *Master Techniques in Orthopaedic Surgery: Knee Arthroplasty.* Philadelphia: Lippincott Williams & Wilkins, 2002, Figure 22–29 A–C.)

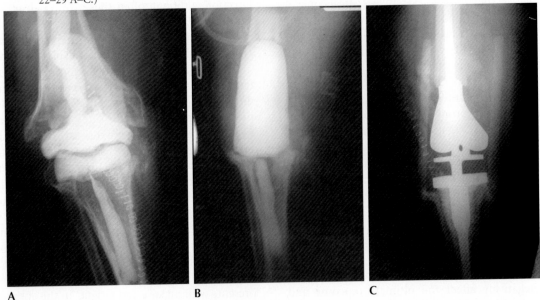

A   B   C

an infection is present. Nonetheless, when taken in concert, several studies can be helpful. Considering the cost of treating the infected TKA, which may be 3 to 4 times that of a primary knee arthroplasty, it is important that unnecessary diagnostic tests be avoided when evaluating the knee for deep infection.[7] Despite our best intentions, approximately 10% to 15% of deep infections after total joint arthroplasty are undetected by standard preoperative diagnostic tools.[22]

Some serologic studies are more useful than others. The peripheral white blood cell count is rarely elevated in the setting of infections after total knee arthroplasty unless there is clear bacteremia. Windsor et al.[23] reported that only 28% of cases had peripheral white blood cell counts greater than 11 000 in the presence of deep knee infection. In isolation, erythrocyte sedimentation rate is nonspecific for infection and may remain elevated for up to 1 year after surgery.[24,25] Levitsky et al. reported that the erythrocyte sedimentation rate had a specificity of 65% and sensitivity of 60%, rendering this test relatively inaccurate in the evaluation of infection.[26] C-reactive protein tends to normalize by 3 to 4 weeks after total knee arthroplasty; its persistent elevation can be reflective of infection. Spangehl et al.[27] found that the diagnostic utility is enhanced by analyzing the erythrocyte sedimentation rate and C-reactive protein together when evaluating the painful joint arthroplasty. In the series by Spangehl et al., the likelihood of both positive C-reactive protein and sedimentation rate in predicting infection was 83%, and when both study results were negative, they were nearly 100% accurate at predicting the absence of deep joint infection.[27]

Radioisotope scanning has been used in the evaluation of the painful joint arthroplasty, with variable results. Technetium scans have proven ineffective in the majority of cases, with a sensitivity of 60% and specificity of 65%.[26] In general, technetium scans are unnecessary in the evaluation of the failed total knee arthroplasty, because they are ineffective in distinguishing between mechanical and septic loosening. Technetium scans, however, may be effective in identifying occult loosening of a painful total knee arthroplasty, and a total body technetium scan might be considered in the evaluation of other joint arthroplasties to rule out metachronous polyarticular infection. Indium scans are moderately more accurate than technetium scans. One study by Rand and Brown, which evaluated 38 total knee arthroplasties, found that indium scans had a sensitivity of 83%, specificity of 85%, and accuracy of 84%.[28] Scher et al. subsequently reported on 153 indium scans that were done to evaluate painful total hip, knee, or resection arthroplasties. In that series there were 41 total knee arthroplasties evaluated, and the indium scans had a sensitivity of 88%, specificity of 78%,

positive predictive value of 75%, negative predictive value of 90%, and accuracy of 83%.[29] This study showed a high percentage false-positive indium scan results in knees that were loose but not infected. It is not clear whether the tendency for false-positive scan results is related to the indiscriminant labeling of both acute and chronic inflammatory white cells, which may be present in infection or chronic inflammation of osteolysis, respectively, ongoing postsurgical inflammation, persistent joint inflammatory disease, or a combination of these factors.[29] The accuracy of indium scans may be enhanced by combining this study with a technetium-99M sulfur colloid scan.[30,31] The technetium-99M sulfur colloid scan can detect increased density of bone marrow elements, which in the case of periprosthetic infection are replaced by inflammatory mediators, including leukocytes, that inhibit the uptake of the technetium sulfur colloid. Matched areas on the indium and sulfur colloid scans are indicative of marrow packing and the absence of infection, thereby reducing the number of false-positive scan results.[30] In a study by Joseph et al., the combined indium/colloid scan was found to have 100% specificity, 46% sensitivity, 100% positive predictive value, 84% negative predictive value, and 88% accuracy. Sensitivity improved to 66%, negative predictive value to 89%, and accuracy to 90%, and specificity was reduced to 98% and positive predictive value to 91% when blood pooling and flow phase data were included.[30] The low sensitivity of these combined studies makes their routine use in the evaluation of the potentially infected total knee arthroplasty imprudent.

Aspiration of the knee is probably the most valuable diagnostic tool in determining the presence of deep knee infection.[32,33] Aspirated fluid can be sent for cell count and culture. Historically, more than 25 000 white blood cells per cubic millimeter with a preponderance of polymorphonuclear leukocytes was considered highly suggestive of infection,[34] and less than this was considered noninfected. However, more recently infections have been noted to occur with substantially lower white blood cell counts in the aspirate. Therefore, the absolute number of white cells within the aspirated fluid is less reliable. A preponderance of acute inflammatory cells, however, should be considered suspicious for infection. Of greater value is the culture result. In a retrospective study by Morrey et al., aspiration of 73 infected total knee arthroplasties had a sensitivity of only 45%; however, it was not clear in that study how many patients were still on antibiotics or what interval of time had passed between terminating antibiotics and aspirating the knees.[35] In a more recent study by Barrack et al., assessing the results of aspiration of 69 symptomatic total knee arthroplasties, 20 knees were determined to be infected. Preoperative aspiration had an overall sensitivity of 55%, specificity of 96%, accuracy of 84%, positive predictive value of 85%, and negative predictive value of 84%. There were 2 false-positive aspirations, which grew on liquid media only, and these were considered contaminants since sedimentation rate was normal, intraoperative cultures were negative, and intraoperative histological analysis showed no evidence of acute inflammatory cells. Nine aspirations were falsely negative in the setting of infection. The sensitivity of aspiration increased from 55% to 61% if the initial aspiration was delayed at least 2 weeks after discontinuing antibiotics.[36] A second aspiration enhanced the sensitivity of the test to 75%, specificity 96%, and accuracy 90%. Clearly then, the aspiration should be delayed at least 2 weeks after discontinuing antibiotics to avoid the potential effect of suppression. The gross appearance of the fluid should be assessed as well, although turbid fluid can be found in total knee arthroplasties affected by noninfectious processes such as gout or calcium pyrophosphate disease. When the diagnosis is in doubt, serial aspirations can be a useful approach.

In situations in which the diagnosis of infection is unclear, molecular diagnostic techniques or intraoperative frozen section histoanalysis can provide further clues regarding the presence of infection. Polymerase chain reaction (PCR) has been used to detect bacterial pathogens within synovial fluid after total knee arthroplasty. PCR amplifies bacterial DNA, but unfortunately is extremely sensitive and at the present time has a high rate of false-positive results.[37] Evolving methods to enhance the specificity of PCR and other molecular techniques will potentially make these important diagnostic tools in the future.

Histological analysis is extremely important in a number of patients in whom the presence of infection is equivocal or uncertain. A prospective study of 100 consecutive total joint arthroplasties was performed to determine the reliability of analysis of intraoperative frozen sections for the identification of infection.[38] Using an index of 10 polymorphonuclear leukocytes per high-power field (HPF) as a determinant of infection, the authors reported a sensitivity of 84%, specificity of 99%, positive predictive value of 89%, and a negative predictive value of 98%. Unlike previous reports on the value of frozen section, the authors concluded that between 5 and 9 polymorphonuclear leukocytes was not necessarily consistent with infection.[39] If there were fewer than 5 PMNs per HPF, infection was unlikely. When 5 to 9 PMNs per HPF are identified, additional scrutiny of granulation tissue from within the wound and analysis of other sections of the tissue should be performed, as frequently foci of additional PMNs per HPF could be identified. In equivocal situations, it is advised that the frozen section

be considered in the overall context of the preoperative evaluation and the ultimate decision to reimplant a new knee arthroplasty or to perform an interval spacer block procedure should be based on the preoperative tests that had been performed as well as the overall appearance of the tissue and the surgeon's impression at the time of surgery. The technique of harvesting and analysis of frozen sections is subject to error, and therefore strict sampling protocols should be followed when using this means of investigation. Granulation tissue is preferentially harvested. Dense fibrous or fibrin-rich tissue is often of no value. At least 2 small tissue samples are analyzed and the 5 most cellular fields are assessed based on the number of PMNs. Cell count is performed under high-power magnification of 40 times, and only PMNs identified within the tissue with well-defined cytoplasmic borders are counted, as cells with isolated nuclear fragmentation cannot be definitely characterized as PMNs.[38,39] The reliability of analysis of frozen sections for the guidance of intraoperative decision making has been questioned, because errors in specimen collection and analysis may confound the ultimate interpretation of results.[40]

No single test can identify infection in all painful or failing total knee arthroplasties. It is important that a careful history be taken in all cases and a high index of suspicion maintained. Sedimentation rate, C-reactive protein (CRP), and aspiration can be invaluable in many patients. It is important, however, that patients be off antibiotics for at least 2 weeks before aspirating the knee joint. Serial aspirations should be considered in those patients in whom infection is clearly suspected despite negative culture results. In equivocal cases or those in which the diagnosis is uncertain, intraoperative frozen section can be helpful in establishing whether the joint is infected.

V. Classification of Infection

Classifying infection after TKA based on symptom duration and the interval from surgery is important because it puts into perspective the potential treatment options. Acute postoperative or late hematogenous infections with acute onset are often treated with methods that attempt to retain the components, while more chronic infections frequently require component removal. In an effort to classify the clinical presentation of an infected TKA, three main categories have been described[6,21] (Table 16.2).

Early postoperative infections become evident within 4 weeks after index TKA. They may have started at the time of surgery or by hematogenous means. Aspiration should be done to rule out hematoma, the most common alternate diagnosis. CRP and ESR will likely still be elevated, as a result of the surgery, but very high values

TABLE 16.2. Classification of Prosthetic Joint Infection.

Positive intraoperative culture
Early postoperative infection
    Superficial
    Deep
Acute hematogenous
Late chronic

From Tsukayama, Goldberg, and Kyle (6), by permission of *J Bone Joint Surg Am.*

TABLE 16.3. Criteria Necessary for Successful Antibiotic Suppression.

Surgical intervention contraindicated (patient health)
Low virulence organism
Organism sensitive to antibiotics
Patient can tolerate antibiotic
No component loosening

should raise concern. Gram's stain and culture are sent to identify the presence of organisms. Do not assume that bacterial growth in broth only is a contaminant; when in doubt, reaspirate.

Acute hematogenous infections are those that present with a short duration of acute symptoms in a previously well-functioning knee. These may occur after invasive procedures, such as dental or genitourinary interventions, after abrasions or lacerations, or after remote or unrelated infections, but often there is no identifiable source of infection. While an acute hematogenous infection with 4 weeks or less of symptoms is often considered amenable to open debridement and retention of components, the results are optimized when patients present within 1 week of the onset of the infection.

Late chronic infections present with greater than 4 weeks of symptoms and may be associated with osteomyelitis, sinus tracts, and loose components. These patients often have a long insidious course of pain, swelling, and stiffness. Patients with chronic infections often present with a history of antibiotic use that decreases the sensitivity of cultures, making accurate diagnosis difficult, or limiting the identification of all organisms, in the case of polymicrobial infections.[41] Chronic infections involve organisms that have penetrated interfaces and tissues. They have often been subjected to a number of antibiotics and may have formed biofilms that resist nonoperative treatments. Therefore, these infections almost always require debridement with component removal and at least 4 to 6 weeks of intravenous antibiotics for complete eradication.

VI. Treatments That Retain Prostheses

A. Antibiotic Suppression Antibiotic treatment alone will fail to eradicate infection from a surrounding total joint arthroplasty. However, in specific clinical scenarios, antibiotics may be used to suppress an infection (Table 16.3). Antibiotic suppression may be appropriate for patients who are poor candidates for surgical intervention. These patients are usually at a high risk of local or systemic complications, and often have other medical issues that preclude an operative procedure. For successful antibiotic suppression, the organism must have low virulence and demonstrate susceptibility to an orally available and tolerable antibiotic. Patients with signs of advanced infection, such as loosening and sinuses, are unlikely to respond well to antibiotic suppression.[1,2,42,43] Attempting to suppress a deep prosthetic infection in the presence of other joint arthroplasties or artificial implants (e.g., heart valves) puts the patient at risk for metastatic implant infection and should be avoided if possible.

Patients treated with antibiotic suppression should be routinely followed for signs of advancing infection. Failed treatment may manifest with either acute or insidious symptoms, such as increased pain, swelling, drainage, and erythema. Constitutional signs of bacteremia are a clear indication of failure of suppression.

B. Open Debridement with Component Retention
Open debridement of acute TKA infections is an attractive option, given the possibility of retaining a stable implant, avoiding revision, and preserving a functional limb. The currently accepted indications for this treatment option include acute postoperative or hematogenous TKA infections that are identified within weeks from the onset of symptoms (Table 16.4). The presence of loosening, sinus tracts, or osteomyelitis suggests more chronic infection and is associated with a high rate of failed debridement. This option is less desirable when other joint implants are present, unless performed within 1 to 2 weeks of the onset of symptoms.

An open arthrotomy and a complete synovectomy are performed to remove the proliferative, inflamed, and

TABLE 16.4. Criteria Necessary for Successful Open Debridement with Component Retention.

Low-virulence organism
Organism sensitive to antibiotics
Acute infection (<4 weeks)
No component loosening
No osteomyelitis
No sinus tracts

sometimes necrotic tissue. A polyethylene insert exchange provides access to interfaces and also assists with exposure of the posterior capsule. Four to 6 liters of saline, with antibiotics, are then used to irrigate the knee and a standard closure using a heavy deep monofilament suture is completed over drains. Multiple intraoperative tissue and fluid samples are sent for the identification of infecting organisms. Four to 6 weeks of appropriately directed intravenous antibiotics are administered, followed by chronic oral antibiotics in select cases. Multiple debridements may enhance the outcome.

Numerous published series have evaluated the capability of early debridement at eradicating infection.[14,44-51] Despite the use of various methodologies, these reports reveal common themes that provide guidelines for the debridement of infected TKA (Table 16.4). The combined published results (561 knees) reveal a rate of success approximating 33% (184 of 561).[14,52]

The most important factor determining its success is the timing of debridement after the onset of infection.[44,45,49,50] Retrospective case series have demonstrated a statistically significant difference in outcome when comparing patients debrided soon after symptoms from those patients debrided after prolonged symptoms.[44,50] Burger[45] found a correlation between successful outcome and debridement within 2 weeks after the onset of symptoms. It is likely that prolonged infections establish deeper penetration within tissues and interfaces and are more difficult to successfully debride. The development of protective mechanisms such as biofilms may be generated by the organism and contribute to failure.[16] Evidence of chronic infection such as sinuses, loosening, or osteomyelitis are generally considered contraindications to attempting component retention. In general, the literature supports component retention if debridement is done within 2 to 4 weeks after the onset of symptoms, but it is best done within days. Some authors suggest that successful debridement is more likely when treating an early acute postoperative infection than a late acute hematogenous infection,[46,47,50] but this is not routinely supported.[44,52]

Patients who are young and healthy with an infection after primary knee arthroplasty are also more likely to have a successful debridement.[48,52] Some authors have suggested that patients with multiple medical problems or immunocompromise are more difficult to treat with debridement and component retention.[48] Additionally, although exceptions have been reported, generally poor results have been found after debridement of hinged and multiply revised components.[48]

Debridement is more likely to succeed with less virulent organisms such as streptococcal species and *Staphylococcus epidermidis*, whereas failed debridement has been associated with more virulent organisms such as *Staphylococcus aureus* and gram-negative organisms and in the setting of antibiotic resistance.[44,48,52,53] Recently, a statistically significant difference was found in outcome after the debridement of *S. aureus* infections versus infection with other gram-positive organisms.[52] Only 1 of 13 TKAs infected with *S. aureus* were successfully debrided in that series, compared with 10 of 18 successful debridements in patients infected with other gram-positive organisms. Multiple debridements, as recommended by Mont and Hungerford,[47] can sometimes be useful. Using indicators of persistent infection after the first debridement, including signs, symptoms, and repeated aspirations, they chose a strategy of multiple debridements when treating certain patients. Of 24 infected TKAs in the series, 12 had multiple debridements and a total of 20 were successfully treated (83% compared with 41% after single debridement).

Arthroscopic debridement[2,14,51,54-56] generally has unacceptably poor results and should be avoided. Waldman et al.[51] reported on the arthroscopic irrigation and debridement of 16 infected TKAs. Despite a strict definition of acute infection (< or = 7 days of knee symptoms), only 6 infected knees (38%) were successfully treated using this method. They recommend reserving arthroscopic treatment of the acutely infected TKA to patients who are medically unstable or anticoagulated.

VII. Exchange Arthroplasty

Exchange arthroplasty involves removal of the infected TKA, thorough debridement, and reimplantation. Direct exchange (one-stage) arthroplasty involves open debridement of the infected TKA followed by immediate revision. Two-stage reimplantation involves open debridement, removal of the infected prosthesis, and delayed reimplantion, with an intervening time for antibiotic therapy.

Exchange arthroplasty is preferred for infections present for greater than 2 to 4 weeks, or persistent infections that could not be eradicated with debridement alone. In order to successfully use exchange arthroplasty, the patient should be medically stable for multiple operative procedures, with an intact immune system that will aid in eradicating the infection. Furthermore, the inherent elements of the knee, such as bone stock, extensor mechanism, and soft tissue envelope, should be amenable to eventual TKA function.

Direct exchange arthroplasty with primary reimplantation[57-61] has been described by Goksan and Freeman.[62] Thorough debridement of synovial tissue and devitalized bone is completed after component removal. One proposed technique includes irrigation with saline, packing with iodine-soaked sponges, and a one-layer wound closure, followed by deflation of the tourniquet to allow for antibiotic perfusion for 30 minutes. After a complete replacement of all gowns, drapes, and gloves, the knee is prepared again with sterile technique, and the components are reimplanted with antibiotic-impregnated cement.[62] Goksan and Freedman[62] reported successful eradication of infection in 16 of 18 patients treated with direct exchange arthroplasty, but clinical follow-up was short. Overall there have been few series of patients managed with direct exchange arthroplasty. With proper patient selection, direct exchange has been associated with a rate of success comparable to two-stage exchange arthroplasty.[14] This is particularly reassuring in those patients who undergo revision arthroplasty in the setting of previously undetected infection, and highlights the importance of using antibiotic-impregnated polymethylmethacrylate (PMMA) in all revision TKAs, with or without known infection.

A two-stage approach is preferred by many[23,41,63–67] when treating long-standing or late TKA infections, with a reported success rate greater than 85 to 90%.[41,50,64,66,68–73] There are different opinions about whether to use a spacer, the type of spacer (static vs. articulating), the route and length of antibiotic treatment, the timing of reimplantation, and the details of revision surgery.

At the time of implant removal, a complete debridement must be performed to provide an optimal environment for eventual reimplantation. This includes not only an extensive synovectomy, but also removal of necrotic and infected bone. The previous incision can almost always be used. Sinuses should be excised, and muscle flaps used if coverage is a potential problem. On entering the joint, several samples of synovial fluid should be sent for culture and analysis. Synovial tissue, interface tissues, and tissue from the canals (when removing stemmed components) should also be sent for culture and pathologic analysis. When removing components, it is critical to preserve maximal bone stock. However, one must be sure to remove all fragments of cement and necrotic bone in an effort to reduce the interfaces available to organisms. Irrigation of the joint with several liters of antibiotic saline is performed, and a spacer is implanted. The capsular closure is performed over drains using a running monofilament suture.

Early reports of two-stage exchange described an intervening resection arthroplasty before reimplantation.[23,67,71,74] However, in an effort to facilitate component reimplantation, some surgeons began using antibiotic-impregnated cement blocks[63,70] (Figure 16-3). The intervening spacer has a dual role of delivering antibiotics to the knee environment and preserving the joint space and reducing soft tissue contracture. Although the use of antibiotic cement blocks has become widespread, interval

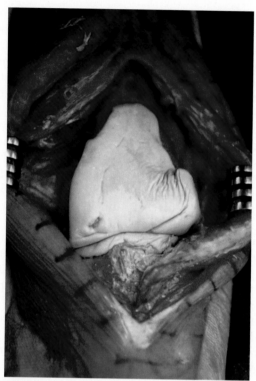

FIGURE 16-3. Intraoperative photograph of a static spacer. (By permission of Lotke PA, Lonner JH, eds. *Master Techniques in Orthopaedic Surgery: Knee Arthroplasty.* Philadelphia: Lippincott Williams & Wilkins, 2002, Figure 22–28.)

bone loss and stiffness due to scarring have been identified as undesirable consequences.[75,76] The use of articulating spacers has been described in an effort to minimize these problems, while ensuring the local delivery of antibiotics[66,68,77] (Figure 16-4). The PROSTALAC system

FIGURE 16-4. Intraoperative photograph of an articulating spacer. (By permission of Lotke PA, Lonner JH, eds. *Master Techniques in Orthopaedic Surgery: Knee Arthroplasty.* Philadelphia: Lippincott Williams & Wilkins, 2002, Figure 22–25.)

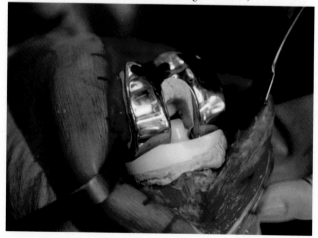

provides one option for an articulating spacer, but it is not universally available in the United States.[68,78] Alternatively, a more accessible option is that described by Hoffman et al.,[77] in which the components removed at debridement are reused to construct an articulating spacer. In short, the femoral component is debrided, cleared of adherent bone and cement, autoclaved for 20 minutes, and coated with antibiotic-impregnated cement on its nonarticulating surface. A fresh polyethylene insert is opened, and it too is coated on its nonarticulating surface, and both are implanted with the cement in a doughy stage, so that there is limited interdigitation with bone. A reasonable mixture is detailed by Emerson et al.[75] using Palacos impregnated with 3.6 g of tobramycin and 2 g of vancomycin per 40-g package of cement. Haddad et al.[68] reported on 45 patients treated with an articulating functional spacer. Only 9% became reinfected, and motion was preserved after reimplantation. Comparison between static spacer blocks and articulating spacers by Emerson et al.[75] and Fehring et al.[76] has shown no difference in the reinfection rate; however, the articulating spacer was found to limit bone loss, facilitate the surgical exposure at the time of reimplantation, and enhance motion after reimplantation. Additionally, patients tend to be more functional in the intervening period with an articulating spacer than with a static spacer.

The ideal time interval between debridement and reimplantation is another controversy yet to be resolved. Many surgeons prefer at least 6 weeks of intravenous antibiotics,[41,64,71,73,75,79] although some have postulated that 4 weeks of antibiotics are ample. Some allow additional time for oral antibiotics, antibiotic-free intervals, and diagnostic testing to confirm the eradication of infection.[72,80,81] Rand and Bryan[74] reported a relatively low success rate (57%) after retrospectively reviewing the treatment of patients who were given antibiotics for 2 weeks before reimplantation. Success rates above 85% to 90%[23,41,64,71] have been reported for treatment that used a 6-week interval of intravenous antibiotics before reimplantation. The decision to proceed with reimplantation should be dependent on the presence of a healthy soft tissue envelope that does not have substantial inflammation after antibiotics have been terminated. The use of antibiotic-impregnated bone cement at the time of reimplantation has been shown by Hanssen et al.[65] to significantly reduce the rate of reinfection.

Attempts to use diagnostic testing to identify persistent infection before proceeding with reimplantation have had mixed results. Nuclear studies have failed to show significant value in the identification of persistent infection.[29,80] However, laboratory studies may be of use. Although the ESR may be persistently elevated after debridement, the CRP value should trend toward normal

after 6 weeks of intravenous antibiotics. Frozen sections[82] from synovial tissues at reimplantation have proven marginally useful at this stage. Variability due to tissue sampling and normal inflammation creates inconsistent results. However, a relatively recent report by Banit et al.[83] suggests that frozen section of knees at implantation may be associated with a sensitivity of 100% and specificity of 96% for infection when applying careful sampling technique and handled by experienced pathologists. Their standard for infection was a positive culture at reimplantation, not reinfection after reimplantation. Aspiration of the knee before reimplantation has been used to identify patients who have persistent infection. False-negative culture results are common when sending an aspirate for culture within 3 weeks after the completion of intravenous antibiotics.[84] However, Mont et al.[85] reported a protocol that used aspiration for culture 4 weeks after the discontinuation of intravenous antibiotics. All patients with a positive culture underwent a second round of debridement, intravenous antibiotics, and aspiration before reimplantation. This protocol significantly reduced the rate of recurrent infection when compared with a control group and has been the only reported method that appears to identify and treat patients who are persistently infected after one round of debridement and antibiotics. Only 1 of 34 (3%) patients in their study had a reinfection after negative aspiration and reimplantation.

The authors' preferred method includes debridement of the infected TKA and implantation of an articulating spacer, when feasible, with antibiotic-impregnated cement. Articulating spacers cannot be used when there is extensive bone loss or incompetence of ligamentous support. After 6 weeks of intravenous antibiotics, 4 weeks are allowed to pass without any antibiotic treatment. Aspiration is performed, and the synovial fluid is sent for culture. Positive samples indicate the need for a second round of debridement and intravenous antibiotics. ESR and CRP are assessed to ensure normalization or a trend toward normalcy. During reimplantation, frozen sections of tissue may be sent, depending on the gross tissue appearance. If the results of these tests are favorable, then reimplantation is performed (Figure 16-5).

VIII. Salvage Procedures

Patients with persistent infection are sometimes unable to retain a functional TKA. Repeated surgical procedures lead to bone loss and soft tissue compromise, necessitating a salvage procedure to relieve pain. Hanssen et al.[59] studied a series of 24 knees that became reinfected following reimplantation for an infected TKA. The average number of procedures per patient, including the index TKA, was 9.3. Only one patient had an uninfected TKA at most recent follow-up. The outcomes included 10

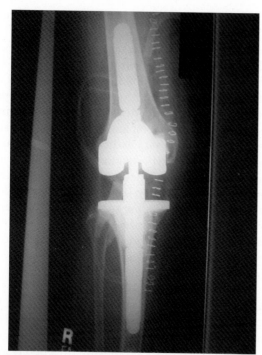

FIGURE 16-5. Anteroposterior radiograph after successful reimplantation.

patients with a successful arthrodesis, 5 with infected TKA on suppressive antibiotics, 4 patients with an above-the-knee amputation, 3 persistent pseudoarthroses, and 1 resection arthroplasty. Salvage procedures are sometimes necessary to eradicate infection and relieve pain.

A. Resection Arthroplasty

The use of resection arthroplasty as a definitive treatment for infected TKAs is generally reserved for patients who are medically ill and sedentary. These patients do not require the full function of a TKA and are served well by an extremity that accommodates transfers and can be flexed. However, resection arthroplasty results in a significant loss of function, instability, and potentially persistent pain.

Falahee et al.[86] retrospectively reviewed the results of resection arthroplasty in 26 patients (28 knees). Those with severe disabilities found resection arthroplasty to be a tolerable procedure and were satisfied with their outcomes. Those with a minimal presurgical disability were more likely to experienced unacceptable instability and persistent pain, and eventually required arthrodesis.[86]

B. Arthrodesis

Certain clinical situations preclude the ability to reliably reimplant components with good results. Patients with irreparable extensor mechanism disruption, an inade-

quate soft tissue envelope, and multiple recurrent infections may be more appropriately treated with arthrodesis. In general, when it is thought that reimplantation will have a high rate of failure, due to inadequate joint mechanics, soft tissue envelope, or immune system, then arthrodesis may be the treatment of choice. The relative contraindications to arthrodesis include significant contralateral limb dysfunction, coexistent ipsilateral ankle or hip disease, or inadequate bone stock for fusion. Wound coverage should be optimized with a muscle flap if necessary.

Different techniques have been described for arthrodesis after TKA infection. Subsequent to a thorough debridement and creation of a sterile environment, a method of internal or external fixation is used. Knees are fused in full extension to maximize osseous apposition; the limb shortening common in fusion for a failed TKA will ensure that foot clearance during gait is not a problem. In fact, patients commonly require shoe lifts. The success of arthrodesis is closely associated to the bone stock available for fusion.[87,88] The minimum amount of bone necessary should be cut to preserve bone stock for fusion. The proximal tibia is cut perpendicular to the longitudinal axis, and posterior slope is introduced as necessary. The femur is cut to provide a limb alignment of 0 to 5 degrees of valgus. When positioned in apposition, the femoral and tibial surfaces should provide an adequate base of support with a vascular osseous bed to facilitate fusion. If the opposing surfaces of the femur and tibia do not have more than 50% contact, a variety of strategies for bone grafting may be used to augment the fusion.

Intramedullary nailing provides many advantages in certain clinical situations. Most surgeons perform nailing with a two-stage approach to prevent the propagation of organisms through the medullary canals.[88–92] However, a one-stage approach has yielded successful results when used to treat nonpurulent, gram-positive infections.[93,94] Intramedullary nailing provides the advantage of rigid fixation, immediate weightbearing, and success in the setting of severe bone loss. Currently used intramedullary nails include long nails that extend from the greater trochanter of the femur to the distal tibia, or short modular nails inserted through the knee (Figure 16-6). Nails may need to be removed if there is persistent or recurrent infection. If short modular nails are used, the fusion must be osteotomized to remove the nail; longer nails may be removed at the hip, with the fusion left undisturbed.

External fixation for arthrodesis of the infected TKA avoids the need for further soft tissue manipulation after debridement and has the advantage of leaving the joint free of interfaces that may serve as a nidus for reinfec-

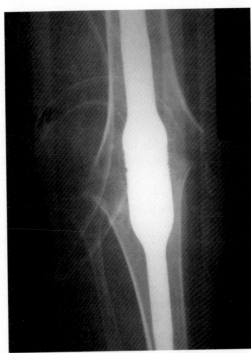

FIGURE 16-6. Radiograph after successful fusion with a short modular intramedullary nail.

tion.[88,95,96] Furthermore, the exact alignment of the extremity is more easily achieved. Although not attaining the success rate of intramedullary nailing, external fixation may be used in the setting of acute infection. Biomechanical studies have demonstrated that when a biplanar fixator is used with sagittal pins and a ventral frame, added rigidity is provided to counter the bending forces at the knee,[97] and this can enhance successful union.[88] The clinical signs of union are usually evident by 10 to 12 weeks, when the external fixator is removed and a cast is applied for 4 to 12 weeks as necessary to achieve radiologic union.

The results reported for arthrodesis after infected TKA depend on the bone stock present before fixation. Brodersen et al.[87] demonstrated an 81% rate of union when treating patients with minimally constrained prostheses, compared with 56% in patients with prostheses that sacrificed more bone stock. With less bone stock, the ability to attain stable bone apposition is diminished, creating a more difficult situation for eventual union. Therefore, in cases with severe bone loss, the more rigid fixation provided by intramedullary nailing is preferred, yielding a fusion rate of 80% to 100%.[89–92,94,98] Both single and biplane external fixators have shown a low rate of fusion under these circumstances.[88,95,99] Use of a circular small wire or hybrid external fixator has yielded very successful results (93% to 100%); however, the complica-

tions involving pin tract infection and loosening are high.[100,101]

Use of dynamic compression plates for arthrodesis has been described, but very few cases have been reported.[102] The rate of union after external fixation ranges from 17% to 100%. When comparing single-plane external fixation with biplane external fixation, a multicenter study revealed that biplane fixation provides superior results (66% union vs. 33% union).[88] Biplane external fixation has also been reported to result in a 71% rate of union out of 28 knees.[96] The results after intramedullary fixation have revealed more consistent results, which is likely a function of providing superior fixation. Numerous studies have demonstrated a success rate of 80% to 100%.[89–92,94,98] The newer nailing system was recently reported to have a 96% (51 of 53 knees) rate of successful fusion.[103]

C. Amputation

Some persistent infections that have been treated with multiple revisions, and consequent bone loss may create a situation in which further reconstructive options would be futile. This is particularly true in the setting of a compromised soft tissue envelope, a disrupted extensor mechanism, or overwhelming sepsis. Amputation is indicated when other attempts at salvaging the knee have failed and when further salvage procedures would likely be ineffective. Functional outcomes after above-the-knee amputation (AKA) for infection after TKA are poor. Sierra et al. reported on 25 AKA after TKA. Many patients in their series were never fitted with a prosthesis, and those who were seldom regained functional independence.[104]

REFERENCES

1. Bengtson S, Knutson K. The infected knee arthroplasty. A 6-year follow-up of 357 cases. *Acta Orthop Scand.* 1991; 62(4)301–311.
2. Grogan TJ, Dorey F, Rollins J, Amstutz HC. Deep sepsis following total knee arthroplasty. ten-year experience at the University of California at Los Angeles Medical Center. *J Bone Joint Surg Am.* 1986;68(2):226–234.
3. Rand JA, Bryan RS, Morrey BF, Westholm F. Management of infected total knee arthroplasty. *Clin Orthop.* 1986; 205:75–85.
4. England SP, Stern SH, Insall JN, Windsor RE. Total knee arthroplasty in diabetes mellitus. *Clin Orthop.* 1990;260: 130–134.
5. Greene KA, Wilde AH, Stulberg BN. Preoperative nutritional status of total joint patients. Relationship to postoperative wound complications. *J Arthroplasty.* 1991;6(4): 321–325.

6. Tsukayama DT, Goldberg VM, Kyle R. Diagnosis and management of infection after total knee arthroplasty. *J Bone Joint Surg Am*. 2003;85-A(Suppl 1):S75–80.

7. Hebert CK, Williams RE, Levy RS, Barrack RL. Cost of treating an infected total knee replacement. *Clin Orthop*. 1996;331:140–145.

8. Sculco TP. The economic impact of infected total joint arthroplasty. *Instr Course Lect*. 1993;42:349–351.

9. Bezwada HP, Nazarian DG, Booth RE Jr. Haemophilus influenza infection complicating a total knee arthroplasty. *Clin Orthop*. 2002;402:202–205.

10. Cierny G III, DiPasquale D. Periprosthetic total joint infections: staging, treatment, and outcomes. *Clin Orthop*. 2002;403:23–28.

11. McPherson EJ, Woodson C, Holtom P, Roidis N, Shufelt C, Patzakis M. Periprosthetic total hip infection: outcomes using a staging system. *Clin Orthop*. 2002;403:8–15.

12. Paulsen F, Pufe T, Petersen W, Tillmann B. Expression of natural peptide antibiotics in human articular cartilage and synovial membrane. *Clin Diagn Lab Immunol*. 2001; 8(5):1021–1023.

13. Paulsen F, Pufe T, Conradi L, Varoga D, Tsokos M, Papendieck J, Petersen W. Antimicrobial peptides are expressed and produced in healthy and inflamed human synovial membranes. *J Pathol*. 2002;198(3):369–377.

14. Silva M, Tharani R, Schmalzried TP. Results of direct exchange or debridement of the infected total knee arthroplasty. *Clin Orthop*. 2002;404:125–131.

15. Wyman J, McGough R, Limbird R. Fungal infection of a total knee prosthesis: successful treatment using articulating cement spacers and staged reimplantation. *Orthopedics*. 2002;25(12):1391–1394.

16. Stewart PS, Costerton JW. Antibiotic resistance of bacteria in biofilms. *Lancet*. 2001;358(9276):135–138.

17. Davies DG, Parsek MR, Pearson JP, Iglewski BH, Costerton JW, Greenberg EP. The involvement of cell-to-cell signals in the development of a bacterial biofilm. *Science*. 1998;280(5361):295–298.

18. Ramage G, Tunney MM, Patrick S, Gorman SP, Nixon JR. Formation of Propionibacterium acnes biofilms on orthopaedic biomaterials and their susceptibility to antimicrobials. *Biomaterials*. 2003;24(19):3221–3227.

19. Fitzpatrick F, Humphreys H, Smyth E, Kennedy CA, O'Gara JP. Environmental regulation of biofilm formation in intensive care unit isolates of Staphylococcus epidermidis. *J Hosp Infect*. 2002;52(3):212–218.

20. Kilgus DJ, Howe DJ, Strang A. Results of periprosthetic hip and knee infections caused by resistant bacteria. *Clin Orthop*. 2002;404:116–124.

21. McPherson EJ, Tontz W Jr, Patzakis M, Woodsome C, Holtom P, Norris L, Shufelt C. Outcome of infected total knee utilizing a staging system for prosthetic joint infection. *Am J Orthop*. 1999;28(3):161–165.

22. Garvin KL, Hanssen AD. Infection after total hip arthroplasty. past, present, and future. *J Bone Joint Surg Am*. 1995;77(10):1576–1588.

23. Windsor RE, Insall JN, Urs WK, Miller DV, Brause BD. Two-stage reimplantation for the salvage of total knee arthroplasty complicated by infection. further follow-up and refinement of indications. *J Bone Joint Surg Am*. 1990; 72(2):272–278.

24. Aalto K, Osterman K, Peltola H, Rasanen J. Changes in erythrocyte sedimentation rate and C-reactive protein after total hip arthroplasty. *Clin Orthop*. 1984;184:118–120.

25. Shih LY, Wu JJ, Yang DJ. Erythrocyte sedimentation rate and C-reactive protein values in patients with total hip arthroplasty. *Clin Orthop*. 1987;225:238–246.

26. Levitsky KA, Hozack WJ, Balderston RA, Rothman RH, Gluckman SJ, Maslack MM, Booth RE Jr. Evaluation of the painful prosthetic joint. relative value of bone scan, sedimentation rate, and joint aspiration. *J Arthroplasty*. 1991;6(3):237–244.

27. Spangehl MJ, Masri BA, O'Connell JX, Duncan CP. Prospective analysis of preoperative and intraoperative investigations for the diagnosis of infection at the sites of two hundred and two revision total hip arthroplasties. *J Bone Joint Surg Am*. 1999;81(5):672–683.

28. Rand JA, Brown ML. The value of indium 111 leukocyte scanning in the evaluation of painful or infected total knee arthroplasties. *Clin Orthop*. 1990;259:179–182.

29. Scher DM, Pak K, Lonner JH, Finkel JE, Zuckerman JD, Di Cesare PE. The predictive value of indium-111 leukocyte scans in the diagnosis of infected total hip, knee, or resection arthroplasties. *J Arthroplasty*. 2000;15(3): 295–300.

30. Joseph TN, Mujtaba M, Chen AL, Maurer SL, Zuckerman JD, Maldjian C, Di Cesare PE. Efficacy of combined technetium-99m sulfur colloid/indium-111 leukocyte scans to detect infected total hip and knee arthroplasties. *J Arthroplasty*. 2001;16(6):753–758.

31. Palestro CJ, Swyer AJ, Kim CK, Goldsmith SJ. Infected knee prosthesis: diagnosis with In-111 leukocyte, Tc-99m sulfur colloid, and Tc-99m MDP imaging. *Radiology*. 1991;179(3):645–648.

32. Barrack RL, Harris WH. The value of aspiration of the hip joint before revision total hip arthroplasty. *J Bone Joint Surg Am*. 1993;75(1):66–76.

33. Duff GP, Lachiewicz PF, Kelley SS. Aspiration of the knee joint before revision arthroplasty. *Clin Orthop*. 1996;331: 132–139.

34. Windsor RE, Bono JV. Infected total knee replacements. *J Am Acad Orthop Surg*. 1994;2(1):44–53.

35. Morrey BF, Westholm F, Schoifet S, Rand JA, Bryan RS. Long-term results of various treatment options for infected total knee arthroplasty. *Clin Orthop*. 1989;248: 120–128.

36. Barrack RL, Jennings RW, Wolfe MW, Bertot AJ. The Coventry Award. the value of preoperative aspiration before total knee revision. *Clin Orthop.* 1997;345:8–16.

37. Mariani BD, Martin DS, Levine MJ, Booth RE Jr, Tuan RS. The Coventry Award. Polymerase chain reaction detection of bacterial infection in total knee arthroplasty. *Clin Orthop.* 1996;331:11–22.

38. Lonner JH, Desai P, Dicesare PE, Steiner G, Zuckerman JD. The reliability of analysis of intraoperative frozen sections for identifying active infection during revision hip or knee arthroplasty. *J Bone Joint Surg Am.* 1996;78(10):1553–1558.

39. Feldman DS, Lonner JH, Desai P, Zuckerman JD. The role of intraoperative frozen sections in revision total joint arthroplasty. *J Bone Joint Surg Am.* 1995;77(12):1807–1813.

40. Fehring TK, McAlister JA Jr. Frozen histologic section as a guide to sepsis in revision joint arthroplasty. *Clin Orthop.* 1994;304:229–237.

41. Lonner JH, Beck TD Jr, Rees H, Roullet M, Lotke PA. Results of two-stage revision of the infected total knee arthroplasty. *Am J Knee Surg.* 2001;14(1):65–67.

42. Johnson DP, Bannister GC. The outcome of infected arthroplasty of the knee. *J Bone Joint Surg Br.* 1986;68(2):289–291.

43. Marsh PK, Cotler JM. Management of an anaerobic infection in a prosthetic knee with long-term antibiotics alone: a case report. *Clin Orthop.* 1981;155:133–135.

44. Brandt CM, Duffy MC, Berbari EF, Hanssen AD, Steckelberg JM, Osmon DR. Staphylococcus aureus prosthetic joint infection treated with prosthesis removal and delayed reimplantation arthroplasty. *Mayo Clin Proc.* 1999;74(6):553–558.

45. Burger RR, Basch T, Hopson CN. Implant salvage in infected total knee arthroplasty. *Clin Orthop.* 1991;273:105–112.

46. Hartman MB, Fehring TK, Jordan L, Norton HJ. Periprosthetic knee sepsis. the role of irrigation and debridement. *Clin Orthop.* 1991;273:113–118.

47. Mont MA, Waldman B, Banerjee C, Pacheco IH, Hungerford DS. Multiple irrigation, debridement, and retention of components in infected total knee arthroplasty. *J Arthroplasty.* 1997;12(4):426–433.

48. Schoifet SD, Morrey BF. Treatment of infection after total knee arthroplasty by debridement with retention of the components. *J Bone Joint Surg Am.* 1990;72(9):1383–1390.

49. Tattevin P, Cremieux AC, Pottier P, Huten D, Carbon C. Prosthetic joint infection: when can prosthesis salvage be considered? *Clin Infect Dis.* 1999;29(2):292–295.

50. Teeny SM, Dorr L, Murata G, Conaty P. Treatment of infected total knee arthroplasty. Irrigation and debridement versus two-stage reimplantation. *J Arthroplasty.* 1990;5(1):35–39.

51. Waldman BJ, Hostin E, Mont MA, Hungerford DS. Infected total knee arthroplasty treated by arthroscopic irrigation and debridement. *J Arthroplasty.* 2000;15(4):430–436.

52. Deirmengian CA, Greenbaum J, Lotke PA, Booth REJ, Lonner JH. Limited success with open debridement and retention of components in the treatment of acute S. aureus infections after total knee arthroplasty. *J Arthroplasty.* 2003. (Awaiting publication).

53. Wilson MG, Kelley K, Thornhill TS. Infection as a complication of total knee-replacement arthroplasty. risk factors and treatment in sixty-seven cases. *J Bone Joint Surg Am.* 1990;72(6):878–883.

54. Flood JN, Kolarik DB. Arthroscopic irrigation and debridement of infected total knee arthroplasty: report of two cases. *Arthroscopy.* 1988;4(3):182–186.

55. Vidil A, Beaufils P. [Arthroscopic treatment of hematogenous infected total knee arthroplasty: 5 cases.] *Rev Chir Orthop Reparatrice Appar Mot.* 2002;88(5):493–500.

56. Wasielewski RC, Barden RM, Rosenberg AG. Results of different surgical procedures on total knee arthroplasty infections. *J Arthroplasty.* 1996;11(8):931–938.

57. Borden LS, Gearen PF. Infected total knee arthroplasty. a protocol for management. *J Arthroplasty.* 1987;2(1):27–36.

58. Freeman MA, Sudlow RA, Casewell MW, Radcliff SS. The management of infected total knee replacements. *J Bone Joint Surg Br.* 1985;67(5):764–768.

59. Hanssen AD, Trousdale RT, Osmon DR. Patient outcome with reinfection following reimplantation for the infected total knee arthroplasty. *Clin Orthop.* 1995;321:55–67.

60. Lu H, Kou B, Lin J. [One-stage reimplantation for the salvage of total knee arthroplasty complicated by infection]. *Zhonghua Wai Ke Za Zhi.* 1997;35(8):456–458.

61. von Foerster G, Kluber D, Kabler U. [Mid- to long-term results after treatment of 118 cases of periprosthetic infections after knee joint replacement using one-stage exchange surgery.] *Orthopade.* 1991;20(3):244–252.

62. Goksan SB, Freeman MA. One-stage reimplantation for infected total knee arthroplasty. *J Bone Joint Surg Br.* 1992;74(1):78–82.

63. Booth RE Jr, Lotke PA. The results of spacer block technique in revision of infected total knee arthroplasty. *Clin Orthop.* 1989;248:57–60.

64. Goldman RT, Scuderi GR, Insall JN. 2-stage reimplantation for infected total knee replacement. *Clin Orthop.* 1996;331:118–124.

65. Hanssen AD, Rand JA, Osmon DR. Treatment of the infected total knee arthroplasty with insertion of another prosthesis. the effect of antibiotic-impregnated bone cement. *Clin Orthop.* 1994;309:44–55.

66. Masri BA, Kendall RW, Duncan CP, Beauchamp CP, McGraw RW, Bora B. Two-stage exchange arthroplasty

using a functional antibiotic-loaded spacer in the treatment of the infected knee replacement: the Vancouver experience. *Semin Arthroplasty.* 1994;5(3):122–136.

67. Wilde AH, Ruth JT. Two-stage reimplantation in infected total knee arthroplasty. *Clin Orthop.* 1988;236:23–35.

68. Haddad FS, Masri BA, Campbell D, McGraw RW, Beauchamp CP, Duncan CP. The PROSTALAC functional spacer in two-stage revision for infected knee replacements. Prosthesis of antibiotic-loaded acrylic cement. *J Bone Joint Surg Br.* 2000;82(6):807–812.

69. Henderson MH Jr, Booth RE Jr. The use of an antibiotic-impregnated spacer block for revision of the septic total knee arthroplasty. *Semin Arthroplasty.* 1991;2(1):34–39.

70. Hirakawa K, Stulberg BN, Wilde AH, Bauer TW, Secic M. Results of 2-stage reimplantation for infected total knee arthroplasty. *J Arthroplasty.* 1998;13(1):22–28.

71. Insall JN, Thompson FM, Brause BD. Two-stage reimplantation for the salvage of infected total knee arthroplasty. *J Bone Joint Surg Am.* 1983;65(8):1087–1098.

72. McPherson EJ, Patzakis MJ, Gross JE, Holtom PD, Song M, Dorr LD. Infected total knee arthroplasty. two-stage reimplantation with a gastrocnemius rotational flap. *Clin Orthop.* 1997;341:73–81.

73. Rosenberg AG, Haas B, Barden R, Marquez D, Landon GC, Galante JO. Salvage of infected total knee arthroplasty. *Clin Orthop.* 1988;226:29–33.

74. Rand JA, Bryan RS. Reimplantation for the salvage of an infected total knee arthroplasty. *J Bone Joint Surg Am.* 1983;65(8):1081–1086.

75. Emerson RH Jr, Muncie M, Tarbox TR, Higgins LL. Comparison of a static with a mobile spacer in total knee infection. *Clin Orthop.* 2002;404:132–138.

76. Fehring TK, Odum S, Calton TF, Mason JB. Articulating versus static spacers in revision total knee arthroplasty for sepsis. The Ranawat Award. *Clin Orthop.* 2000;380: 9–16.

77. Hofmann AA, Kane KR, Tkach TK, Plaster RL, Camargo MP. Treatment of infected total knee arthroplasty using an articulating spacer. *Clin Orthop.* 1995;321:45–54.

78. Masri BA, Duncan CP, Beauchamp CP. Long-term elution of antibiotics from bone-cement: an in vivo study using the prosthesis of antibiotic-loaded acrylic cement (PROSTALAC) system. *J Arthroplasty.* 1998;13(3): 331–338.

79. Nelson CL. Primary and delayed exchange for infected total knee arthroplasty. *Am J Knee Surg.* 2001;14(1):60–64.

80. Lonner JH. Identifying ongoing infection after resection arthroplasty and before second-stage reimplantation. *Am J Knee Surg.* 2001;14(1):68–71.

81. Pellegrini VD Jr. Management of the patient with an infected knee arthroplasty. *Instr Course Lect.* 1997;46: 215–219.

82. Della Valle CJ, Bogner E, Desai P, Lonner JH, Adler E, Zuckerman JD, Di Cesare PE. Analysis of frozen sections of intraoperative specimens obtained at the time of reoperation after hip or knee resection arthroplasty for the treatment of infection. *J Bone Joint Surg Am.* 1999;81(5): 684–689.

83. Banit DM, Kaufer H, Hartford JM. Intraoperative frozen section analysis in revision total joint arthroplasty. *Clin Orthop.* 2002;401:230–238.

84. Lonner JH, Siliski JM, Della Valle C, DiCesare P, Lotke PA. Role of knee aspiration after resection of the infected total knee arthroplasty. *Am J Orthop.* 2001;30(4): 305–309.

85. Mont MA, Waldman BJ, Hungerford DS. Evaluation of preoperative cultures before second-stage reimplantation of a total knee prosthesis complicated by infection. a comparison-group study. *J Bone Joint Surg Am.* 2000;82-A(11): 1552–1557.

86. Falahee MH, Matthews LS, Kaufer H. Resection arthroplasty as a salvage procedure for a knee with infection after a total arthroplasty. *J Bone Joint Surg Am.* 1987;69(7): 1013–1021.

87. Brodersen MP, Fitzgerald RH Jr, Peterson LF, Coventry MB, Bryan RS. Arthrodesis of the knee following failed total knee arthroplasty. *J Bone Joint Surg Am.* 1979;61(2): 181–185.

88. Knutson K, Hovelius L, Lindstrand A, Lidgren L. Arthrodesis after failed knee arthroplasty. a nationwide multicenter investigation of 91 cases. *Clin Orthop.* 1984; 191:202–211.

89. Donley BG, Matthews LS, Kaufer H. Arthrodesis of the knee with an intramedullary nail. *J Bone Joint Surg Am.* 1991;73(6):907–913.

90. Ellingsen DE, Rand JA. Intramedullary arthrodesis of the knee after failed total knee arthroplasty. *J Bone Joint Surg Am.* 1994;76(6):870–877.

91. Incavo SJ, Lilly JW, Bartlett CS, Churchill DL. Arthrodesis of the knee: experience with intramedullary nailing. *J Arthroplasty.* 2000;15(7):871–876.

92. Waldman BJ, Mont MA, Payman KR, Freiberg AA, Windsor RE, Sculco TP, Hungerford DS. Infected total knee arthroplasty treated with arthrodesis using a modular nail. *Clin Orthop.* 1999;367:230–237.

93. Lai KA, Shen WJ, Yang CY. Arthrodesis with a short Huckstep nail as a salvage procedure for failed total knee arthroplasty. *J Bone Joint Surg Am.* 1998;80(3): 380–388.

94. Puranen J, Kortelainen P, Jalovaara P. Arthrodesis of the knee with intramedullary nail fixation. *J Bone Joint Surg Am.* 1990;72(3):433–442.

95. Hak DJ, Lieberman JR, Finerman GA. Single plane and biplane external fixators for knee arthrodesis. *Clin Orthop.* 1995;316:134–144.

96. Rand JA, Bryan RS, Chao EY. Failed total knee arthroplasty treated by arthrodesis of the knee using the Ace-Fischer apparatus. *J Bone Joint Surg Am.* 1987;69(1):39–45.

97. Knutson K, Bodelind B, Lidgren L. Stability of external fixators used for knee arthrodesis after failed knee arthroplasty. *Clin Orthop.* 1984;186:90–95.

98. Harris CM, Froehlich J. Knee fusion with intramedullary rods for failed total knee arthroplasty. *Clin Orthop.* 1985; 197:209–216.

99. Bengston S, Knutson K, Lidgren L. Treatment of infected knee arthroplasty. *Clin Orthop.* 1989;245:173–178.

100. Garberina MJ, Fitch RD, Hoffmann ED, Hardaker WT, Vail TP, Scully SP. Knee arthrodesis with circular external fixation. *Clin Orthop.* 2001;382:168–178.

101. Oostenbroek HJ, van Roermund PM. Arthrodesis of the knee after an infected arthroplasty using the Ilizarov method. *J Bone Joint Surg Br.* 2001;83(1):50–54.

102. Nichols SJ, Landon GC, Tullos HS. Arthrodesis with dual plates after failed total knee arthroplasty. *J Bone Joint Surg Am.* 1991;73(7):1020–1024.

103. Christie MJ, DeBoer DK, McQueen DA, Cooke FW, Hahn DL. Salvage procedures for failed total knee arthroplasty. *J Bone Joint Surg Am.* 2003;85-A(Suppl 1):S58–62.

104. Sierra RJ, Trousdale RT; Pagnano MW. Above-the-knee amputation after a total knee replacement: prevalence, etiology, and functional outcome. *J Bone Joint Surg Am.* 2003;85-A(6):1000–1004.

CHAPTER 17

Periprosthetic Fractures After Total Knee Arthroplasty

Michael E. Ayers, Richard Iorio, and William L. Healy

Periprosthetic fractures of the femur, tibia, or patella around a knee replacement are relatively uncommon. However, when these fractures occur, they are associated with considerable discomfort and disability. These fractures can be difficult to treat, and the rate of complications is high, ranging from 25% to 75% for both operative and nonoperative treatment.[1,2]

The Mayo Clinic Joint Registry documented 573 periprosthetic fractures following 19810 primary and revision knee replacement operations for an incidence of 2.8%.[3] Following primary total knee arthroplasty (TKA), the incidence of periprosthetic fracture was 2.3%, and after revision TKA, the incidence of periprosthetic fracture was 6.3%.[3]

The reported incidence of periprosthetic distal femur fractures ranges from 0.3% to 2.5%.[4] The prevalence of proximal tibial fractures is less than the distal femur. Thirty-two tibia fractures around knee replacements were reported from 1970 to 1992,[5] and the prevalence has been reported from 0.4% to 1.7%.[1] The incidence of periprosthetic patellar fractures has been reported at 0.05% when the patella is not resurfaced,[6] and with patella resurfacing, the incidence ranges from 0.2% to 21%.[6–21] The Mayo Clinic series documents 85 patella fractures out of 12464 consecutive TKAs, for an incidence of 0.68%.[21]

During the next decade, it is likely that the number of TKA operations in the United States will increase. The population is growing and aging; the prevalence of arthritic knees is increasing; and the success of knee replacements in patients of all ages is well documented.[22] The volume of TKA operations is predicted to nearly double by 2030 to 474319 knee replacement operations.[23] Considering that elderly patients are having more knee replacements, these patients are maintaining active lifestyles, and elderly patients have risks of osteopenia and falls, it is reasonable to predict an increase in periprosthetic fractures around knee replacements in the next decade.

An understanding of several factors involved with periprosthetic fractures can help in prevention, diagnosis, and treatment of these fractures and their potential complications. These factors include deformity, osteoporosis and osteopenia, rheumatoid arthritis, steroid use, neuromuscular disorders, previous surgery, revision surgery, surgical technique, component positioning, component design, stress risers from screw holes, and osteolysis.[24] Major concerns with treatment of these fractures are timing of the fracture (intraoperative or postoperative), type of fracture (condylar, intercondylar, supracondylar), stability of component fixation, and the activity and medical condition of the patient.

In this chapter, we discuss fractures of the femur, proximal tibia, and patella adjacent to a total knee arthroplasty. The discussion of fractures is subdivided by anatomic location and whether they occur intraoperatively or postoperatively. Postoperative fractures can be further divided into traumatic and stress-related fractures. Intraoperative fractures occur less often than postoperative fractures, and they are more common with revision TKA operations than during primary total knee arthroplasty. These fractures are often minimally displaced and lack extensive soft tissue trauma. If recognized they can be adequately stabilized, and neither the rehabilitation nor the outcome need be significantly impacted.[5]

PROXIMAL AND MIDSHAFT FEMUR FRACTURES

Although uncommon, proximal femur fractures in the femoral head, femoral neck, or intertrochanteric area can be caused during TKA by exuberant impaction of femoral trials or implants in an osteopenic patient.[25,26] These fractures are rare; they can occur in patients with osteopenic bone; and they are apt to be missed if not suspected. A delay in postoperative mobilization or pain with weightbearing in the groin or thigh should evoke suspicion for a proximal femur fracture. These fractures must be treated appropriately to progress to weightbearing and rehabilitation of the total knee arthroplasty.

Femoral shaft fractures occurring during knee replacement operations can be related to intramedullary guide rod insertion or insertion of oversized stems on femoral implants. Enlargement of the distal femoral drill hole and careful, slow placement of the intramedullary guide rod can usually avert perforation of the femoral shaft. Analysis of preoperative radiographs ensures proper placement of the distal femoral hole, especially in cases of bony deformity. If femoral canal perforation occurs and goes undetected it can affect the alignment of the reconstruction and create a stress riser in the femur. Fluoroscopy or intraoperative radiographs can be helpful in preventing femoral shaft perforation and fracture when placing large stemmed implants in osteopenic patients. When these fractures occur, supplementary fixation using plates, wires and or cortical strut bone grafts may be necessary to ensure stability.

DISTAL FEMUR FRACTURES

Intraoperative Distal Femur Fractures

The occurrence of condylar and supracondylar fractures during TKA can be associated with surgical technique, bone stock, and component design. Femoral notching decreases the torsional strength of the distal femur by 29% to 39%,[27,28] and osteopenia further decreases torsional load to failure in notched femurs[29] (Figure 17-1). However, there is controversy regarding whether femoral notching increases the incidence of periprosthetic fracture of the distal femur.[30,31]

The intercondylar box cut in posterior stabilized knee implant designs can be a source of fracture. If the notch is not deep enough or wide enough to accommodate the implant, a fracture can occur when the femoral trial or implant is impacted.[32] Medial placement of the femoral component can increase this risk, and most of these fractures occur at the medial condyle. Failure to enlarge the depth of the box when changing to a more constrained implant requiring a deeper box can also predispose to fracture on component insertion.

Treatment of intraoperative distal femur fractures requires radiographic definition of the fracture and sufficient surgical exposure of the fracture to achieve stable fixation. During revision knee replacement operation,

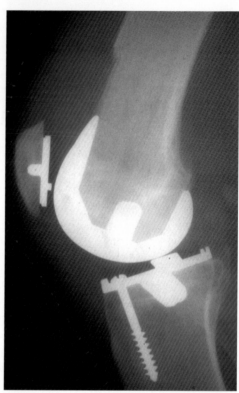

FIGURE 17-1. Lateral radiograph shows a worrisome anterior notch on the distal femur, which could place this patient at higher risk for fracture. The surgical technique was also compromised by an asymmetric patella osteotomy.

intraoperative fracture should be anticipated as a possible challenge and, implants to bypass the metaphyseal area should be available. Compression screw fixation of a condylar or transcondylar fracture may be adequate for nondisplaced fractures. A stemmed femoral component is usually indicated to stabilize the condyle to the diaphysis in displaced or comminuted fractures.[5] Stems should be long enough to reach the metaphyseal/diaphyseal narrowing and wide enough so that flutes can provide rotational stability. Bone cement may be used to augment stem fixation, but it may also interfere with fracture healing, and cement use should be limited at or proximal to the fracture. When fracture of the distal femur is encountered, protected weightbearing should be considered during the early postoperative period.[5]

Postoperative Distal Femur Fractures

The etiology of most periprosthetic fractures of the femur is trauma. Older patients with osteoporosis are susceptible to injury with low-energy accidents such as falls or twisting. Younger more active patients with knee replacements are more likely to encounter high-energy trauma causing a periprosthetic fracture. Restricted knee range of flexion increases the risk of periprosthetic fracture of the distal femur.[33]

Several classification systems describe periprosthetic distal femur fractures. In the Lewis and Rorabeck[34] classification (Figure 17-2), type I is a nondisplaced fracture with a well-fixed intact knee implant; type II is a displaced fracture with an intact implant; and type III is either a displaced or nondisplaced fracture, but the prosthesis is loose or failing due to instability or bearing surface wear.

Pain-free function is the goal of treatment of periprosthetic fractures of the distal femur. A well-healed fracture, with appropriate coronal (+/– 5 degrees) and

FIGURE 17-2. Lewis and Rorabeck classification of supracondylar periprosthetic fractures proximal to total knee arthroplasty. (A) Type I: Undisplaced fracture—prosthesis intact. (B) Type II: Displaced fracture—prosthesis intact. (C and D) Type III: Displaced or undisplaced fracture—Prosthesis loose or failing (i.e., significant instability or polyethylene wear). (Adapted from Rorabeck, Taylor,[35] by permission of *Orthop Clin North Am.*)

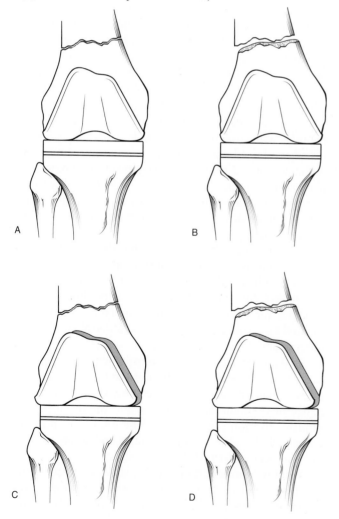

sagittal (+/– 10 degrees) alignment and adequate range of motion (90 degrees), represents successful treatment. Some shortening (up to 2 cm) of the femur may be accepted.[33] Nonoperative and operative methods of treatment have been reported.[1,2,4,5,35] Unfortunately, with many studies, small numbers of patients, long study intervals up to 20 years, and varied techniques, it is difficult to draw firm conclusions regarding optimal treatment. Three review studies [2,4,36] looked at displaced fracture treatment in the 1980s and found generally mediocre results; 56% to 68% satisfactory results were reported for nonoperative treatment and 66.7% to 69% for operative treatment. A recent summary of results of nonoperative and surgical management in 393 periprosthetic distal femur fractures in the English language literature demonstrates surgical management to be preferable with 70% to 80% good results compared with less than 60% good results for nonoperative treatment.[37] Improvements in surgical techniques and numerous studies support a more recent trend toward operative treatment.[35]

The stability of knee implant fixation is a key factor in selection of treatment of periprosthetic distal femur fractures, and stability should be determined preoperatively. Adequate radiographs are essential. If the prosthesis is stable, treatment can focus on appropriate fixation of the specific fracture. If the femoral implant is not stable and well fixed to bone, revision of the component must accompany fracture fixation, and the possibility of using allograft or tumor type, constrained prosthetic reconstruction should be considered.

Nonoperative treatment with a cast or brace can be considered for Lewis-Rorabeck type I fractures. The patient must have suitable strength to safely maintain protected weightbearing until the fracture is healed. Early range of motion exercises are key to optimal outcome but also greatly increase the chances of malunion or nonunion. Close radiographic follow-up is essential. Nonoperative treatment of nondisplaced periprosthetic distal femur fractures produced 83% successful outcomes in a literature review of 30 fractures.[2] However, many of these results were not reported in terms of knee motion. The results of bracing with early limited motion have not been adequately reported.[5]

Operative treatment should be considered if fracture position becomes unacceptable during nonoperative treatment, if the patient is unable to perform protected weightbearing in a type I fracture, or for a type II fracture. Fracture fixation devices include extramedullary plates, intramedullary rods, and external fixators. Adjuncts to operative treatment include bone graft or polymethylmethacrylate (PMMA) to augment fixation of the fracture fragments and allograft femoral bone struts (Figure 17-3). When operative treatment includes frac-

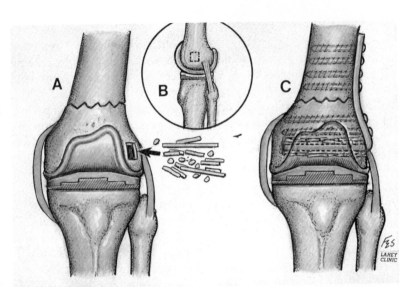

FIGURE 17-3. For patients with extreme osteopenia in the distal condylar fragment, polymethyl-methacrylate or bone graft may be used to augment distal fixation of the fracture implant. (A) A window is made in the lateral distal condyle, and bone graft is packed into the metaphysis. (B) Lateral view. (C) Fracture fixation with implant in place and augmentation of distal fixation with bone graft.

ture fixation and revision TKA, combinations of fracture fixation devices and stemmed femoral implants can be used to achieve a stable reconstruction of the knee.

Open reduction and internal fixation of periprosthetic fractures of the distal femur offer the potential for anatomic reduction of the fracture and a stable reconstruction of the knee to allow early motion and functional rehabilitation. The challenge of osteosynthesis with plates and screws is to respect the biology of fracture healing. All of these devices are placed in an extramedullary position that can disrupt the vascular supply of fracture fragments. The technique of surgical approach and fracture reduction is critical to achieving bony union. Options for fracture fixation include blade plates, condylar screw plates, condylar buttress plates, and locked condylar plates. Condylar buttress plates offer the most flexible fixation with multiple variable angle screws; however, condylar plates are not as stable as fixed-angle plates, and they can be associated with early fracture motion and failure. Double plating can enhance fracture stability, but it can also lead to extensive devascularization. The dynamic condylar screw was shown to be the strongest device in a biomechanical study using synthetic bone.[38] This strength requires firm purchase of the large screw in the distal condyle, which can be difficult in elderly patients with osteoporosis. The blade plate is a fixed-angle device with a low profile, which is preferred in distal fractures. The blade plate also has a large surface area of contact that is helpful in osteoporotic bone. However, insertion of the blade plate can be technically challenging. Locked condylar plating combines the flexibility of a condylar buttress plate with the strength of a fixed angle device. Screws can be locked to the plate both proximally and distally. The LISS (Less Invasive Stabilization System, Synthes, Oberdorf, Switzerland) takes this a step further. It can be placed through a minimally invasive technique, which has the potential to reduce blood loss and operative time. The device is designed to be placed percutaneously with the use of multiple fixed-angle screws distally and fixed-angle unicortical screws proximally. All screws are placed through an accurate guide system. The percutaneous nature of this system limits its ability to aid in reduction and significant efforts to align the fracture with traction and manipulation must be carried out before its use.

Periprosthetic fractures of the distal femur can present technical challenges during operative treatment, which requires special techniques in addition to plates and screws. Insufficient bone stock of the distal femoral condyles for fixation of fracture implants can be augmented by a cortical window in the femoral condyle for the introduction of bone graft or cement[39,40] (Figure 17-3). Anterior-to-posterior interfragmentary lag screws can be used to enhance fixation of the fracture. In some cases, a blade plate can be wedged between the anterior flange of the femoral component and the distal lugs to improve fixation (Figure 17-4). The use of an intramedullary fibular graft to enhance plate and screw fixation has also been described.[41]

Potential complications with plate and screw treatment of the distal femur include loss of fixation, malunion, nonunion, hardware migration, poor motion, and infection. Early studies of ORIF showed a high incidence of fixation failure and complications.[42–45]

More recent studies have shown improved results, likely related to the use of fixed-angle devices and adjuncts to fixation.[39,40] The use of cerclaged cortical allograft struts medially and posteriorly along with a lateral blade plate or dynamic condylar screw (DCS) provided satisfactory results in 9 of 10 patients in one study. Five of these patients had failed a previous fixation attempt, and average healing time was 17.6 weeks. One infection was reported.[46] A preliminary study of the LISS system was conducted in 13 patients. One required secondary bone graft and one required revision TKA due to loosening. No cases of varus collapse or distal condylar screw loosening and no infections were reported. Mean time to full weightbearing was 13 weeks.[47]

Flexible intramedullary devices have been suggested as satisfatory treatment for periprosthetic fracture of the distal femur by Ritter et al.[48] These rods can be inserted with a minimally invasive technique with limited morbidity. Flexible intramedullary rods are internal splints, and they do not offer adequate rotational or axial stability for unstable fracture patterns. While this technique can be successful, fracture reduction, stable fixation, and early motion may be difficult to achieve with flexible intramedullary rods.

Rigid intramedullary devices with locking screw capability offer an attractive alternative for type I and II periprosthetic fractures of the distal femur in which the femoral implant is well fixed to bone. They can be inserted with a less invasive technique than open reduction and internal fixation with plates and screws. Furthermore, orthopedic surgeons who use the retrograde intramedullary devices in trauma surgery are familiar with this technique. The fracture hematoma can be avoided, there is minimal periosteal stripping, and the

FIGURE 17-4. (A and B) A healed fracture in a woman with severe osteopenia and ankylosing spondylitis 6 months after open reduction internal fixation and bone grafting. Fracture is healed. To achieve fixation of the blade in the distal condylar fragment, femoral head allograft was packed into the condyles and the blade was wedged between the anterior femoral flange and the lugs. The bone graft can be seen as sclerotic bone distal to the blade plate.

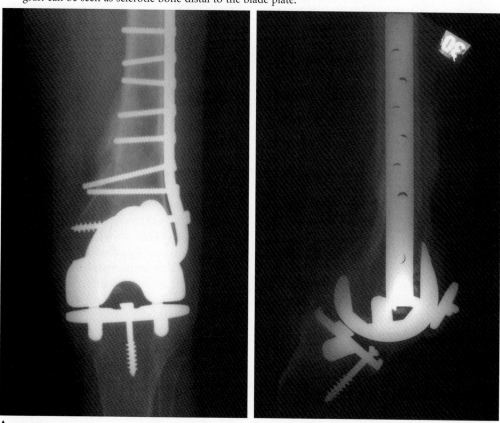

A   B

zone of injury is bridged, allowing optimal biology for healing.[1,36] The insertion of the rod can also often aid in achieving satisfactory reduction and alignment. When adequate proximal and distal locking are possible, axial, angular, and rotational stability can be attained. The most distal transcondylar fractures and fractures in osteopenic bone may not be successfully treated with this technique. Newer devices offer very distal locking holes that can be helpful. Extreme distal locking screw fixation can also be achieved by leaving the locked rod 1 cm proud within the knee and cutting it off with a bur.[36] Distal locking bolts are also available that can enhance distal fixation in the osteoporotic patient.

When locked intramedullary rods are used for periprosthetic distal femur fractures, the surgeon must know the manufacturer and dimensions of the existing well-fixed femoral component. The intercondylar distance of the posterior cruciate retaining total knee determines the size rod that can be placed. In a well-fixed posterior stabilized component the intercondylar box blocks access to the medullary canal. A technique of opening the box with a diamond-tip metal-cutting bur to allow access for an intramedullary rod has been described.[49]

When stable fixation is achieved with an intramedullary rod, early range of motion and ambulation with protected weightbearing are possible. In osteopenic patients, early motion may be possible, but weightbearing should be delayed. A recent review of 4 studies and 19 cases revealed 100% union, no malalignment, and minimal complications with the use of IM fixation.[1] Complications can include loss of fixation, malunion, shortening, and/or migration of the rod into the knee, and infection. Contraindications include the presence of a long stem hip prosthesis and very distal fractures.

External fixation has also been reported as a successful treatment for periprosthetic distal femur fractures.[50,51] However, the inherent risks of external fixation make it a less than optimal choice for this indication. The need to place pins intra-articularly can lead to infection, and pin placement in the quadriceps muscle can reduce motion.

Type III periprosthetic distal femur fractures involve a loose or failing implant. These fractures can be nondisplaced or displaced. If the fracture can be stabilized to achieve union, it may be advantageous to fix the fracture and revise the knee implants at a later date. The advantage of this approach is the relative ease of a revision in the face of a healed and thus nonmobile distal femur as well as conservation of bone stock and avoidance of the need for allografts and constrained prostheses.[5] Unfortunately, many type III fractures are very distal, and they

occur in elderly patients with osteoporosis. When stable fixation allowing mobilization in the face of a loose or failing component is unlikely, the possibility of revision knee replacement must be planned for and appropriate implants and grafts must be available at the time of operation.

Revision TKA in the face of periprosthetic fracture is a considerable technical challenge. Care must be taken to restore the tibiofemoral joint line and normal rotation of the femoral component. Stable patellar and tibial components can be retained if they are compatible with the design of the revised femur. Revision options depend on the bone stock of the distal femur. As more condylar bone is lost to fracture comminution or attempts to remove the existing femoral component, allograft-prosthesis can be considered to replace bone loss in the distal femur. When possible, implant fixation can be obtained in the diaphysis with press-fit stems. The use of cement in the diaphysis is discouraged because it may interfere with fracture healing. Wedges and blocks allow for reconstruction of smaller defects, and bone graft should be used. As the amount of bone and soft tissue injured increases, stability becomes a major concern and constrained or rotating hinge prostheses become a necessity. Another option in the face of severe bone loss is the use of a hinged prosthesis. When cemented, this can allow for immediate range of motion and weightbearing in a very elderly and low-demand patient.

Most studies of revision TKA for periprosthetic fractures are small and while satisfactory results can be obtained, complications are common.[52,53] A meta-analysis reported 10 satisfactory results out of 11 patients treated with revision TKA for periprosthetic supracondylar femur fracture.[2] This same study reported a 30% complication rate for both nonsurgical and surgical management all types of these fractures. Nonunion and malunion were common, and infection was reported as high as 8%. This is a devastating complication, possibly leading to amputation or loss of life.

In summary, periprosthetic distal femur fractures greater than 4 cm above a well-fixed femoral implant can be successfully treated with extramedullary fixed metal plates or intramedullary locking rods. The use of intramedullary rods is increasing and can produce successful outcomes when used appropriately. When the femoral canal, the femoral component, or the fracture pattern is not *rod friendly* or if the fracture is very distal, blade plate treatment is preferred, and the surgeon should have a low threshold for bone grafting. The early results of newer techniques like LISS plates are encouraging and await further study. In cases of femoral component loosening, revision TKA is generally required to treat periprosthetic fracture of the distal femur.

PROXIMAL TIBIAL FRACTURES

The Mayo Clinic classification of periprosthetic tibial fractures (Figure 17-5) describes the anatomic location in relation to the anterior tibial tubercle, timing of the fracture (intraoperative or postoperative) and whether the component is well fixed or loose.[54] A type 1 fracture is at the tibial plateau; type 2 fractures involve the area adjacent to the stem of the tibial component; a type 3 fracture is distal to the stem; and a type 4 fracture involves the tibial tubercle. The fracture subtype is based on when the fracture occurs and whether or not the component is stable. Subtypes A and B proximal tibial fractures occur postoperatively. In subtype A the prosthesis is well fixed and in subtype B the prosthesis is loose. Subtype C fractures of the proximal tibia occur interoperatively.

Intraoperative Proximal Tibia Fractures

Intraoperative proximal tibia periprosthetic fractures can occur with aggressive positioning of bone retractors, during cement removal in revision TKA, during medullary preparation for a stemmed component, with insertion of the stemmed component, at trial reduction, during impaction of the tibial implant or with torsional stress on the lower leg.[54] Type 1C tibial plateau fractures and type 2C metaphyseal fractures are generally treated with a longer-stem prosthesis to bypass the fracture when recognized. Type 1C fractures can often be stabilized with a cancellous bone screw. Type 2C fractures occur during cement removal in revisions or at stem insertion. These are often vertical and nondisplaced. If nondisplaced, they can be treated with protected weightbearing, and early motion with or without a brace.[5] Type 3 fractures distal to the stem need to be individualized based on the location. They often need ORIF if displaced. If nondisplaced and stable these fractures can often be treated with bracing and nonweightbearing[54] or weightbearing in a patella tendon bearing cast.[5] Tibial tubercle fractures are best avoided with careful techniques including medial dissection to the midcoronal plane and consideration of a quadriceps snip or tubercle osteotomy. If a type 4 tibial tubercle fracture occurs, it needs to be securely fixed with screws or wires and protected for 6 weeks.[33] In the revision setting these can be quite severe due to extensive osteolysis, and salvage with an extensor tendon allograft is a possible option.[55]

Postoperative Proximal Tibia Fractures

Tibial stress fractures were reported by Rand and Coventry in 1980. They described 15 medial tibial plateau fractures occurring distal to Geomedic and Polycentric knee implants (Howmedica, Mahwah, NJ). These type 1B tibial plateau fractures were associated with axial malalignment due to incorrect component positioning. The tibial components loosened and revision was required in all cases.[56] While mostly related to older designs, these fractures have

FIGURE 17-5. Classification of periprosthetic fractures whereby selection of anatomic location combined with a subtype provides description of a specific fracture treatment group. Determination of subtypes includes timing of the fracture and the status of prosthesis fixation. Postoperative subtypes A and B are determined by whether the prosthesis is well fixed or loose, whereas subtype C shows the fracture that occurs during surgery. (From Felix, Stuart, Hanssen,[60] by permission of *Clin Orthop.*)

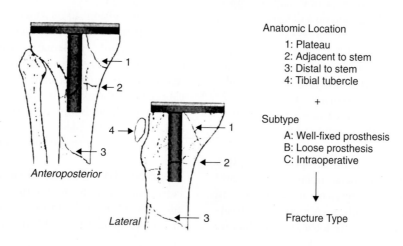

Mayo Classification of Periprosthetic Tibial Fractures

Anteroposterior

Lateral

Anatomic Location

   1: Plateau
   2: Adjacent to stem
   3: Distal to stem
   4: Tibial tubercle

+

Subtype

   A: Well-fixed prosthesis
   B: Loose prosthesis
   C: Intraoperative

Fracture Type

been reported with modern condylar knee designs. Stress fractures have also been reported in osteopenic women with neutral or valgus preoperative alignment receiving press-fit LCS knee implants (DePuy, Warsaw, IN).[57] Revision with a stemmed component, and augments or graft as necessary, is the recommended treatment.[54]

Type 2A metaphyseal fractures, adjacent to a well-fixed tibial stem, can occur with modern condylar knee designs. These are generally related to a fall or other traumatic event. They are often minimally displaced, and nondisplaced fractures can be treated with rigid cast immobilization until fracture healing.[55] Displaced type 2A fractures are a challenging problem, and open reduction and internal fixation is the preferred treatment. However, axial and rotational alignment must be maintained and there is limited proximal bone for fixation. Revision may be necessary, but this adds the risk of additional bone loss while removing the well-fixed tibia from the proximal bone.[55]

Type 2B fractures are metaphyseal fractures associated with a loose component. These require revision with stemmed components. Bone loss can be extensive, and both structural and morselized grafting is often necessary.[55] Ghazavi and associates reported the successful use of proximal tibial allografts in three cases.[58] Another option in the elderly is use of a hinged oncology prosthesis, which when cemented, allows for early mobilization.

Type 3 tibial shaft fractures are usually associated with trauma in a well-fixed component (Figure 17-6). They can also be associated with poor alignment or with a prior tubercle osteotomy, creating a stress riser through which a fracture occurs.[55,59] Treatment must be individualized based on stability and can often be nonoperative. Cast immobilization and limited weightbearing were successful in 14 of 15 reported cases.[60]

Type 3B fractures involve the tibial shaft and a loose stem. Revision is required but the sequence of treatment should be individualized. In some cases it may be appropriate to treat the fracture first, then do a delayed revision once healing has occurred.[55]

Type 4 fractures involve the tibial tubercle. These can be the result of trauma or related to a nonunion of an osteotomy.[59,61] Nondisplaced fractures may be successfully treated by immobilization in extension. Displaced fractures require ORIF with a tension band wiring technique. Reinforcing this repair with a semitendinosus graft is described.[54]

In general, if the knee implant components are well fixed, nondisplaced periprosthetic tibial fractures and those fractures that can be reduced to a stable and anatomic position are amenable to nonoperative treatment. If the knee components are loose, or the fracture

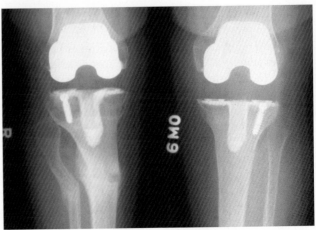

FIGURE 17-6. Radiograph shows a type IIIA postoperative tibia fracture that was successfully treated with cast immobilization.

pattern is unstable, long-stemmed revision is often necessary. Such revisions may need to be accompanied by open reduction and internal fixation with extramedullary plating as well as bone grafting. Finally, displaced tibial tubercle fractures require open reduction and internal fixation to maintain the integrity of the extensor mechanism.

PATELLAR FRACTURES

Intraoperative Patellar Fractures

Intraoperative patella fractures can occur in primary TKA and are usually a result of overresection and/or a deep hole for a fixation peg or an inset design. These are frequently vertical or marginal fractures and do not disrupt the extensor mechanism.[34] Vertical fractures can be observed, and small marginal fragments can be excised to avoid potential pain.

The challenges of removing a well-fixed patellar component in revision surgery increase the likelihood of fracture. During revision TKA, vertical fractures are usually stable and not problematic. Transverse fractures that disrupt the extensor mechanism must be stabilized. A tension band construct may allow early motion. If surgical repair of the extensor mechanism is required in revision, it is not advisable to replant the patella.[5] If a stable construct is not achievable, the patella should be excised and the extensor mechanism reinforced with graft.[5]

Postoperative Patellar Fractures

Periprosthetic patellar fractures can be traumatic or fatigue/stress related. Trauma is usually secondary to a fall or violent quadriceps contraction and often results in a displaced transverse fracture through the body of the patella or an avulsion of the superior or inferior pole.[5,34] Fatigue-related failure is multifactorial in nature and more commonly results in an asymptomatic, vertical, or transverse fracture that is seen incidentally on radiography.

Many factors predispose the patella to fracture following TKA. Several factors are related to surgical technique and are presumable. Initial patella osteotomy weakens the bone, then resurfacing subjects it to altered stresses.[17] Excessive resection resulting in a bone thickness <15 mm can increase anterior patellar strain and predispose to fracture.[62,63] Designs using a large central hole for fixation also increase anterior patellar strain more than smaller peripheral peg designs.[64,65] *Overstuffing* the patellofemoral joint can increase the likelihood of fracture. Insufficient patellar resection, oversized AP femoral dimension, and flexion of the femoral component all increase patellofemoral joint reaction force and quadriceps tendon tension.[1,66] Symmetric resection, especially overresection of the lateral facet, causes weakness and predisposes to fracture.[1] Other factors associated with periprosthetic patellar fracture include increased flexion,[11] thermal necrosis due to PMMA, and revision TKA.[6]

Patellofemoral malalignment and component position can increase the chance of patellar fracture. Biomechanical studies have shown an increase in contact force with malalignments, and clinical studies show a relationship between alignment and fracture risk.[9,67] Extremes of joint line position and coverage of the resected patella are factors, and major malalignment has been linked to more severe fracture and worse prognosis.[1]

Compromise of patellar blood supply and subsequent osteonecrosis have been implicated as a predisposing factor for fracture. Patellar blood supply is both intraosseous and extraosseous. The medial superior and inferior geniculate arteries are sacrificed in the medial parapatellar approach. The lateral inferior geniculate can be damaged with fat pad excision and lateral meniscectomy. The lateral superior geniculate is at risk with lateral retinacular release. Finally the intraosseous supply can be injured while drilling fixation pegs.[1] The implication of lateral release on patellar blood supply and fracture is controversial. Scuderi et al. demonstrated a 56.4% incidence of reduced blood flow by bone scan after lateral release.[18] Ritter et al. were unable to duplicate these results and showed a higher incidence of patellar fracture in those without a lateral release.[19] Histological evaluations after patellar fracture have shown osteonecrosis.[17,68] Whether this alone is enough to lead to fracture is unclear, but it certainly appears to be a contributing factor.

Several series of periprosthetic patellar fractures have described a variety of different classification systems. Insall[69] classified periprosthetic patella fractures based on fracture pattern: horizontal, vertical or comminuted, and displacement (<2 cm). Hozak et al.[7] reported on 21 periprosthetic patella fractures and classified them based on location, displacement, and extensor lag. Goldberg et al.[8] looked at 36 periprosthetic patellar fractures. They included location, status of the extensor mechanism, and stability of implant fixation as well as dislocation in their classification. Le et al.[20] looked at 22 nontraumatic fractures and classified them based on patterns of radiographic change (sclerosis and fragmentation) and displacement. The largest and most recent series was reported by Ortiguera and Berry[21] and included 85 fractures. Their system for classification includes the major elements that must be considered in treatment: disruption of the extensor mechanism, fixation of the patellar prosthesis, and quality of remaining bone stock. Type I is a stable implant and an intact extensor mechanism. Type II is a disrupted extensor mechanism, whether the implant is stable or not. Type III is a loose patellar implant with an intact extensor mechanism (Figure 17-7) and is further defined as IIIA, indicating reasonable remaining bone stock, and IIIB, poor bone stock (<10 mm).

Treatment of periprosthetic patellar fractures is controversial. Recommendations can be based on classification, but treatment must be individualized to the functional status and medical condition of the patient.[21] Type I fractures with stable implants and intact extensor mechanism are the most common, constituting 38 out of 85 or 49% of fractures in the Mayo group. This group includes the asymptomatic stress fracture found incidentally at follow-up as well as more serious but nondisplaced (<2 cm) vertical or transverse fractures with intact extensor mechanism and stable implant. Asymptomatic stress fractures can be treated with observation. Other type I fractures can be treated with immobilization in slight

FIGURE 17-7. Tangential radiograph shows a vertical patella fracture. While the extensor mechanism is intact, the implant appears loose. Revision will be required.

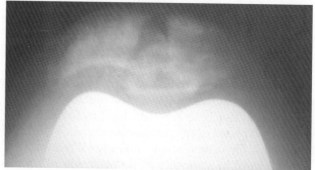

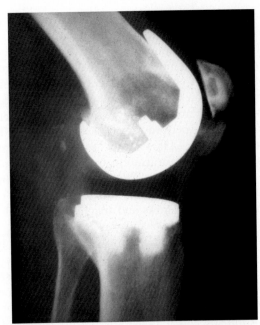

FIGURE 17-8. Lateral radiograph showing a transverse patella fracture with disruption of the extensor mechanism. The implant appears stable. Open reduction will be necessary to restore integrity of the extensor mechanism.

flexion (cast or brace) and weightbearing as tolerated for 6 weeks. Nonoperative treatment leads to satisfactory results in the overwhelming majority of these fractures. Problems reported with nonoperative treatment include a slight decrease in knee score, and slight increase in need for walking aids, but little change in range of motion.[7,8,10] Ortiguera and Berry[21] reported 1 failure out of 38 treated nonoperatively. This was due to a painful, nonunited marginal fracture requiring excision.

Surgical treatment is generally recommended for most type II fractures with extensor mechanism disruption (Figure 17-8) and symptomatic type III fractures with loose implants (Figure 17-7). If the implant is fixed and there is adequate bone stock, tension band fixation is attempted. Ideally this treatment allows early motion. In type III fractures with good bone stock, revision can be attempted. Where bone stock is poor or fixation not feasible, patelloplasty or complete patellectomy may be considered.

Overall, results for surgical treatment have been poor and complications rates high.[7,8] Ortiguera and Berry reported a 50% complication rate and a 42% reoperation rate for operative treatment of type II fractures. The outcome of nonoperative treatment for these difficult fractures has not been reported, but functional deficits would be expected due to extensor insufficiency.[21] In light of the risk for complications, nonsurgical treatment is recommended by some in type II fractures in which the

implant is stable. It is thought that 4 to 6 weeks of immobilization can result in satisfactory restoration of extensor function.[1]

In summary, periprosthetic patella fractures in the setting of a stable patella implant and an intact extensor mechanism can be treated nonoperatively. When the extensor mechanism is compromised but the implant is stable, controversy exists. Operative treatment is recommended to avoid extensor lag, but complications are common. When the implant is loose and adequate bone stock remains, it should be revised.

REFERENCES

1. Dennis D. Periprosthetic fractures following total knee arthroplasty. *AAOS Instr Course Lect.* 2001;50:379–389.
2. Chen F, Mont MA, Bachner RS. Management of ipsilateral supracondylar femur fractures following total knee arthroplasty. *J Arthroplasty.* 1994;9:521–526.
3. Berry D. Epidemiology: hip and knee. *Orthop Clin North Am.* 1999;30:183–190.
4. Healy WL, et al. Femoral fractures above total knee arthroplasty. In: Siliski JM, ed. *Traumatic Disorders of the Knee.* New York: Springer-Verlag; 1994:409–415.
5. Engh GA, Ammeen DJ. Periprosthetic fractures adjacent to total knee implants treatment and clinical results. *AAOS Instr Course Lect.* 1998;47:437–448.
6. Grace JN, Sim FH. Fracture of the patella after total knee arthroplasty. *Clin Orthop.* 1988;230:168–175.
7. Hozack WJ, Gall SR, Lotke PA, Rothman RH, Booth RE. Treatment of patella fractures after total knee arthroplasty. *Clin Orthop.* 1988;236:123–127.
8. Goldberg VM, Figgie HE, Inglis AE, et al. Patella fracture type and prognosis in condylar total knee arthroplasty. *Clin Orthop.* 1988;236:115–122.
9. Figgie HE, Goldberg VM, Figgie MP, et al. The effect of alignment of the implant on fractures of the patella after condylar total knee arthroplasty. *J Bone Joint Surg Am.* 1989; 71(7):1031–1039.
10. Tria AJ, Harwood DA, Alicea JA, et al. Patella fractures in posterior stabilized knee arthroplasties. *Clin Orthop.* 1994; 299:131–138.
11. Windsor RE, Scuderi GR, Insall JN. Patella fractures in total knee arthroplasty. *J Arthroplasty.* 1989;4(suppl):563–567.
12. Brick GW, Scott RD. The patello-femoral component of total knee arthroplasty. *Clin Orthop.* 1988;231:163–178.
13. Lynch AF, Rorabeck CH, Bourne RB. Extensor mechanism complications following total knee arthroplasty. *J Arthroplasty.* 1987;2(2):135–140.
14. LeBlanc JM. Patellar complications in total knee arthroplasty: a literature review. *Orthop Rev.* 1989;18(3): 296–304.

15. Healy WL, Wasilewski SA, Takei R, et al. Patello-femoral complications following total knee artroplasty. correlation with implant design and patient risk factors. *J Arthroplasty.* 1995;10(2):197–201.

16. Cameron HU, Fedorkow DM. The patella in total knee arthroplasty. *Clin Orthop.* 1982;165:197–199.

17. Scott RD, Turoff N, Ewald FC. Stress fractures of the patella following duopatellar total knee arthroplasty with patella resurfacing. *Clin Orthop.* 1982;170:147–151.

18. Scuderi G, Scharf SC, Meltzer LP, et al. The relationship of lateral release to patella viability in total knee arthroplasty. *J Arthroplasty.* 1987;2(3):209–214.

19. Ritter MA, Campbell ED. Post-operative patella complications with or without lateral release during total knee arthroplasty. *Clin Orthop.* 1987;219:163–168.

20. Le AX, Otsuka NY, Bhargava M, Cameron HU, Harrington IJ. Fractures of the patella following total knee arthroplasty. *Orthopedics.* 1999;22(4):395–398.

21. Ortiguera CJ, Berry DJ. Patellar fracture after total knee arthroplasty. *J Bone Joint Surg Am.* 2002;84A(4):532–540.

22. Birdsall PD, Hayes JH, Cleary R, Pinder IM, Moran CG. Health outcome after total knee replacement in the very elderly. *J Bone Joint Surg Br.* 1999;81(4):660–662.

23. Frankowski JJ, Watkins-Castiello S. *Primary Total Knee and Hip Arthroplasty: Projections for the U.S. Population to the Year 2030.* Rosemont, IL: AAOS Dept of Research and Scientific Affairs; 2002:1–8.

24. Haddad FS, Masri BA, Garbuz DS, Duncan CP. The prevention of periprosthetic fractures in total hip and knee arthroplasty. *Orthop Clin North Am.* 1999;30(2):191–206.

25. Hardy DC, Delince PE, Yasik E, Lafontaine MA. Stress fracture of the hip. an unusual complication of total knee arthroplasty. *Clin Orthop.* 1992;281:140–144.

26. Flipp G. Stress fractures of the femoral neck following total knee arthroplasty. *J Arthroplasty.* 1988;3(4):347–350.

27. Culp RW, Schmidt RG, Hanks G, et al. Supracondylar fracture of the femur following prosthetic knee arthroplasty. *Clin Orthop.* 1987;222:212–222.

28. Lesh ML, Schneider DJ, Deol G, et al. The consequences of anterior femoral notching in total knee arthroplasty. A biomechanical study. *J Bone Joint Surg Am.* 2000;82:1096–1101.

29. Shawen SB, Belmont PJ Jr., Klemme WR, et al. Osteoporosis and anterior femoral notching in periprosthetic supracondylar femoral fractures. a biomechanical analysis. *J Bone Joint Surg Am.* 2003;85:115–121.

30. Aaron RK, Scott R. Supracondylar fracture of the femur after total knee arthroplasty. *Clin Orthop.* 1987;219:136–139.

31. Ritter MA, Faris PM, Keating EM. Anterior femoral notching and ipsilateral supracondylar femur fracture in total knee arthroplasty. *J Arthroplasty.* 1988;3:185–187.

32. Lombardi AV, Mallory TH, Waterman RA, et al. Intercondylar distal femur fracture: an unreported complication of posterior stabilized total knee replacement. *J Arthroplasty.* 1995;10:643–650.

33. Rorabeck CH, Angliss RD, Lewis PL. Fractures of the femur, tibia, and patella after total knee arthroplasty: decision making and principles of management. *AAOS Instr Course Lect.* 1998;47:449–458.

34. Lewis PL, Rorabeck CH. Periprosthetic fractures. In: Engh GA, Rorabeck CH, eds. *Revision Total Knee Arthroplasty.* Baltimore: Williams & Wilkins; 1997:275–294.

35. Rorabeck CH, Taylor JW. Periprosthetic fractures of the femur complicating total knee arthroplasty. *Orthop Clin North Am.* 1999;30(2):265–276.

36. McLaren AC, Dupont JA, Scrober DC. Open reduction internal fixation of supracondylar fractures above total knee arthroplasties using intramedullary supracondylar rod. *Clin Orthop.* 1994;302:194–198.

37. McAliden GM, Massi BA, Garbuz DS, et al. Periprosthetic fractures after total knee arthroplasty. In: Callahan JJ, ed. *The Adult Knee.* Philadelphia: Lippincott Williams & Wilkins; 2003:1359–1375.

38. Cusick RP, Lucas GL, McQueen DA, Graber CD. Construct stiffness of different fixation methods for supracondylar femoral fractures above a total knee prosthesis. *Am J Orthop.* 2000;29(9):695–699.

39. Healy WL, Siliski JM, Incavo SJ. Operative treatment of distal femoral fractures proximal to total knee replacements. *J Bone Joint Surg Am.* 1993;75:27–34.

40. Zehntner MK, Ganz R. Internal fixation of supracondylar fractures after condylar total knee arthroplasty. *Clin Orthop.* 1993;293:219–224.

41. Tani Y, Inoue K, Kaneko H, Nishioka J, Hukuda S. Intramedullary fibular graft for supracondylar fracture of the femur following total knee arthroplasty. *Arch Orthop Trauma Surg.* 1998;117:103–104.

42. Moran MC, Brick GW, Sledge CB, et al. Supracondylar femoral fracture following total knee arthroplasty. *Clin Orthop.* 1996;324:196–209.

43. Figgie MP, Goldberg VM, Figgie HE III, et al. The results of supracondylar fracture above total knee arthroplasty. *J Arthroplasty.* 1990;5:267–276.

44. Cordeiro EN, Costa RC, Carazzato JG, et al. Periprosthetic fractures in patients with total knee arthroplasties. *Clin Orthop.* 1990;252:182–189.

45. Nielsen BF, Petersen VS, Varmarken JE. Fracture of the femur after knee arthroplasty. *Acta Orthop Scand.* 1988;59:155–157.

46. Wang JW, Wang CJ. Supracondylar fractures of the femur above total knee arthrolpasties with cortical allograft struts. *J Arthroplasty.* 2002;17(3):365–371.

47. Kregor PJ, Hughes JL, Cole PA. Fixation of distal femoral fractures above total knee arthroplasty utilizing the Less Invasive Stabilization System. *Injury.* 2001;32(Suppl 3):64–75.

48. Ritter MA, Keating M, Faris PM, Meding JB. Rush rod fixation of supracondylar fractures above total knee arthroplasties. *J Arthroplasty.* 1995;10(2):213–216.

49. Maniar RN, Umlas ME, Rodriguez JA, Ranawat CS. Supracondylar femoral fracture above a PFC posterior cruciate-substituting total knee arthroplasty treated with supracondylar nailing: a unique technical problem. *J Arthroplasty.* 1996;11:637–639.

50. Merkel KD, Johnson EW Jr. Supracondylar fracture of the femur after total knee arthroplasty. *J Bone Joint Surg Am.* 1986;68:29–43.

51. Biswas SP, Kurer MH, Mackenney RP. External fixation for femoral shaft fracture after Stanmore total knee replacement. *J Bone Joint Surg Br.* 1992;74:313–314.

52. Kraay MJ, Goldberg VM, Figgie MP, et al. Distal femoral replacement with allograft/prosthetic reconstruction for treatment of supracondylar fractures in patients with total knee arthroplasty. *J Arthroplasty.* 1992;7:7–16.

53. Wong P, Gross AE. The use of structural allografts for treating periprosthetic fractures about the hip and knee. *Orthop Clin North Am.* 1999;30(2):259–264.

54. Stuart SJ, Hanssen AD. Total knee arthroplasty, periprosthetic tibial fractures. *Orthop Clin North Am.* 1999;30(2):279–286.

55. Hanssen AD, Stuart MJ. Treatment of periprosthetic tibial fractures. *Clin Orthop Rel Res.* 2000;380:91–98.

56. Rand JA, Coventry MB. Stress fractures after total knee arthroplasty. *J Bone Joint Surg Am.* 1980;62:226–233.

57. Thompson NW, McAlinden MG, Breslin E, et al. Periprosthetic tibial fractures after cementless low contact stress total knee arthroplasty. *J Arthroplasty.* 2001;16(8):984–990.

58. Ghazavi MT, Stockley I, Yee G, et al. Reconstruction of massive bone defects with allograft in revision total knee arthroplasty. *J Bone Joint Surg Am.* 1997;79:17–25.

59. Ritter MA, Carr K, Keating EM, et al. Tibial shaft fracture following tibial tubercle osteotomy. *J Arthroplasty.* 1996;11:117–119.

60. Felix NA, Stuart MJ, Hanssen AD. Periprosthetic fractures associated with total knee arthroplasty. *Clin Orthop.* 1997;345:113–124.

61. Whiteside LA: Exposure in difficult total knee arthroplasty using tibial tubercle osteotomy. *Clin Orthop.* 1995;321:32–35.

62. Josechak RG, Finlay JB, Bourne RB, Rorbeck CH. Cancellous bone support for patellar resurfacing. *Clin Orthop.* 1987;220:192–199.

63. Reuben JD, McDonald CL, Woodard PL, Hennington LJ. Effect of patella thickness on patella strain following total knee arthroplasty. *J Arthroplasty.* 1991;6:251–258.

64. Rand JA, Gustilo RB. Technique of patellar resurfacing in total knee arthroplasty. *Tech Orthop.* 1988;3:57–66.

65. Goldstein SA, Coale E, Weiss AP, et al. Patellar surface strain. *J Orthop Res.* 1986;4:372–377.

66. Ranawat CS. The patellofemoral joint in total condylar knee arthroplasty: Pros and Cons based on ten-year follow-up observations. *Clin Orthop.* 1986;205:93–99.

67. Kaufer H. Mechanical function of the patella. *J Bone Joint Surg Am.* 1971;53:1551–1560.

68. Insall JN, Scott WN, Ranawat CS. The total condylar prosthesis: a report of two hundred and twenty cases. *J Bone Joint Surg Am.* 1979;61:173–180.

69. Insall JN, Haas SB. Complications of total knee arthroplasty. In: Insall JN, ed. Surgery of the Knee. 2nd ed. New York: Churchill Livingstone; 1993:891–934.

CHAPTER 18

Total Knee Arthroplasty After Failed High Tibial Osteotomy

Michael C. Dixon and Richard D. Scott

High tibial osteotomy (HTO) is a good alternative to arthroplasty in selected cases of medial compartment osteoarthritis because it enables high activity levels for the patient and delays the need for total knee arthroplasty (TKA). With the passage of time these results deteriorate, and the most common means of treating a failed HTO is with revision to a TKA. As a result, the surgeon performing an HTO must be mindful of the potential need for subsequent TKA and avoid compromising its outcome. The available literature on this issue is divided. There are studies that show favorable results similar to primary TKA[1–5] and other studies that show inferior results[6–8] similar to those associated with revision TKA. There is an overall consensus, however, that an HTO does often make TKA more technically demanding, with a higher level of postoperative complications and less postoperative range of movement.[1] This chapter reviews the literature on TKA after a failed HTO, the factors that influence the outcome of the TKA, and the associated intraoperative technical factors and complications.

HIGH TIBIAL OSTEOTOMY

The first reported HTO for osteoarthritis of the knee was in 1958.[9] This procedure was then popularized by Coventry[10] and Jackson and Waugh.[11] Since this time there have been many reports in the literature documenting the success of this procedure.[12–14] In the short term there is a high level of satisfaction, with reports of 80% to 90% satisfactory results.[15–18] However, at 6 to 10 years only 45% to 65% of patients are reported to have satisfactory results.[5,15,18] Those patients requiring further surgical intervention usually require a TKA. The results of a TKA post HTO are therefore an important consideration, as

are the factors that influence the outcome of a TKA in this situation.

Coventry reported that the factors that influenced a successful outcome of HTO were correction of anatomical alignment, the maintenance of this correction in at least 8 degrees of anatomical valgus, and a body mass index (BMI) less than 132% of the patient's ideal body weight.[19] Berman et al. reported favorable results in those younger than 60 years of age, with less than 12 degrees of angular deformity, pure unicompartmental disease, ligamentous stability, and a preoperative range of motion of at least 90 degrees.[20]

The factors that had no effect on the outcome of HTO were age, height, gender, preoperative weightbearing pain, preoperative varus angulation, and severity of degenerative change in the patellofemoral and medial compartments, and previous surgical intervention.[19]

The reported early complications associated with HTO include peroneal nerve palsy, malunion, nonunion, intraoperative fracture, compartment syndrome, and infection. The incidence of reported complications varies considerably from 10%–50%.[17–19] Late adverse sequelae include joint line distortion, patella infera, offset tibial shafts, problematic prior incisions, and retained hardware.

A well-corrected and maintained HTO in the ideal patient has a high likelihood of long-term success, is less likely to require a TKA, and would pose the least troublesome scenario at the *time* of conversion to a TKA. An HTO that fails early, due to malunion or nonunion, is most likely to present technical difficulties.

There is an ongoing controversy about the frequency with which the results of TKA are compromised after HTO. There are studies that show favorable results similar to primary TKA[1–5] and other studies that show inferior results, similar to results associated with revision TKA.[6–8]

The majority of research on this issue uses matched pair analysis comparing the results of primary TKA with those having TKA after failed tibial osteotomy.[3] Mont et al.[21] recommended more appropriate comparison groups, such as patients who have undergone revision TKA or ideally a group matched on multiple criteria.

Several authors have reported good or excellent results in 64% to 81% of their post-osteotomy patients at 2.9- to 6-year follow-up.[6–8,22] These results are significantly less than their control groups of primary TKA with 88% to 100% good or excellent results at the same follow-up. Katz[6] reported an increased average operating time due to an increased incidence of technical difficulties, including difficulty with exposure and patellar eversion. A decrease in the average arc of motion with a flexion contracture and limited flexion post-osteotomy has been reported.[1,6,23] Nizard et al.[22] reported a statistically significant difference in the Knee Society Score and pain relief, but not in the function score between the primary TKA group matched with the post-osteotomy group. Using the Western Ontario and McMaster Universities (WOMAC) Osteoarthritis Index, which is a reliable and validated instrument to assess the functional outcome in knee arthritis, Karabatsos et al.[24] found a trend toward a significant difference in pain ($p = 0.07$), function ($p = 0.18$), and stiffness ($p = 0.14$), suggesting a poorer outcome in patients undergoing TKA for a failed HTO.

By including the cases with significant complications in the osteotomy group there should be a tendency toward an overall less favorable outcome with TKA. Even with these cases excluded from the post-osteotomy group, Laskin[23] reported statistically inferior results and an increase in tibial radiolucent lines compared with primary TKA patients. This is in contrast to several studies that showed no increase in adverse outcome in the post-osteotomy arthroplasty patients.[1–3,5] Meding et al.[2] acknowledged that in those patients with a previous osteotomy there were important differences preoperatively, including valgus alignment, patella infera, and decreased bone stock in the proximal part of the tibia. However, the clinical and radiographic results of TKA with and without a previous HTO were not substantially different.[2] Amendola et al.[1] found comparable percentages of successful outcomes in those patients having a primary TKA (90%) and those having a TKA after a failed HTO (88%) at an average of 37 months. Staeheli et al.[5] reported an 89% successful outcome, at 4 years follow-up, in an unmatched group of 35 patients with TKA post-osteotomy, but also somewhat surprisingly reported that the intraoperative and postoperative rates of complications were not higher, and no untoward technical difficulties were encountered at surgery.

Mont et al.[21] report that for 60% to 80% of patients requiring a TKA for a failed HTO, the arthroplasty presents no significant difficulty. However, for the remaining 20% to 40% of patients, there are a variety of intraoperative challenges that require careful preoperative clinical and radiological evaluation, as well as intraoperative technical difficulties that need to be understood and addressed by the attending surgeon (Figure 18-1).

The key issues that potentially influence the outcome of a TKA post-osteotomy are reviewed. These issues include previous surgical incisions, intraoperative exposure, retained hardware, patella infera (baja), limited range of motion, joint line angle distortion, lateral tibial plateau deficiency, tibial rotational deformity, an offset tibial shaft, malunion, nonunion, collateral ligament imbalance, flexion and extension gaps, implant choice, peroneal nerve palsy, and reflex sympathetic dystrophy and infection.

Previous Surgical Incisions

Planning for surgery and avoiding potentially catastrophic skin necrosis require an awareness of the previous incisions used at previous knee surgery. A laterally based incision from the previous HTO should not provide

FIGURE 18-1. An AP radiograph of a previous HTO with nonunion, retained broken hardware, proximal tibial bone loss, and a sloping joint line.

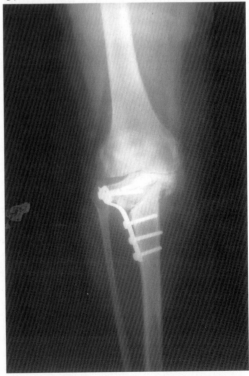

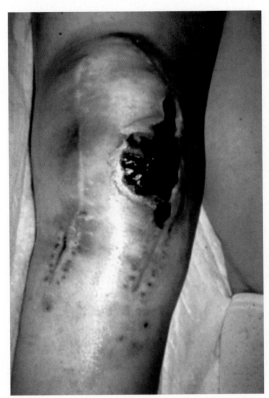

FIGURE 18-2. Wound breakdown in a case with parallel incisions, a narrow skin bridge, and the medial incision parallel to previous lateral incision.

significant difficulties as long as a skin bridge of at least 8 cm can be achieved. This may require a slightly medially based skin incision rather than a true midline incision. A previous transverse incision should pose no problem as long as the new incision is perpendicular to it. Where parallel incisions are present, the more lateral incision is recommended, as the blood supply to the extensor surface is medially dominant. Very rarely, a *sham* incision can be used before the definitive surgery, to more safely assess the potential wound healing. Jackson et al.[25] noted a 30% rate of primary wound healing in TKA after failed HTO, with a 20% incidence of deep infection (Figure 18-2).

Intraoperative Exposure

Scar tissue between the patellar tendon and the proximal anterior tibia often makes eversion of the patella after a previous HTO more difficult.[22] Release of this scar tissue and excision of a thickened fat pad can improve exposure. The patellofemoral ligament should be routinely released to improve lateral exposure. Meding et al.[2] reported that this was adequate to complete the tibial exposure in each case.

If difficulty with exposure is still encountered, then an early lateral release can be performed.[8,21] Personal experi-

ence of the senior author (RDS) in 74 consecutive conversions of failed HTO to TKA is of a lateral release rate of 38% compared with a 30% lateral release rate in 1000 consecutive arthroplasties from the same era. Nizard et al.[22] reported a lateral release rate of 24% in their post-osteotomy group compared with just 2% in their control group. If exposure is still compromised, then a quadriceps snip is recommended. A tibial tubercle osteotomy should rarely be required for exposure, although Nizard et al.[22] used a tibial tubercle osteotomy in 7 of 63 post-osteotomy cases. Finally, a pin through the patella tendon insertion intraoperatively is strongly recommended, as a prophylactic measure to protect it from avulsing (Figure 18-3).

Retained Hardware

Various fixation devices are usually used in HTO. Options include staples, a compression plate and screws, a blade plate, and other similar hardware. Preoperative planning is required to assess whether the hardware will interfere with the TKA (Figures 18-4 and 18-5). If not, then the HTO fixation device does not require removal unless its presence is symptomatic to the patient.

If the hardware will interfere with the tibial jigs or implant, then the decision as to whether to perform the TKA in one stage or two would depend on whether a separate incision is required for hardware removal, the size and placement of the hardware, and the site of previous incisions.

For 2-stage arthroplasty, an interval of 6 to 12 weeks after hardware removal should be used to enable good wound healing before the TKA. Also, cultures of the osteotomy site should always be obtained at the first-stage procedure.

FIGURE 18-3. A pin inserted in the tibial tubercle (*arrow*) to protect against patella tendon avulsion.

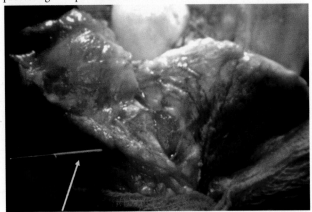

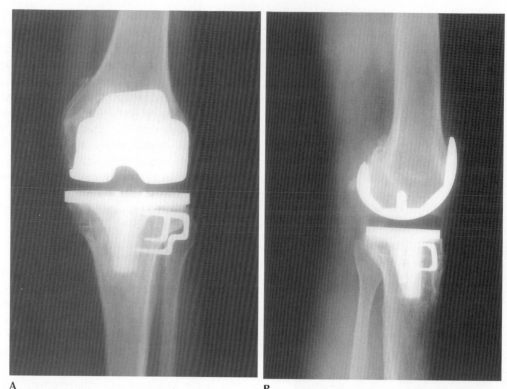

FIGURE 18-4. Postoperative A-P (A) and lateral (B) radiographs of a TKA with retained hardware.

Patella Infera

Patella infera is often seen after a closing wedge osteotomy where shortening of the distance between the tibial tubercle and the tibial plateau occurs, which results in secondary shortening of the patella tendon.[2,8,21,22] This can easily

FIGURE 18-5. Weightbearing AP radiographs of bilateral closing wedge HTOs with retained fixation devices.

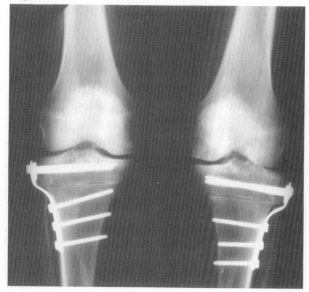

be assessed with preoperative radiographs using the Insall-Salvati ratio, which is the ratio of the patella height to the length of the tibial patella tendon.[26] Patella infera is defined as a ratio of 0.8 or less.

Patella infera is also a problem with respect to elevation of the joint line. The easiest way to compensate for this intraoperatively is to resurface the patella with a smaller than templated patella button placed as proximally as possible. Alternatively, up to 5 mm of extra proximal tibia can be resected, while minimizing the bone resection from the distal femur. This lowers the joint line, or at least insures that the joint line is not elevated, which can improve the patella infera.[27] Finally, at capsular closure, an attempt should be made to advance the medial capsule distally on the lateral capsule, pulling the patella proximally. Patella infera is associated with a decreased arc of motion and potential impingement between the inferior pole of the patella against the anterior flange of the tibial prosthesis. Several studies have shown the presence of patella infera is not necessarily associated with a less successful outcome of TKA for failed HTO[2,21] (Figure 18-6).

Limited Range of Motion

Many studies, including reports that show no significant difference between primary TKA and TKA after failed

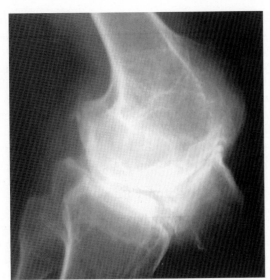

FIGURE 18-6. A lateral radiograph of patella infera.

HTO, report less flexion in the postosteotomy group.[1,3,6] Amendola et al.[1] reported an average 14-degree decrease in flexion in the post-osteotomy group, but believed that this did not compromise the overall functional outcome. Poor preoperative flexion and/or poor intraoperative flexion against gravity after capsular closure warns of this possibility.

A fixed flexion deformity (FFD) can occur in patients after an HTO. The majority of cases of FFD can be addressed intraoperatively. Care must be taken if the patient has patella infera and a FFD, because the former requires a minimal distal femoral resection to avoid elevating the joint line, while a FFD is often addressed by resecting more distal femur than usual. Careful removal of all posterior osteophytes with the addition of capsular stripping from the femur and tibia can be helpful.

Joint Line Angle Distortion and Deficient Lateral Tibial Bone

The post-osteotomy joint line is invariably distorted. First, after a closing wedge osteotomy, there is a valgus angulation of the tibia on the coronal view. Second, there is sometimes a loss of the normal posterior slope of the proximal tibial joint line on the sagittal view. In contrast to the anatomical deformity expected with a varus knee, the post-osteotomy valgus angulation of the joint line results in a thicker medial tibial resection than on the lateral side. The tibial cut should resect minimal or no bone from the lateral tibia, with any remaining bony defect managed with lateral augmentation or a structural bone graft if the defect is uncontained. A contained defect can be managed with morsellized graft or cement as

required. With preoperative radiographic templating for the appropriate tibial cut this should be identified hence eliminating intraoperative error (Figure 18-7).

An osteoarthritis-induced valgus deformity of the knee will be due to a valgus deformity in both the femur and the tibia, whereas a valgus deformity post-osteotomy will be solely due to the tibial deformity. The tibial valgus deformity is compensated for by the varus deformity of the femur due to the initial medial compartment osteoarthritis that necessitated the original HTO. Mont et al.[21] stress the practical implication of this for the surgeon who, after making the routine valgus femoral cut, will make the valgus deformity worse.

The loss of the normal posterior tibial slope can present as either a neutral slope or in fact as an upsloping joint line (Figure 18-8). The posterior slope must be recreated, necessitating minimal bony resection from the anterior proximal tibia to avoid excess posterior bony resection. Otherwise the potential for flexion and extension gap mismatch can occur, with resultant flexion instability. Once again, radiographic templating will prepare the surgeon for this unusual situation.

FIGURE 18-7. An AP radiograph of a sloping lateral joint line (*arrow*).

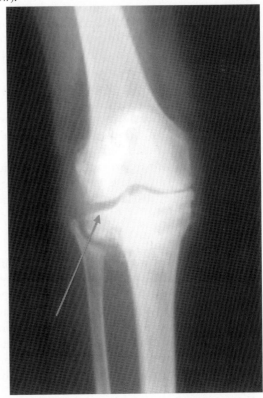

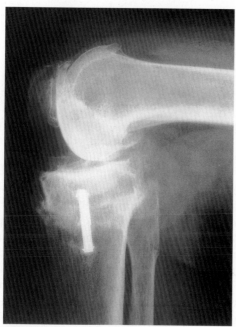

FIGURE 18-8. A lateral radiograph of an upsloping joint line.

Tibial Rotational Deformity

A closing wedge osteotomy has no inherent rotational stability other than that provided by the internal fixation. Inadvertent intraoperative tibial rotation or loss of fixation can result in either internal or external rotation of the tibia. As a result the medial one-third of the tibial tubercle may not necessarily be an accurate or reliable guide to tibial rotation. This will necessitate rotation to be determined from more distal landmarks, including the tibialis anterior tendon, the bony ridge of the tibial diaphysis, or the midpoint of the talus. It should be noted that external rotation of the distal tibia increases the Q-angle, which accentuates abnormal patellofemoral mechanics. Difficulty of surgical exposure also produces a tendency to internally rotate the tibial component, which increases the likelihood of patellofemoral subluxation.

An Offset Tibial Shaft

A closing wedge HTO will result in a lateral step-off at the osteotomy site due to the resultant disparity in the medial-lateral metaphyseal bone width. This will be accentuated if there is any secondary lateral collapse. Careful preoperative templating will help determine whether the chosen prosthesis will impinge on the lateral tibial cortex. Cutting the proximal tibia in slight valgus can help accommodate for a standard tibial prosthesis (Figure 18-9).

If a stemmed implant is required, then it is important to confirm that medial offset stems are available to prevent potential medialization of the tibial tray, or a potential iatrogenic fracture of the proximal tibia (Figure 18-10). Whether an intramedullary or extramedullary alignment guide is used is at the discretion of the surgeon.[27,28] However, an extramedullary guide is recommended because the medullary canal may be offset medially, such that an intramedullary guide will have difficulty being positioned correctly.

Malunion of Osteotomy Site

A malunion at the osteotomy site is less common with rigid internal fixation. It is more common for a malunion to result in excess valgus than excess varus, due to the propensity of a closing wedge osteotomy to collapse on the lateral side at the level of the truncated metaphysis. Preoperative planning will determine whether correction of the mal-union can be incorporated into the TKA. If not, then a one- or two-stage procedure incorporating an osteotomy of the tibia with a stemmed tibial prosthesis will be required. A dome or opening wedge osteotomy of the tibia is preferred over a closing wedge osteotomy in

FIGURE 18-9. An AP radiograph of a truncated lateral tibial cortex.

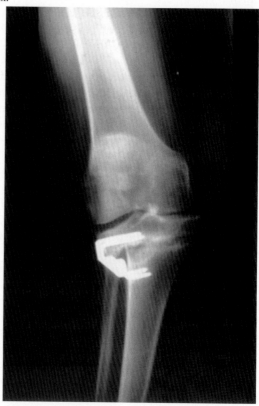

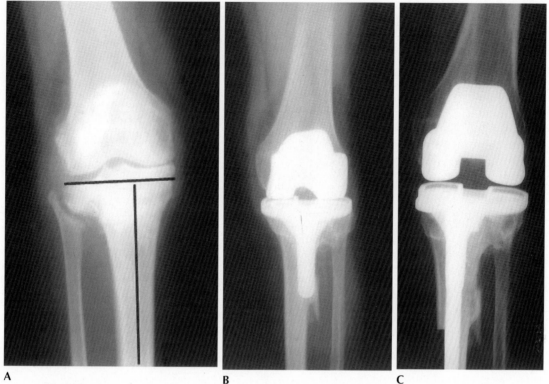

FIGURE 18-10. An AP radiograph showing an offset tibial shaft post HTO (A), an iatrogenic fracture of the proximal tibia with a standard tibial stem (B), and the revision TKA with an offset stem bypassing the cortical defect (C).

this situation to preserve lateral tibial metaphyseal bone stock before performing a TKA. However, a dome osteotomy is a difficult option if correction is required in 2 planes, as is seen in Figure 18-11 (See also Figure 18-12).

Nonunion of the Osteotomy Site

Nonunion of the osteotomy is a rare complication, but poses a difficult challenge to the arthroplasty surgeon. The management of the nonunion and the arthroplasty can be performed separately or incorporated into a single procedure. It is imperative to determine whether the nonunion is septic or aseptic and atrophic or hypertrophic. A single-stage correction of the malalignment, bone grafting of the defect, and the use of a long-stem tibial prosthesis can address this difficult problem (Figure 18-13).

Collateral Ligament Imbalance

The potential for lateral ligament balancing to is to be expected during a TKA postosteotomy.[2,29,30] This is especially the case if there has been a malunion into further valgus or severe overcorrection. Meding et al.[2] reported no significant increase in the rate of lateral ligament release in post osteotomy TKA compared with a con-

tralateral TKA in 39 consecutive patients. However, if there is a trapezoidal extension space that is tight laterally, then a lateral release in extension at the level of the joint line is performed.[31] Conversely, a trapezoidal flexion space that is tight laterally would require extension of the lateral release proximally above the level of the superior genicular artery.

If a valgus deformity of more than 20 degrees is present, then a complex ligamentous reconstruction of advancing the lax medial collateral ligament, the medial hamstring tendons, and the posterior cruciate ligament[30] or a more constrained prosthesis may be required.[31] However, despite the benefit of a lateral release in cases with difficult exposure, the lateral release rate is not significantly higher in TKA post-osteotomy than in primary TKA.[2]

Flexion and Extension Gaps

The general principles of balancing flexion and extension gaps apply in post-osteotomy TKA (Figure 18-14). However, the routine external rotation of the femoral component, as referenced from the anteroposterior axis or the transepicondylar axis, does not routinely produce a quadrangular flexion space, because of the abnormal valgus angulation of the joint line.

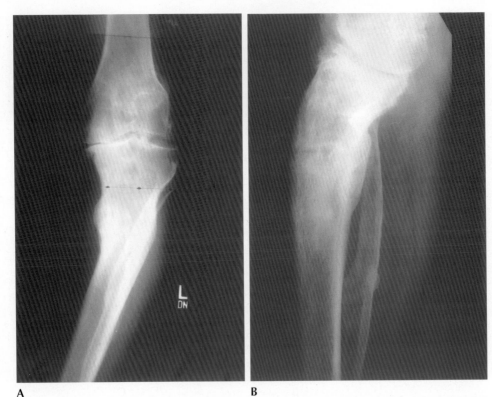

A   **B**

FIGURE 18-11. (A) AP and (B) lateral radiographs of a left knee showing tibial malunion subsequent to a previous HTO using an external fixation device.

FIGURE 18-12. Postoperative (A) AP and (B) lateral radiographs of a one-stage TKA and osteotomy for proximal tibial malunion.

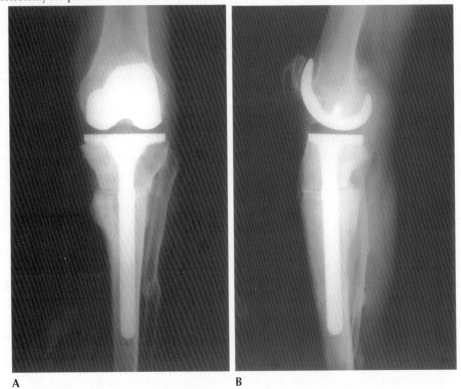

A   **B**

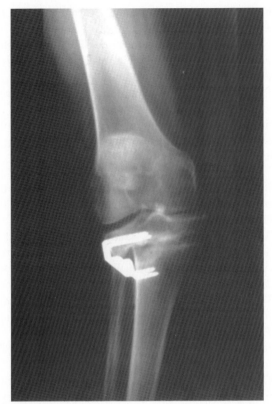

FIGURE 18-13. An AP radiograph of nonunion of HTO.

alternatively an extensive lateral release in flexion could be considered, but this complicates flexion and extension gap balancing.

As previously mentioned, an upsloping tibial joint line post-osteotomy needs to be converted into the normal joint line slope. Even with a minimal anterior proximal tibial resection this can result in a thick posterior proximal tibial resection that can potentially create a larger gap in flexion than in extension. In these cases, a less pronounced initial posterior slope on the tibial cut is recommended. If the flexion gap is still larger than the extension gap, then the principles of using a larger femoral component with posterior augmentation or resecting more distal femur to increase the extension gap to match the flexion gap are required. The latter option requires a thicker polyethylene insert, which raises the joint line and exacerbates patella infera if present.

Implant Choice
Preoperative planning helps determine whether the surgeon's preferred implant will result in any impingement between the prosthesis and the lateral cortex. The selected implant should have standard and offset stem options available. Whether to substitute or preserve the posterior cruciate is the surgeon's decision. The senior author (RDS) has used a cruciate retaining prosthesis in 74 consecutive cases of TKA for failed osteotomy.

Peroneal Nerve Palsy
The reported incidence of post-osteotomy peroneal nerve palsy is approximately 5%.[21] A failed osteotomy with an unresolved peroneal nerve palsy needs careful clinical

When the tibial resection is made perpendicular to the longitudinal axis, the flexion gap will potentially be asymmetrical. To correct this, the femur must sometimes be internally rotated to create a symmetrical flexion gap;

FIGURE 18-14. Intraoperative photographs showing the valgus joint line post HTO (A), and the asymmetrical flexion gap that would result if femoral rotation was measured from the AP or transepicondylar axes (B).

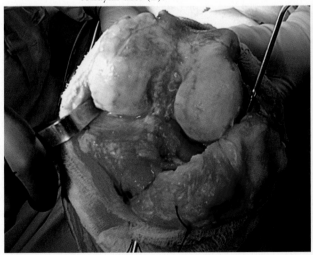

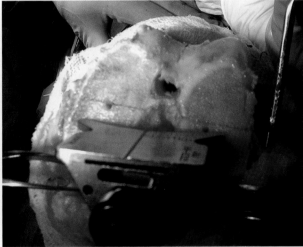

A   B

assessment to differentiate neurogenic from mechanically induced pain. The surgeon then needs to consider whether decompression of the nerve is warranted. Thereafter, the decision is whether to primarily decompress the nerve or to do this at the same time as the TKA.

Reflex Sympathetic Dystrophy

Total knee arthroplasty in the presence of reflex sympathetic dystrophy (RSD) increases the likelihood of a fair or poor outcome. Cases in which features of RSD are present or in which there was no pain relief from the HTO should make the surgeon cautious to proceed with TKA. Even if previous RSD symptoms are quiescent, there is a high risk of recurrence (47%) of symptoms with further surgery.[6]

Infection

Although the incidence of deep infection in TKA after failed HTO is not significantly higher than in primary TKA,[2,5] there is a tendency toward an increase in deep infections.[22] Of concern is a report by Jackson et al.[25] that noted 6 out of 20 patients with a TKA for a failed osteotomy had a failure of primary wound healing resulting in 4 cases of deep infection. In contrast, no wound healing problems or deep infections occurred in 23 patients requiring a TKA for a failed unicompartmental arthroplasty.

CONCLUSION

The available literature is divided as to the effect that a previous HTO has on the overall outcome of TKA. However, it is hard to refute that TKA after a failed HTO does present potential challenges to the surgeon. The key issues that potentially influence the outcome of a TKA post-osteotomy have been reviewed. An HTO is a good alternative to arthroplasty in selected cases of medial compartment osteoarthritis; however, with the passage of time these results deteriorate, and the most common means of treating a failed HTO is with revision to a TKA. As a result, the surgeon performing an HTO must be mindful of the potential need for subsequent TKA and avoid compromising its outcome.

REFERENCES

1. Amendola A, Rorabeck CH, Bourne RB, Apyan PM. Total knee arthroplasty following high tibial osteotomy for osteoarthritis. *J Arthroplasty.* 1989;4(Suppl):S11–S17.
2. Meding JB, Keating EM, Ritter MA, Faris PM. Total knee arthroplasty after high tibial osteotomy. a comparison study in patients who had bilateral total knee replacement. *J Bone Joint Surg Am.* 2000;82:1252–1259.
3. Bergenudd H, Sahlström A, Sanzén L. Total knee arthroplasty after failed proximal tibial valgus osteotomy. *J Arthroplasty.* 1997;12:635–638.
4. Ritter MA, Fechtman RA. Proximal tibial osteotomy. a survivorship analysis. *J Arthroplasty.* 1988;3:309–311.
5. Staeheli JW, Cass JR, Morrey BF. Total knee arthroplasty after failed proximal tibial osteotomy. *J Bone Joint Surg Am.* 1987;69:28–31.
6. Katz MM, Hungerford DS, Krackow KA, Lennox DW. Results of total knee arthroplasty after failed proximal tibial osteotomy for osteoarthritis. *J Bone Joint Surg Am.* 1987; 69:225–233.
7. Mont MA, Antonaides S, Krackow KA, Hungerford DS. Total knee arthroplasty after failed high tibial osteotomy. A comparison with a matched group. *Clin Orthop.* 1994; 299:125–130.
8. Windsor RE, Insall JN, Vince KG. Technical considerations of total knee arthroplasty after proximal tibial osteotomy. *J Bone Joint Surg Am.* 1988;70:547–555.
9. Jackson JP. Osteotomy for osteoarthrosis of the knee. *J Bone Joint Surg Br.* 1958;40:826–830.
10. Coventry MB. Osteotomy of the upper portion of the tibia for degenerative arthritis of the knee: a preliminary report. *J Bone Joint Surg Am.* 1965;47:984–990.
11. Jackson JP, Waugh W. Tibial osteotomy for osteoarthritis of the knee. *J Bone Joint Surg Br.* 1961;53:746–751.
12. Coventry MB. Osteotomy about the knee for degenerative and rheumatoid arthritis. *J Bone Joint Surg Am.* 1973;55: 23–48.
13. Slocum DB, Larson RL, James SL, Greiner R. High tibial osteotomy. *Clin Orthop.* 1974;104:239–243.
14. Odenbring S, Egund N, Knutson K, Lindstrand A, Larsen ST. Revision after osteotomy for gonarthrosis: a 10- to 19-year follow up of 314 cases. *Acta Orthop Scand.* 1990; 61(2):128–130.
15. Coventry MB. Upper tibial osteotomy for gonarthrosis. *Orthop Clin North Am.* 1979;10:191–210.
16. Coventry MB. Current concepts review: Upper tibial osteotomy for osteoarthritis. *J Bone Joint Surg Am.* 1985;67: 1136–1140.
17. Hernigou PH, Medevielle D, Debeyre J, Goutallier D. Proximal tibial osteotomy for osteoarthritis with varus deformity. *J Bone Joint Surg Am.* 1987;69:332–354.
18. Insall JN, Joseph DM, Msika C. High tibial osteotomy for varus gonarthritis. a long-term follow-up study. *J Bone Joint Surg Am.* 1984;66:1040–1048.
19. Coventry MB, Ilstrup DM, Wallrichs SL. Proximal tibial osteotomy: a critical long-term study of eighty-seven cases. *J Bone Joint Surg Am.* 1993;75:196–201.
20. Berman AT, Bosacco SJ, Kirschner S, Avolio A Jr. Factors influencing long term results in high tibial osteotomy. *Clin Orthop.* 1991;272:192–198.

21. Mont MA, Alexander N, Krackow KA, Hungerford DS. Total knee arthroplasty after failed high tibial osteotomy. *Orthop Clin North Am.* 1994;25:515–525.

22. Nizard RS, Cardinne L, Bizot P, Witvoet J. Total knee replacement after failed tibial osteotomy: results of a matched-pair study. *J Arthroplasty.* 1998;13:847–853.

23. Laskin RS. Total knee replacement after high tibial osteotomy. American Academy of Orthopedic Surgeons 60th Annual Meeting. San Francisco, February, 1993.

24. Karabatsos B, Mahomed NN, Maistelli GL. Functional outcome of total knee arthroplasty after high tibial osteotomy. *Can J Surg.* 2002;45(2):116–119.

25. Jackson M, Sarangi PP, Newman JH. Revision total knee arthroplasty. comparison of outcome following primary proximal tibial osteotomy or unicompartmental arthroplasty. *J Arthroplasty.* 1994;9:539–542.

26. Insall JN, Salvati E. Patella position in the normal knee joint. *Radiology.* 1971;101:101.

27. Johnson BP, Dorr LD. Total knee arthroplasty after high tibial osteotomies. In: Lotke PA, ed. *Master Techniques in Orthopaedic Surgery.* New York: Raven Press; 1995.

28. Nelson CL, Windsor RE. Total knee arthroplasty following high tibial osteotomy. In: Scuderi GR, Tria AJ Jr, eds. *Surgical Techniques in Total Knee Arthroplasty.* New York: Springer-Verlag; 2002.

29. Cameron HU, Welsh RP. Potential complications of total knee replacement following tibial osteotomy. *Orthop Rev.* 1988;17:39–43.

30. Krackow KA, Holtgrewe JL. Experience with a new technique for managing severely overcorrected valgus high tibial osteotomy at total knee arthroplasty. *Clin Orthop.* 1990;258:213–224.

31. Insall JN. Surgical techniques and instrumentation in total knee arthroplasty. In: Insall JN, et al., eds. *Surgery of the Knee.* New York: Churchill Livingstone, 1993.

CHAPTER 19

Total Knee Arthroplasty Following Prior Unicompartmental Replacement

William P. Barrett

While the role of unicompartmental knee arthroplasty (UKA) in the treatment of arthritis of the knee has evolved since its introduction in the 1950s, the controversy regarding its use has been constant. For UKA to be a viable alternative in the treatment of degenerative arthritis involving one compartment of the knee, the results should be similar to total knee arthroplasty (TKA), with revisions that are easier than revising a failed TKA. In this chapter we review a brief history of unicompartmental arthroplasty, technical factors that lead to failure of these procedures, mechanisms of failure, techniques for revision of failed UKA, and results of revision of failed UKA.

HISTORICAL PERSPECTIVE

In the 1950s, one-piece interposition metal prostheses were introduced to prevent bone-on-bone articulation of the joint surface and partially restore alignment of the knee (Figure 19-1). These enjoyed moderate success.[1,2] Scott et al. reported 70% good/excellent results at 8-year follow-up. Two-piece designs with a metal femoral runner and polyethylene tibial component were introduced in the 1970s. These were implanted with minimal instrumentation and limited sizes (Figure 19-2). These first-generation implants yielded mixed results. Some authors reported poor results,[3,4] but included patients who were not ideal candidates for UKA, while others reported success rates comparable with those of TKA, in that era.[5–8] Lessons learned from these first-generation procedures included overcorrection leading to opposite compartment degeneration; narrow component subsidence leading to contained defects; medial-lateral component malposition leading to iatrogenic subluxation of the knee; lack of secure posterior prosthetic fixation leading to

femoral loosening. Failure was primarily due to loosening, the majority on the tibial side.[9]

Second-generation implants were introduced in the 1980s, and corrected many of the problems noted with first-generation procedures. The implants were made wider to resurface the involved compartment and resist subsidence. The tibial implants were metal-backed to decrease focal stresses on the tibial bone. This led to a resultant thinning of the overall poly thickness of the tibial components. In some designs, peripheral polyethylene was only 2 mm thick (Figure 19-3). Good results were noted with a variety of these implants, but there was noted to be an increased rate in polyethylene wear, particularly after 5 years of function (Scott RD, personal communication). Concerns over polyethylene wear led to modifications of the tibial implants. The articular geometry was made more congruent with thicker polyethylene and/or use of all-polyethylene tibial implants. This increased conformity in fixed-bearing knees led to increased interface stresses, particularly on the femoral side, and an increased rate of femoral loosening was noted with these implants.[10] However, increased conformity, when associated with mobile bearing implants, performed well, both at early as well as long-term follow-up.[11,12]

Currently used designs feature resurfacing implants with minimally constrained geometry in fixed-bearing implants, and a minimum 6 mm polyethylene thickness for metal-backed implants. Mobile bearing implants are available; the minimum thickness of the tibial implant is 9.5 mm and thus requires a less conservative tibial resection.

The surgical technique for implantation of UKAs has evolved over the last 3 decades from primarily a freehand procedure to current techniques that use highly instrumented systems that facilitate proper alignment of the

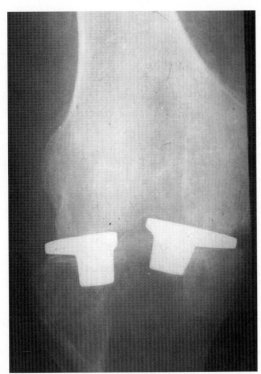

FIGURE 19-1. Medial and lateral McKeever hemiarthroplasty implants.

incision does increase the technical difficulty and raises the possibility of higher failure rates.

Where UKA fits into the treatment of the patient with knee arthritis continues to evolve. In comparison with high tibial osteotomy (HTO), it offers the following advantages: higher early and late success, fewer complications, and restoration of neutral mechanical axis rather than creation of a secondary deformity.[15,16] The advantages of UKA, when compared with TKA, include better proprioception, increased range of motion, more normal

FIGURE 19-3. (A) Radiograph of second-generation metal-backed tibial UKA. (B) Metal-backed tibial implant demonstrating the thin polyethylene at the peripheral margin of the implant.

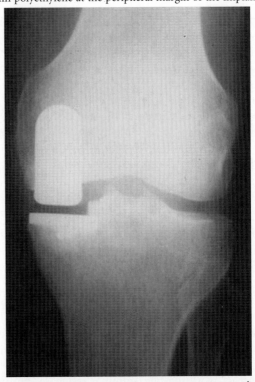

A

limb, as well as implant-to-implant alignment. This is accomplished using both intramedullary and extramedullary alignment guides and jigs that mate the tibial and distal femoral resections. Recently, the evolution of minimally invasive surgery has led to smaller incisions, less dissection, and new instruments for implanting UKAs. These changes have decreased hospital stays and costs and have sped the recovery following surgery.[13,14] However, performing this procedure through a 3-inch

FIGURE 19-2. Two-piece first-generation UKA implant.

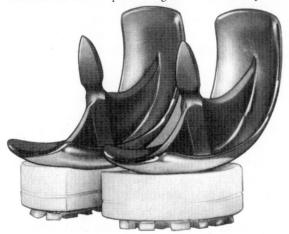

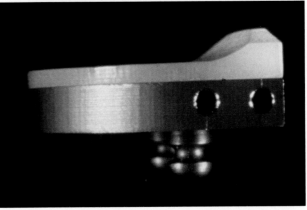

B

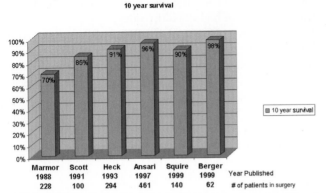

FIGURE 19-4. Studies with documented 10-year survivorship of UKA, ranging from 70% to 98%.

gait, preservation of bone stock, and restoration of more normal knee kinematics with preservation of both the anterior cruciate ligament (ACL) and the posterior cruciate ligament (PCL). Preference for UKA in patients with a UKA in one knee and TKA in the opposite knee has been documented by several authors.[17–21]

Several studies have documented 10-year survivorship of UKA ranging from 70% to 98% (Figures 19-4 and 19-5). While a handful of 10-year follow-ups of UKA exceed the results of 10-year follow-ups of TKA, the majority of reported series approach—but do not equal—the results of long-term follow-up of TKA.[11,12,22–26]

INDICATIONS FOR UNICOMPARTMENTAL KNEE ARTHROPLASTY

The indications for UKA have evolved and have had an impact on the failure rate of the procedure. The classic indications, as noted by Kozen and Scott,[27] include patients with degenerative arthritis in one compartment, age greater than 60 years old, weight less than 82 kg, low-impact work/lifestyle, minimal rest pain, minimum

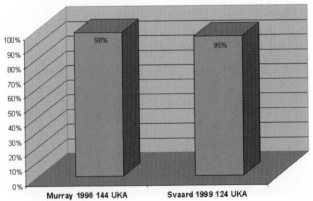

FIGURE 19-5. Ten-year survival of UKAs in 2 studies.

flexion of 90 degrees with less than 5 degrees of flexion contracture, angular deformity less than 10 degrees of varus or 15 degrees of valgus, intact anterior cruciate ligament, and intact opposite compartment. Using these criteria, the use of UKA has been reported to vary from 6% to 30% of patients undergoing knee arthroplasty.[12,28,29] Some authors have advocated use of UKA in the younger, more active patient as the first in a series of arthroplasties because of the perceived ease of revisability.[30,31] While the incidence of osteoarthritis has remained constant, the use of UKA has increased in recent years with the popularity of a minimally invasive approach. Whether or not this contributes to a higher failure rate remains to be seen.

FACTORS THAT CONTRIBUTE TO FAILURE

In general, diagnosis, weight, activity of the patient, implant design, and technique all affect outcome of unicompartmental arthroplasty. In various series, errors regarding the above factors have contributed to failure of UKA in 10% to 55% of patients.[24,26,32,33] The ideal diagnosis for use of a unicompartmental arthroplasty is degenerative arthritis or osteonecrosis without extensive metaphyseal involvement, involving one compartment of the knee. Patients with inflammatory arthritis or chondrocalcinosis should be avoided. Some authors have found an increased risk of failure in patients greater than 90 kg,[6,26] whereas others have not noted increased failure rates with excess body weight. Engh and McAuley reported on a group of patients 40 to 60 years of age, noting a success rate of 86% at 7.1-year follow-up in this high-demand population. They concluded that UKA can provide the young active patient pain relief and function with durability of 80% at 10 years of follow-up.[30]

Implant design has evolved since the introduction of 2-piece UKAs in the 1970s. Some design evolutions have led to increased success, whereas others, such as more constrained surface geometries, have led to increased failure rates, particularly on the femoral side.

Polyethylene

First-generation implants had all-polyethylene tibial components. Several authors cited thin polyethylene—less than 6 mm in thickness—as a risk factor for failure in these first-generation implants.[6,7] Second-generation implants with metal backing had overall thinner polyethylene, particularly at the periphery, which led to an increase of polyethylene wear as a failure mode. White et al. reported that the wear pattern of varus osteoarthritic knees with early disease is anterior and peripheral.[34]

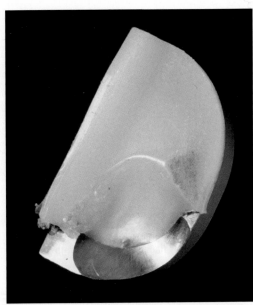

FIGURE 19-6. Metal-backed tibial component with wear through of the peripheral polyethylene in a pattern similar to anteromedial wear in an osteoarthritic varus knee.

Retrieval of these second-generation implants revealed a similar pattern of wear. Thus, the greatest stresses were placed on the thinnest polyethylene (Figure 19-6). Treatment of polyethylene with a heat pressing process, as was done with the porous-coated anatomic (PCA) implant, led to increased rates of failure, particularly when associated with a more constrained surface geometry.[35–37] Polyethylene sterilized with gamma radiation in air and a long shelf life led to early catastrophic failure in a series of UKAs reported by McGovern et al.[38] At a mean of 18 months after index UKA, 49% of the implants were either revised or scheduled for revision secondary to polyethylene wear.

Surgical Technique

Surgical technique is an important factor influencing the outcome of unicompartmental replacement. Some argue that UKA is technically more demanding than TKA, with a larger learning curve.[39] If technical errors do occur, UKA is less forgiving than TKA. The experience of the surgeon and/or center has been associated with the rate of failure for this procedure.[40,41] In one study, a specialty center had a lower failure rate versus results from a multicenter group with less experienced surgeons. Seven of 8 revisions in this series occurred in the first 10 procedures at each hospital. Review of data from the Swedish Knee Registry revealed the risk of revision for failed UKA to be 1.63 times greater for less experienced surgeons versus a more experienced group. In the United States, 70% of TKAs are performed by surgeons who perform 30 or fewer a year.

If the indications for UKA are 10% to 20% of patients considered for arthroplasty, then the question of the minimum number of procedures to maintain proficiency is warranted.

Most authors have advocated slight undercorrection of the deformity in unicompartmental arthroplasty to avoid overload of the unresurfaced opposite compartment.[10–12,22,24,42] The importance of implant-to-implant alignment and proper soft tissue tensioning has also been recognized. Bone cuts are conservative, but the surgeon must avoid overstuffing the compartment with implant. This leads to overcorrection and subluxation of the implants and joint. Extensive soft tissue releases are not necessary in patients undergoing UKA, as deformity is not typically significant. Fixation with cement has led to better short- and long-term results in UKA, versus use of cementless implants, and appears to be the most appropriate fixation at this time.[43]

MECHANISMS OF FAILURE

Mechanisms of failure have varied, depending on implant design. First-generation implants, which were narrow and did not resurface the entire compartment, had a higher incidence of subsidence with associated loosening (Figure 19-7). The femoral component was often laid onto dense

FIGURE 19-7. AP radiograph of loose first-generation tibial component with subsidence into tibial metaphyseal bone.

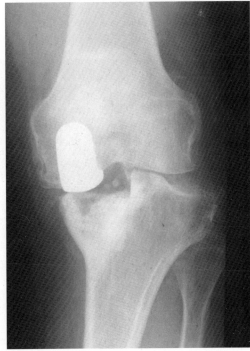

subchondral bone, while the tibial implant required some form of resection, placing the implant on softer cancellous bone. At times, greater tibial resections were required to avoid overstuffing the involved compartment. The combination of increased resection and higher incidence of subsidence led to a greater incidence of defects in failed first-generation implants (Figure 19-8). Second-generation implants resisted subsidence and had more conservative tibial cuts, but design changes led to increased polyethylene wear.

Loosening

Loosening, particularly on the tibial side of UKAs, has been a primary cause of failure since the 1970s. Current designs, which are resurfacing implants, typically use some form of distal femoral resection and a more conservative tibial cut, making revision of the tibial side less challenging. The tibial cut for a medial UKA is very similar to the medial portion of a standard tibial cut for a TKA (Figure 19-8). The incidence of subsidence in association with loosening has also decreased, leading to smaller defects on removal of these implants.

Polyethylene Wear

Wear was rarely encountered in first-generation implants, but with the introduction of metal backing in modular implants and the associated thinning of polyethylene, wear became a predominant form of failure in second-generation implants.[9] These and other design defects mentioned earlier have generally been corrected, and

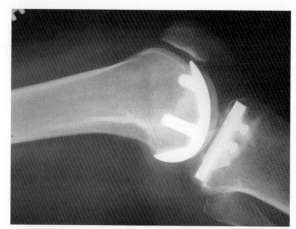

FIGURE 19-9. Lateral radiograph of lateral compartment UKA with prominent anterior flange and patellar impingement.

along with the use of high-quality polyethylene sterilized in a manner to avoid oxidative degradation, should avoid premature failure of the implant secondary to polyethylene wear.

Progression of Disease

Progression of disease has been associated with longer-term follow-up and technical errors, such as overcorrection of deformity. While some authors have reported the presence of patellofemoral degenerative changes at the time of index UKA, failure of UKA secondary to advanced patellofemoral arthrosis is rare. However, a relatively recent report noted a 28% incidence of patellar impingement on the anterior edge of the femoral component. Twenty of 28 patients had erosive changes noted on the patella. This was more common in lateral compartment replacements (40%) versus medial compartment replacements (28%)[44] (Figure 19-9).

REVISION OF FAILED UNICOMPARTMENTAL KNEE ARTHROPLASTY

The initial evaluation of a patient with a painful UKA is similar to that of a patient with a painful TKA, and the approach outlined in Chapter 3 is used. As previously noted, revision for pain without a clear-cut etiology of the pain is only rarely successful. The surgeon must ask: "What has failed?"

Failure of polyethylene in a modular implant can be associated with an intact femoral component and tibial base plate, loosening of one or both implants, and

FIGURE 19-8. Defects in distal femur and proximal tibia from subsidence of first-generation implants. (Photo courtesy of RD Scott, MD.)

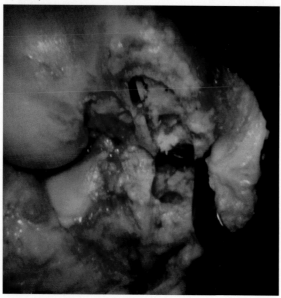

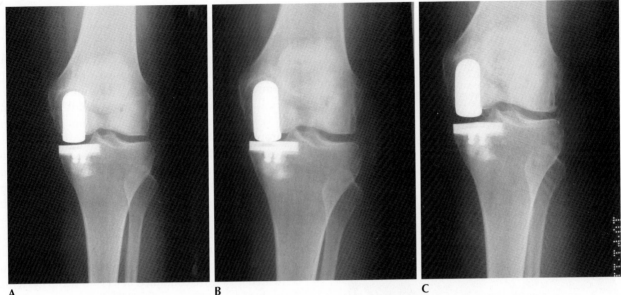

FIGURE 19-10. (A) A 62-year-old patient postoperative medial UKA. (B) Patient 3 years after index UKA presents with pain and swelling secondary to polyethylene wear. (C) Workup negative for infection and loosening. Failure secondary to oxidative degeneration of polyethylene liner. Implant fixation and design satisfactory, so revision of liner performed.

associated osteolysis. Failure of fixation may occur with one or both implants and may be associated with some degree of bone loss. Progression of disease most likely will involve the opposite compartment, but occasionally the patellofemoral joint. This is confirmed with weight-bearing radiographs, as well as a sunrise view of the patella.

Revision Options

Depending on the cause of failure, options range from insert exchange to conversion to total knee arthroplasty.

Insert Exchange Indications include polyethylene wear, modular implant with intact fixation both on the tibial and femoral sides, acceptable implant design, and absence of progression of disease in the opposite compartment and patellofemoral joint (Figure 19-10).

Revision to Unicompartmental Knee Arthroplasty Revision to UKA may be indicated with loosening or failure of one or both implants, indications for UKA still present, no damage to the opposite compartment, and suitable bone stock available for revision.

Conversion to Total Knee Arthroplasty Conversion to TKA is indicated in the majority of failed UKAs. If any doubt exists regarding the indications for lesser procedures noted previously, conversion to TKA should be used.

REVISION TECHNIQUE

Preoperative Evaluation

After a complete history and physical examination, radiographs including standing AP, lateral, and sunrise views are obtained looking for signs of failure and possible bone loss. Three-foot AP views are obtained to check alignment and planned cuts at revision. Templating for revision TKA is performed with attention to joint line restoration, need for augments or stems, and appropriate sizing.

Necessary Equipment

A knee system with both primary and revision options, which include metal augmentation on both the tibial and femoral sides, and a variety of stems, both cemented and uncemented, are required. Cement and implant removal tools including osteotomes, thin-bladed saws, and high-speed burs are useful.

Exposure

Previous incisions are used. If multiple incisions are present, the lateralmost incision is used. If a prior minimally invasive incision was used, this needs to be extended into a more traditional incision and arthrotomy. Exposure of the knee with a failed UKA is rarely difficult, but occasionally a quadriceps snip may be necessary in the tight knee. A synovectomy is carried out, and assessment of the unresurfaced compartment is made. If the decision is made to convert to another UKA, the loose or damaged components are removed. If tibial loosening is noted, a

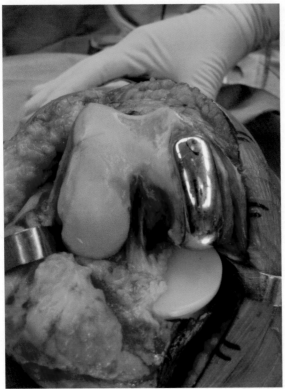

FIGURE 19-11. Exposure for revision of UKA to TKA. Complete synovectomy performed with wide medial exposure for removal of implants.

new tibial cut—using an extramedullary alignment guide—is made, referencing off the femoral component in extension, with appropriate ligament tension to facilitate implant-to-implant alignment. A thicker tibial com-

ponent is used to fill the defect. Femoral component loosening is rare in minimally constrained UKAs. If femoral component loosening in a more constrained system is present, conversion to a total knee arthroplasty is preferable to perpetuating a poor design. In mobile-bearing systems, polyethylene wear is rare. Bearing subluxation or dislocation usually indicates improper soft tissue balance and is better served with a conversion to total knee arthroplasty.

The majority of revisions of failed UKA are converted to a total knee arthroplasty. After appropriate exposure and synovectomy, the implants are removed (Figure 19-11). The femoral component is removed by disrupting the prosthesis-cement interface using flexible or rigid osteotomes or thin-bladed saws. After complete disruption of the interface, the implant can be removed with minimal damage to the underlying bone. Often the cemented lugs leave contained defects in the distal femur. All-poly tibial components can be removed by cutting the cement-implant interface, amputating the polyethylene pegs. The pegs and cement can be removed with curved curets or a pencil-tipped, high-speed bur. Metal-backed implants can be removed by disrupting the cement prosthesis interface, either with osteotomes or thin-bladed saws, and extracting the lugs from the cement bed. This can be accomplished with small extraction tools or wide osteotomes placed under the tibial tray, and axial blows with a mallet. If the cement from the tibial holes is intact, it can be removed as noted previously.

After removal of the implants, defects are assessed and determined to be either contained or noncontained (Figures 19-12 and 19-13). The significance of these

FIGURE 19-12. (A) After removal of the femoral component and initial distal femoral cut is made, a contained defect is noted. (B) After completing the femoral cuts, the residual contained defect is small and easily filled with morsellized autograft.

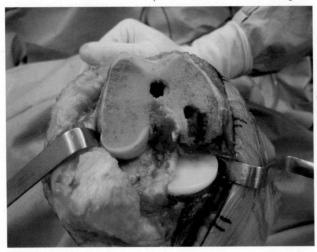

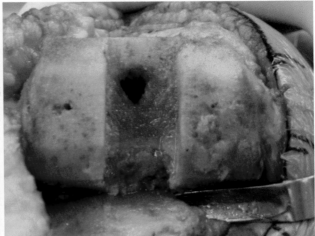

A

B

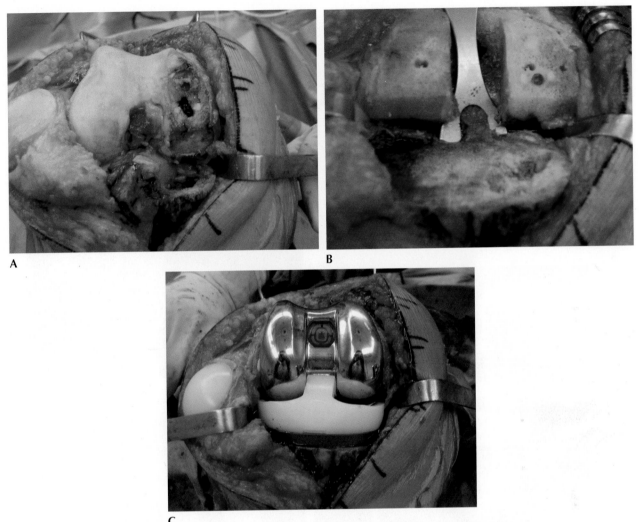

FIGURE 19-13. (A) Initial defects after removal of a third-generation UKA. (B) Standard cuts for a TKA are made and residual small contained defects persist. These are treated with morsalized autograft. (C) Standard cruciate-substituting TKA performed.

defects can be determined after preliminary bony resections are made. A tibial cut to establish a flat tibial platform is performed using either an intramedullary or extramedullary alignment system based on the surgeon's choice. The level of resection is based off the intact opposite plateau. Resecting 8 to 10 mm of proximal tibia from the intact opposite plateau allows you to assess the degree of defect on the involved side. If a small residual defect persists, then increased tibial resection with a thicker polyethylene insert is an option. Alternatively, a slightly thicker layer of cement can be used to deal with a small defect. In the case of a contained defect, particulate autograft obtained locally can be used. In the case of an uncontained defect, either metal augmentation or bulk allograft can be used. The algorithm for defect treatment is as follows: less than 5 mm, defect treated with

increased cement thickness; 5 to 10 mm, metal augmentation; and greater than 10 mm, bulk grafting. If significant defects are present and augments or bone graft support the implant, then modular stems should be used to bypass the defect and offload the surface (Figures 19-14 and 19-15).

Once a flat tibial platform has been established, a distal femoral cut is made, resecting a standard amount of distal femur from the intact condyle, using an intramedullary guide in approximately 5 degrees of valgus. After making a standard distal femoral cut (typically 9 to 11 mm), residual defects on the involved side are assessed. As before, increased resection for minimal defects can be performed but do run the risk of elevation of the joint line, which has greater significance in a cruciate-retaining system versus a cruciate-substituting

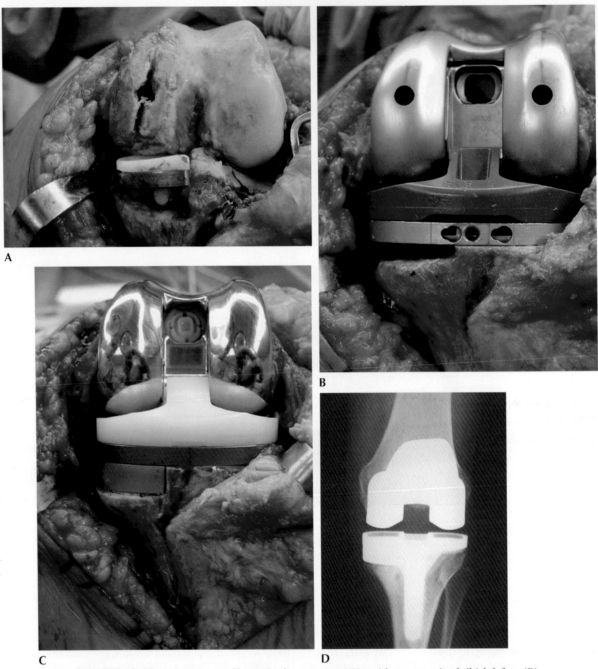

FIGURE 19-14. (A) Revision of loose third-generation UKA with noncontained tibial defect. (B) After standard resections for femur and tibia, a substantial defect on the medial tibial surface persists. (C) Rather than increase the tibial resection, a medial metal augment is used. (D) With the augment supporting the medial plateau, a modular cemented stem extension is used to offload the metaphyseal bone.

system. Larger defects of the distal femur can be treated with either metal augmentation or bulk allograft, based on the previously mentioned algorithm.

Flexion-extension gap balancing is carried out using appropriate spacer blocks or tensor systems. Rotation of the femoral component is determined from several references: the cut tibial surface with appropriate soft tissue tension, the epicondylar axis, and Whiteside's line. Posterior condylar referencing cannot be used, because the posterior condyle on the affected side has been resected

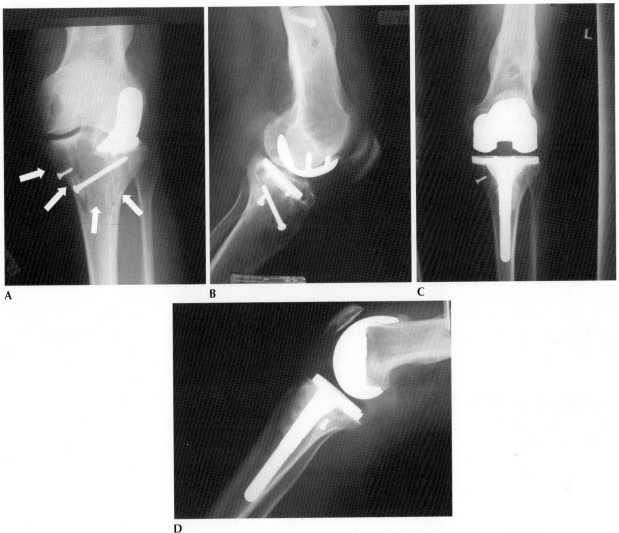

FIGURE 19-15. (A and B) Patient with a failed lateral compartment UKA and failed Gore-Tex ACL reconstruction, producing a large osteolytic defect in the tibial metaphyseal bone. (C and D) After revision, the contained defect is treated with morsellized allograft and tibial stem extension.

with the unicompartmental replacement. Anterior-posterior and chamfer cuts are then made for the appropriate-sized femoral component, based off preoperative templating and intraoperative measurements. Retention or substitution of the posterior cruciate is performed, based on the surgeon's preference. Final medial-lateral soft tissue balancing is confirmed, and definitive defect management is carried out. Use of stems is determined by the degree of defect, the use of augments and/or graft, and the integrity of the metaphyseal bone of the tibial and femur. Stem length and fixation are based on the surgeon's preference and are outlined in previous chapters. Patellar resurfacing is recommended and carried out in a standard fashion for the particular implant system used.

RESULTS

The results of revision of failed UKA are related to the implant and technique used at the initial procedure, the mode of failure, and the experience of the surgeon.

Revision of Unicompartmental Knee Arthroplasty to Unicompartmental Knee Arthroplasty

The Swedish Registry from 1975 to 1995 reported 14 772 primary UKAs were performed. Of these, 1135 (7.7%) were revised.[29] Two hundred thirty-two of the 1135 revisions were to another unicompartmental arthroplasty. At 5 years after revision, the cumulative re-revision rate

(CRRR) for UKA to UKA was 3 times higher than the re-revision rate for the UKA to TKA group. When the data were further stratified to revisions performed after 1986, the CRRR for UKA to UKA was 31% versus 4.9% for UKA to TKA, making a strong case for revision of a failed UKA to TKA as the preferable procedure.

Barrett and Scott reviewed 29 patients who had revision of a failed UKA to TKA, performed between 1974 and 1981.[32] The interval from index UKA to revision averaged 47 months. These were first-generation implants. The mechanism of failure was loosening in 55%, progression of disease in 31%, and patellofemoral symptoms and instability in the remaining patients. In 55% of the patients, technical errors, which led to the failure, were noted. Ninety-three percent of the patients were revised to posterior cruciate-retaining implants. Thirty-one percent had defects requiring treatment. These included cement and screw augmentation, metal augments, and bone graft. Fourteen percent required stems to bypass weak metaphyseal bone. At 4.6 years' average follow-up, 66% of patients had good or excellent results, 27% fair results, and 7% poor.

Padgett and Stern reviewed 19 cases of failed UKA, revised to TKA, performed between 1973 and 1983.[45] The interval from index UKA to revision ranged between 8 months and 8 years. These were first-generation UKA implants. Component loosening and progression of disease accounted for 74% of the revisions. All were converted to primary total knee implants. Major osseous defects were noted in 16 (76%) of the knees. These were treated with cement in 9 knees, autograft in 3 knees, cement plus metal or screws in 3 knees, and a custom implant in one knee.

Lai and Rand reported on 48 failed UKA converted to TKA, performed between 1970 and 1988.[46] The majority were polycentric UKAs. The interval from index procedure to revision averaged 3.7 years. Loosening accounted for 65% of the failures, the majority on the tibial side. Progression of disease was noted in 21%. The remaining causes of failure included instability, broken prosthesis, and fracture of the bone. The majority of implants were revised to a cruciate-retaining total knee. Fifty percent of the patients had bone defects that were treated with cement. No grafts, augments, or stems were used. Results at 5.0 year average follow-up were 81% good or excellent.

Chakrabarty et al. reported on revision of 73 UKA implants performed between 1979 and 1994.[47] The majority of the implants were second-generation devices. The time from index UKA to revision averaged 56 months. Eighty-eight percent of the revisions were with cemented posterior cruciate-retaining or cruciate-substituting implants. Nine percent were UKA to a second

UKA, a practice they now no longer recommend. Forty-two percent of the knees had no defects, 36% had minor defects that were dealt with by cement or local autograft, 22% of the knees had major defects requiring either metal augments or bone graft, and 11% of the reconstructions required stem augmentation. The average tibial insert thickness was 11.5 mm. At average follow-up of 56 months, 79% of the surviving revisions had good or excellent results, 11% fair, and 10% poor.

Levine et al. reported on revision of 31 failed UKAs converted to TKAs.[48] These were primarily second-generation implants, all with metal-backed tibiae. The revision procedures were performed between 1983 and 1991. The interval from index UKA to revision averaged 62 months. The mechanism of failure was polyethylene wear in 68% of the cases. The majority of the revised implants had a thin polyethylene insert that averaged 2 mm at its periphery. Thirty-two percent of knees failed secondary to progression of disease. Thirty of 31 knees were revised to a posterior cruciate-retaining TKA. The average tibial insert thickness ranged from 8 to 15 mm. Twenty-three percent of knees had contained defects dealt with by local autograft, 19% had metal augmentation, and no structural allografts were needed. At an average follow-up of 45 months after revision (range, 2.0 to 5.5 years) the Knee Society scores were 91, which were comparable with the author's series of primary total knee arthroplasty.

McAuley et al. reported on 32 second-generation UKAs that were revised to TKAs.[33] The average time to revision was 67 months (range, 9 to 204 months). The mode of failure was polyethylene wear in 68% and 26% component loosening, the majority of which was on the tibial side. Primary femoral components were used in all the knees, 80% cruciate-retaining knees, 11% cruciate-substituting, and 9% UKA to second UKA. Tibial wedges were used in 26% of cases, tibial stems in 45% of cases, and bone grafting with local autogenous graft was used in 30% of cases. No structural or allografts were required for defects encountered. At average follow-up of 53 months, Knee Society scores were 89.

SUMMARY

The majority of failed UKAs are revised to TKAs. If appropriate indications are met, then liner exchanges or revision to another UKA are possible. The mechanism of failure and potential challenges at revision are influenced by the type and generation of UKA, the presence or absence of technical errors, and patient-related factors. Most revisions can be accomplished using primary TKA implants without the need for augments or bone grafts. However, when planning for a revision of a failed UKA, one should have available a TKA system with complete revision options including tibial and femoral augments, stems, and a variety of insert options, including cruciate-retaining and substituting designs.

REFERENCES

1. Scott RD, Joyce MJ, Ewald FC, Thomas WH. McKeever metallic hemiarthroplasty of the knee in unicompartmental degenerative arthritis. *J Bone Joint Surg.* 1985;67-A: 203–207.

2. Emerson RH Jr, Potter T. The use of the McKeever metallic hemiarthroplasty for unicompartmental arthritis. *J Bone Joint Surg.* 1985;67-A(2):208–212.

3. Insall J, Aglietti P. A five to seven-year follow-up of unicondylar arthroplasty. *J Bone Joint Surg.* 1980;62-A(8): 1329–1337.

4. Laskin RS. Unicompartmental tibiofemoral resurfacing arthroplasty. *J Bone Joint Surg.* 1978;60-A(2):182–185.

5. Scott RD, Santore RF. Unicondylar unicompartmental replacement for osteoarthritis of the knee. *J Bone Joint Surg.* 1981;63-A(4):536–544.

6. Marmor L. Unicompartmental knee arthroplasty, ten- to 13-year follow-up study. *Clin Orthop.* 1988;226:14–20.

7. Bae DK, Guhl JF, Keane SP. Unicompartmental knee arthroplasty for single compartment disease. *Clin Orthop.* 1983; (176):233–238.

8. Jackson RW, Burdick W. Unicompartmental knee arthroplasty. *Clin Orthop.* 1984;190:182–185.

9. Scott RD. Mistakes made and lessons learned after 2 decades of unicompartmental knee replacement. In: Cartier PH, Epinette JA, Deschamps G, Hernigau PH. *Unicompartmental Knee Arthroplasty.* Paris: Expansion Scientifique Francaise; 1997.

10. Schai PA, Suh JT, Thornhill TS, Scott RD. Unicompartmental knee arthroplasty in middle-aged patients. *J Arthroplasty.* 1998;13(4):365–372.

11. Murray DW, Goodfellow JW, O'Connor JJ. The Oxford medial unicompartmental arthroplasty, a ten-year survival study. *J Bone Joint Surg.* 1998;80-B(6):983–989.

12. Svärd UCG, Price AJ. Oxford medial unicompartmental knee arthroplasty. A survival analysis of an independent series. *J Bone Joint Surg.* 2001;83-B(2):191–194.

13. Repicci JA, Eberle RW. Minimally invasive surgical technique for unicondylar knee arthroplasty. *J South Orthop.* 1999;8(1):20–27.

14. Price AJ, Webb J, Topf H, Dodd CAF, Goodfellow JW, Murray DW, et al. Rapid recovery after Oxford unicompartmental arthroplasty through a short incision. *J Arthroplasty.* 2001;16(8):970–976.

15. Broughton NS, Newman JH, Baily RAJ. Unicompartmental replacement and high tibial osteotomy for osteoarthritis of the knee: a comparative study after 5–10 years' follow-up. *J Bone Joint Surg Br.* 1986;68-B:447–452.

16. Weale AE, Newman JH. Unicompartmental arthroplasty and high tibial osteotomy for osteoarthritis of the knee: a comparative study with a 12- to 17-year follow-up period. *Clin Orthop.* 1984;302:134–137.

17. Ackroyd CE, Whitehouse SL, Newman JH, Joslin CC. A comparative study of the medial St. Georg sled and kinematic total knee arthroplasties: ten-year survivorship. *J Bone Joint Surg.* 2002;84-B(5):667–672.

18. Laurencin CT, Zelicof SB, Scott RD, Ewald FC. Unicompartmental versus total knee arthroplasty in the same patient. *Clin Orthop.* 1991;273:151–156.

19. Newman JH, Ackroyd CE, Shah NA. Unicompartmental or total knee replacement? *J Bone Joint Surg.* 1998;80-B(5): 862–865.

20. Rougraff BT, Heck DA, Gibson AE. A comparison of tricompartmental and unicompartmental arthroplasty for the treatment of gonarthrosis. *Clin Orthop.* 1991;273:157–164.

21. Weale AE, Halabi OA, Jones PW, White SH. Perceptions of outcomes after unicompartmental and total knee replacements. *Clin Orthop.* 2000;382:143–152.

22. Berger RA, Nedeff DD, Barden RM, et al. Unicompartmental knee arthroplasty: clinical experience at 6- to 10-year follow-up. *Clin Orthop.* 1999;367:50–60.

23. Argenson JNA, Chevrol-Benkeddache Y, Aubaniac JM. Modern unicompartmental knee arthroplasty with cement: a three to ten-year follow-up study. *J Bone Joint Surg.* 2002; 84-A(12):2235–2239.

24. Squire MW, Callaghan JJ, Goetz DD, Sullivan PM, Johnston RC. Unicompartmental knee replacement: a minimum 15-year follow-up study. *Clin Orthop.* 1999;367:61–72.

25. Ansari S, Newman JH, Ackroyd CE. St. Georg sledge for medial compartment knee replacement: 461 arthroplasties followed for 4 (1–17) years. *Acta Orthop Scand.* 1997;68(5): 430–434.

26. Heck DA, Marmor L, Gibson A, Rougraff BT. Unicompartmental knee arthroplasty: a multicenter investigation with long-term follow-up evaluation. *Clin Orthop.* 1993;(Jan)86: 154–159.

27. Kozin SC, Scott RD. Unicondylar knee arthroplasty. *J Bone Joint Surg.* 1989;71:145.

28. Stern SH, Becker MW, Insall JN. Unicondylar knee arthroplasty: an evaluation of selection criteria. *Clin Orthop.* 1993; 286:143–148.

29. Lewold S, Robertsson O, Knutson K, Lidgren L. Revision of unicompartmental knee arthroplasty: outcome in 1135 cases from the Swedish Knee Arthroplasty Study. *Acta Orthop Scand.* 1998;69(5):469–474.

30. Engh GA, McAuley JP. Unicondylar arthroplasty: an option for high-demand patients with gonarthrosis. *AAOS Instr Course Lect.* 1999;48:143–148.

31. Engh GA. Can we justify unicondylar arthroplasty as a temporizing procedure? In the affirmative. *J Arthroplasty.* 2002;17(4 suppl):54–55.

32. Barrett WP, Scott RD. Revision of failed unicondylar unicompartmental knee arthroplasty. *J Bone Joint Surg.* 1987; 69-A(9):1328–1336.

33. McAuley JP, Engh GA, Ammeen DJ. Revision of failed unicompartmental knee arthroplasty. *Clin Orthop.* 2001(Nov);392:279–282.

34. White SH, Ludkowski PF, Goodfellow JW. Anteromedial osteoartritis of the knee. *J Bone Joint Surg Br.* 1991;73: 582–586.

35. Bernasek TL, Rand JA, Bryan RS. Unicompartmental porous-coated anatomic total knee arthroplasty. *Clin Orthop.* 1988;236:52–59.

36. Skyrme AD, Mencia MM, Skinner PW. Early failure of the porous-coated anatomic cemented unicompartmental knee arthroplasty. *J Arthroplasty.* 2002;17(2):201–205.

37. Hodge WA, Chandler HP. Unicompartmental knee replacement: a comparison of constrained and unconstrained designs. *J Bone Joint Surg.* 1992;74-A(6):877–883.

38. McGovern TF, Ammeen DJ, Collier JP, Currier BH, Engh GA. Rapid polyethylene failure of unicondylar tibial components sterilized with gamma irradiation in air and implanted after a long shelf life. *J Bone Joint Surg.* 2002;84-A(6):901–906.

39. Sculco TP. Can we justify unicondylar arthroplasty as a temporizing procedure? *J Arthroplasty.* 2002;17(4 suppl)(1): 56–58.

40. Lindstrand A, Stenström A, Ryd L, Toksvig-Larsen S. The introduction period of unicompartmental knee arthroplasty is critical: a clinical, clinical multicentered, and radiostereometric study of 251 Duracon unicompartmental knee arthroplasties. *J Arthroplasty.* 2000;15(5):608–616.

41. Robertsson O, Knutson K, Lewold S, Lidgren L. The routine of surgical management reduces failure after unicompartmental knee arthroplasty. *J Bone Joint Surg Br.* 2001;83-B(1):45–49.

42. Kennedy WR, White RP. Unicompartmental arthroplasty of the knee: postoperative alignment and is influence on overall results. *Clin Orthop.* 1987;221:278–285.

43. Bert JM. Ten-year study survivorship of metal-backed unicompartmental arthroplasty. *J Arthroplasty.* 1998;13: 901–905.

44. Hernigou P, Deschamps G. Patellar impingement following unicompartmental arthroplasty. *J Bone Joint Surg.* 2002;84-A(7):1132–1137.

45. Padgett DE, Stern SH, Insall JN. Revision total knee arthroplasty for failed unicompartmental replacement. *J Bone Joint Surg.* 1991;73-A(2):186–190.

46. Lai CH, Rand JA. Revision of failed unicompartmental total knee arthroplasty. *Clin Orthop.* 1993;287:193–201.

47. Chakrabarty G, Newman JH, Adkroyd CE. Revision of unicompartmental arthroplasty of the knee: clinical and technical considerations. *J Arthroplasty.* 1998;13(2):191–196.

48. Levine WN, Ozuna RM, Scott RD, Thornhill TS. Conversion of failed modern unicompartmental arthroplasty to total knee arthroplasty. *J Arthroplasty.* 1996;11(7):797–801.

CHAPTER 20

Hinge Implants

David W. Manning, Peter P. Chiang, and Andrew A. Freiberg

The origin of knee arthroplasty can be traced to 1863 and Vernuil's attempt to relieve arthritic knee pain through the surgical interposition of joint capsule.[1] Soft tissue substrates such as muscle, fat, fascia, and pig bladder were later used. However, the outcomes of each were equally as unsatisfactory as Vernuil's original procedure. Eventually *biologic* or *tissue* arthroplasty substrates were abandoned in favor of acrylics and metal alloys in the form of a hinge.[1] The constraint to motion inherent in the hinge design was thought necessary to allow a stable physiologic range of motion and prevent dislocation of the prosthetic joint.[2] Like soft tissue arthroplasty, the clinical results of early, hinged prosthesis were poor. Prosthetic loosening, fracture, and deep infection were common.[1-17] Newer generations of the hinge design were developed to combat perceived design flaws but met with little success. Continued poor results led to disfavor of the hinge design, and the adoption of newer, more successful, unlinked arthroplasty designs. As total knee arthroplasty has expanded, specific indications for both an unconstrained and a highly constrained arthroplasty design have become apparent, and the development and evolution of the linked hinge prosthesis has continued. Further design modifications include multiple sizing, component modularity, hinge rotation, ingrowth surfaces, polyethylene bearings, and the manufacture of fracture-resistant superalloys. The resultant generation of linked, rotating, hinged prostheses holds promise for improved survivorship in complex knee reconstruction.

HISTORY

The first hinged total knee prosthesis was made from acrylic resin and introduced by Walldius in 1951.[1] The same design was later produced from stainless steel. Other designs soon followed, such as the Shier's metallic hinge in 1953, Young's Vitallium valgus hinge in 1958, and the Stanmore and Guepar hinges in 1969.[1-18] These prostheses, among others, are termed the *first generation*. The first-generation prostheses were highly constrained, allowing only simple flexion and extension. These highly constrained designs transferred high stresses to the implant-cement-bone interfaces, producing early prosthetic loosening. In addition, the majority of first-generation hinges consisted of metal-to-metal articulations and resulted in fretting, fatigue, fracture, and sometimes, dramatic particulate wear debris. Overall, these prostheses were found to have unacceptable complications and early failure rates.

A *second generation* of hinged prostheses followed with design modifications that decreased prosthetic constraint by including axial rotation and varus/valgus motion of the hinge.[19-33] These less constrained designs include the Sheehan, Herbert, Attenborough, Spherocentric, Noiles, and Kinematic rotating hinge prostheses. Like their first-generation counterparts, some early second-generation prostheses suffered unacceptable complication rates and early failure. The Herbert total knee is one such example. Catastrophic failure within 1 year of implantation forced the implant to be pulled from the market soon after its introduction.[21] However, most second-generation rotating hinged knees enjoyed early promising results. The mid- to late-term outcomes were more disappointing.[22-33] As a whole, the second generation of hinged knee designs were a clinical improvement over the first generation, but unacceptably high failure rates and numerous complications continued.[34]

In general, these second-generation implants are no longer used. Design evolution has resulted in the marketing of a *third generation* of implants such as the Finn, S-ROM, and NexGen RHK prostheses.[35-41] In one instance a second-generation implant, the Noiles hinge, is the direct predecessor to the newer, third-generation, S-ROM modular, mobile bearing hinge prosthesis.[39,40] Specific third-generation modifications include prosthetic modularity; deepening of the anterior femoral groove to improve patellar tracking; the manufacture and utilization of *superalloys*; broad polished tibial components; congruent polyethylene bearings; multiple sizing for better metaphyseal fit and fill; long stem extensions; bony ingrowth collars; and distal augments that restore the joint line. These third-generation modular, mobile bearing, hinged prostheses have produced good results in the short- and midterm.[35,39,40] However, additional follow-up is necessary to evaluate the long-term success of these third-generation implants.

FIRST-GENERATION IMPLANTS

Walldius

Borge Walldius is credited with the first attempt at knee arthroplasty using an endoprosthesis. The Vitallium hinged prosthesis was introduced in 1951 and intended for use in patients with rheumatoid arthritis.[1] The design of this prosthesis underwent several modifications and subsequently produced 4 types of designs known as Mark I through Mark IV (Figure 20-1). The 4 designs differed in length, angulation, and stem construction. The Mark I

and II were implanted without the use of methylmethacrylate, whereas the Mark III and IV were designed to be secured with methylmethacrylate. The Mark IV differed further in that stem fenestrations were provided to improve cement fixation. Neutral and 7-degree valgus designs allowed for a range of motion from 5 degrees of hyperextension to 110 degrees of flexion. The uniaxial hinge consisted of a central cylinder fixed with a washer and locking screw. A single 28-mm hinge width was available. Rotation along the longitudinal axis was prevented by both the anterior femoral and posterior tibial lips. In addition, the femoral lip provided an articular surface for the patella.[1–7]

The long-term clinical results with the Walldius hinge were poor. At the time, constraint was thought necessary to provide stability. Axial rotation, a normal part of knee kinematics, was not perceived to be important.[2] However, these design concepts led to excessive stress concentration at the implant-cement-bone interfaces, which in turn led to early loosening. The prosthesis also suffered from significant subsidence in both femoral and tibial bone. Nevertheless, there are several reports in the literature using this prosthesis in rheumatoid patients with short-term follow-up (1 to 3 years) and good results with regard to pain relief, stability, and range of motion.[1–7] These reports, however, also highlight a high rate of complications such as infection, fracture, loosening, subsidence, and peroneal nerve palsy.[1–7] Despite the clinical failure of

Figure 20-1. Walldius Mark IV prosthesis. (From Jones, Blundell,[1] by permission of *Clin Orthop.*)

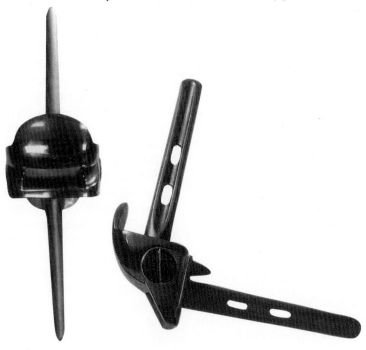

the Walldius experience, it represents the original foundation for prosthetic hinge knee design evolution.

Shiers

The Shiers hinged knee prosthesis (Figure 20-2) was first implanted in 1953.[8,9] The hinge was made of a molybdenum bearing and stainless steel. The actual hinge consisted of a femoral female surface and a tibial male surface united by a main bearing, which was prevented from unwinding by a reverse-threaded locking screw. In addition, tri-flanged stems of varying lengths, accommodating differing femur and tibia lengths, were screwed onto the hinged surfaces. The design concept allowed uniaxial flexion via the hinge, limited extension to 180 degrees, and preserved lateral stability via the large bearing surfaces.[6,8–12]

The operative technique consisted of a lateral parapatellar approach to expose the knee joint. A patellectomy was performed with care to maintain the continuity of the extensor mechanism. Approximately 0.75 inch of distal

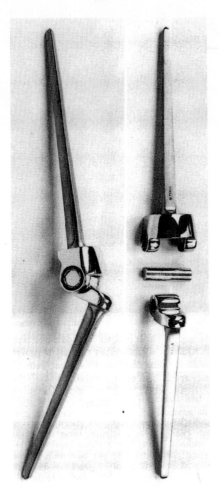

Figure 20-2. The uniaxial Shiers total knee arthroplasty. (From Arden,[8] by permission of *Clin Orthop.*)

femoral condyle was removed with a saw, and the posterior aspects of the condyles were removed with an osteotome. The proximal 0.25 inch of the tibial plateau was resected while preserving the collateral ligaments. The stems of both the female and male components were gently hammered into the medullary cavities of the femur and tibia, respectively. The components were then linked and locked with the main bearing and locking screw. Patients were placed in a cylindrical cast for 10 days, after which full weightbearing was allowed to impact the hinge. The cast was removed on day 12, and formal physical therapy was initiated.[8,9]

A common complication with this early design of the Shiers hinged knee was stem fracture from metal fatigue.[8,9] In Shiers' original series of 17 patients, there were 8 stem fractures in 6 patients. All fractures occurred at the threaded junction of the stem and hinged surface. The fractures occurred at varying intervals ranging from 4 months to 4 years.[9] This complication led to modifications including the elimination of stem modularity. The hinge halves were machined out of a single block of steel, thereby eliminating the easily fatigued stem-hinge modular interface. In addition, the hinges were made a shorter standard length. Finally, the locking screw was made more robust by increasing the diameter.[8,9]

Shiers reported his short-term clinical results in 1961.[10] After modifications to the hinge, Shiers reported no more prosthetic fatigue fractures and concluded that a short-term successful result was possible in 3 cases out of 4. This report was complicated by multiple cases of skin necrosis, deep infection, loosening, and foot drop. Later reports on the Shiers hinged knee also demonstrated short-term improvements in knee pain. However, many authors noted more severe complications, such as skin necrosis and deep infection necessitating amputation, bolt extrusion, extensor lag and tendon rupture, tibia fracture, hematoma, fat embolism, deep vein thrombosis (DVT), and even 4 cases of death within 48 hours. As with the Walldius hinged knee, the Shiers showed degrading results over time with regard to pain and function.[8–12]

Stanmore

The Stanmore hinged knee prosthesis (Figure 20-3) was introduced in 1969.[13] The early designs were constructed of either titanium 160 with Vitallium bearings or entirely of CoCr. The latest designs were made from CoCr with bushings of ultra-high molecular weight polyethylene (UHMWPE), in which a stationary metal axle was retained by a titanium 318 clip. The prosthesis had long, oval, tapered medullary stems that were cemented into place and at a fixed angle of 8 degrees of valgus.[13,14]

The clinical results, as with all the first-generation prostheses, were poor long term because of the highly constrained design. However, inconsistent short-term results were reported. In 1978, Lettin reported pain relief in 94% of patients at an average follow-up of 2.5 years.[13] On the other hand, Karpinski in 1987 had good results in only 23% of his patients at an average follow-up of 44.7 months.[14] The experience with the Stanmore prosthesis was also associated with an unacceptable rate of major complications.[13,14]

Guepar

The Guepar prosthesis (Figure 20-4), introduced in 1969, had several specific design goals and represents the first real attempt to improve on previous design shortcomings.[15] These goals included minimal bone resection, joint stability, valgus alignment, preservation of motion, preservation of patellar tracking, and a dampening effect in extension. The prosthesis had an offset hinge of CoCr that provided 5 degrees of recurvatum and 180 degrees of flexion. There was a choice of either a 7-degree valgus or modified straight femur, both with 13-cm stems. A trochlear plate provided for patellofemoral articulation.

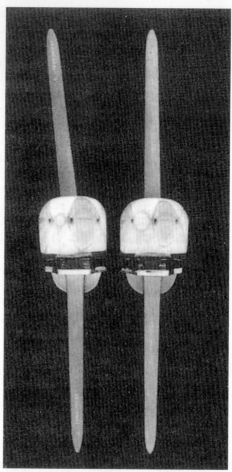

Figure 20-4. The Guepar total knee arthroplasty prosthesis. Fixed neutral and valgus femoral stems are pictured. (From LeNobel, Patterson,[17] by permission of *J Bone Joint Surg Br.*)

Figure 20-3. The Stanmore total knee arthroplasty prosthesis. (From Lettin, Deliss, Blackburne,[13] by permission of *J Bone Joint Surg Br.*)

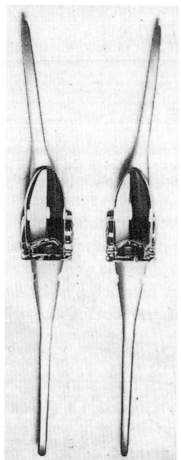

Finally, a silicone rubber bumper was present on the anterior-superior tibia to dampen the femoral-tibial contact by 25% in extension.[15]

The clinical results, as with all the highly constrained first-generation prostheses, were poor in the long term. Le Nobel in 1981 reported on 113 knees in 97 patients with an average follow-up of 19 months.[16] Seventy-four of 97 patients reported little or no pain, and 79 patients believed that surgery was worthwhile. Fifty-five results were graded as excellent or good, but 30 were poor.[15] In addition, the complications associated with this prosthesis, like the other first-generation prostheses, were both numerous and severe.[7,15–17]

SECOND-GENERATION IMPLANTS

In the early 1970s it became apparent that midterm results with the first-generation hinged prostheses were poor, and that early results with unlinked prostheses were promising. As such, designers began attempting to meld the concepts of linked and unlinked knee arthroplasty.[18] The successive design changes throughout the second generation document a newer, more scientific approach to prosthesis design, outcomes analysis, and knee arthroplasty. The newer prostheses were a clear attempt by investigators to decrease joint constraint, decrease bone-cement-prosthesis stress, and improve longevity. As a whole, the design modifications associated with the second generation of hinged knee implants may be summarized as the inclusion of varus/valgus motion and modest axial rotation to a linked design.[19–33]

Sheehan

The Sheehan hinged knee (Figure 20-5) was introduced in 1971.[19] This design was both constrained and unconstrained depending on the degree of flexion and extension of the knee. The prosthesis was made up of femoral and tibial components with intramedullary stems, which were mirror images for the left and right knees. The external surface of the femoral component was designed to have a curvature simulating a normal knee, thus allowing for a constantly changing instant center of rotation. The tibial component had a high-density polyethylene surface mounted on an intramedullary stem. The tibial polyethylene had an expanded intracondylar stud shaped like a rugby football. This polyethylene stud interlocked between the femoral bearing surfaces and engaged the inner radius of the femoral component. When the knee was fully extended, the tibial stud engaged the notch of the femoral component and prevented axial rotation and allowed 2 to 3 degrees of side-to-side motion. With 30 degrees of flexion, the gradual widening of the femoral notch allowed approximately 20 degrees of rotation and 6 to 7 degrees of side-to-side motion. Beyond 90 degrees of flexion, there was no direct linkage between the tibial stud and the femoral component. This allowed femoral rollback and reduced tensile and distraction forces on the components. The prosthesis did not have an accommodating patellar surface; nevertheless, the patella made contact with the prosthesis after 50 degrees of flexion.[19]

Sheehan reported his short-term results in 1978 with 157 knees and an average follow-up of 34 months. He reported good results with regard to pain relief, and had no cases of clinical or radiological loosening. However, there were 4 cases of the plastic-metal interface detaching on the tibial component and 2 cases of fracturing of the tibial stud.[19] Furthermore, long-term results deteriorated, like the rest of the first- and second-generation hinged knees. Rickhuss et al. reported in 1994 the 5- to 10-year follow-up for the Sheehan hinged knee.[20] Using the Hospital for Special Surgery Scoring System, only 15.6% had good results, while 40% had poor results. At review, 31% of the patients had undergone revision surgery or were awaiting such surgery. Therefore, the authors thought that the Sheehan knee replacement should be considered obsolete.[20]

Herbert

One of the earliest second-generation prostheses was described in 1973 by Herbert[21] (Figure 20-6). The ball-in-socket Herbert design consisted of a polyethylene femoral socket and a CoCr tibial sphere on a shank. While providing unrestrained flexion and extension, the ball-in-socket also allowed 10 degrees of varus and valgus and some limited rotation. The surgical technique called for a limited notch resection, posterior femoral condylar resection, and cementing of left or right fixed valgus femoral stems.[21]

Original laboratory testing showed significant shank wear from metal-on-metal gliding between the femoral housing and the tibial shank (Figure 20-7). Shank wear created increased varus and valgus motion at 500,000 flexion/extension cycles. It was assumed that 1 million cycles represented 1 year of expected *in vivo* use. Medial condylar and shank fractures were also observed[21] (Figure 20-6). Clinical experience with 23 prostheses in 22 patients implanted at the Cleveland Clinic from 1973–1974 was disastrous. Three dislocations and 4 medial housing fractures occurred between 5 and 23 months postoperatively.[21]

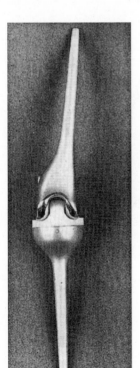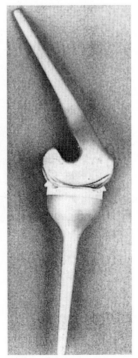

Figure 20-5. The Sheehan total knee arthroplasty prosthesis. (From Sheehan [19], by permission of *J Bone Joint Surg Br.*)

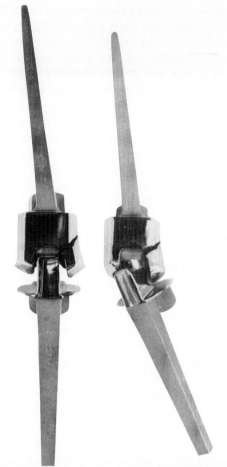

Figure 20-6. The Herbert total knee arthroplasty prosthesis. Pictured are prosthetic medial condylar fractures that resulted in the prosthesis being pulled from market soon after its release. (From Murray, Wilde, Werner,[21] by permission of *J Bone Joint Surg Am.*)

Figure 20-7. Shank etching from metal-metal wear at 1 million cycles. (From Murray, Wilde, Werner,[21] by permission of *J Bone Joint Surg Am.*)

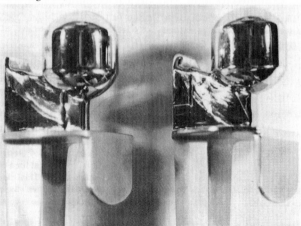

The prosthesis was modified in late 1974 to add metal to the femoral housing and narrow the notch. The ultimate strength of the prosthesis was increased, while decreasing varus/valgus and rotatory motion. Laboratory testing showed significant shank wear at 2 million cycles. Medial housing fracture was noted at 2.8 million cycles. Clinically, one medial housing fracture occurred at 13 months postoperatively in 12 knees. In total, the Herbert prosthesis was found to have a 15% failure by prosthetic fracture within 2 years. The prosthesis was discontinued in April 1976.[21] Although a clinical failure, the Herbert prosthesis experience emphasized the relevance of laboratory assessment in new prosthetic designs.

Spherocentric

The Spherocentric knee (Figure 20-8) was first introduced in 1973 near the same time as the Herbert prosthesis.[22] As in the design of the Herbert knee, the Spherocentric knee was designed to address specific problems experienced with earlier designs. The designers identified 3 main problems with earlier designs: (1) metal-on-metal contact generates extensive wear and fatigue of the implant; (2) uniaxial rotation creates high torsional loads that are transferred from the prosthesis linkage to the prosthesis

Figure 20-8. The Spherocentric total knee arthroplasty prosthesis. (From Mathews, Kaufer,[22] by permission of *Orthop Clin North Am.*)

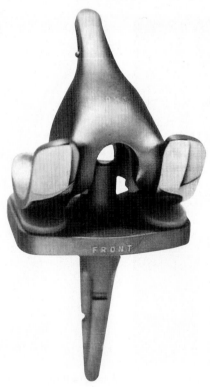

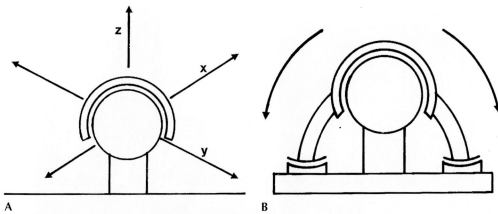

Figure 20-9. (A and B) Schematic of ball and socket articulation of the Spherocentric total knee arthroplasty prosthesis. Design permits motion in all rotatory planes. Condylar outriggers transfer weight-bearing forces and unload the prosthetic link. (From Mathews, Kaufer,[22] by permission of *Orthop Clin North Am.*)

cement or bone interfaces, thus producing early loosening; and (3) mechanical extension stops produce high-impact loads that are also transferred to the prosthesis bone or cement interfaces, creating early loosening.[22] The design of the Spherocentric knee included free motion in all rotational axes through a ball-in-socket articulation (Figure 20-9A), but provided for load sharing with condylar outriggers and tracks (Figure 20-9B). A cam mechanism that provided controlled deceleration reduced end loading in extension. All metal-on-metal contact was eliminated by incorporating replaceable polyethylene bearing surfaces. All prostheses were cemented, and all polyethylene surfaces were loaded in compression. These design features provided for multiaxial motion with decreased prosthesis-cement interface stress, thereby theoretically improving longevity.[22,23]

Before clinical experience with the Spherocentric knee, mechanical testing was performed in extension, flexion, varus, and valgus, and compression on implants in cadaveric knees. The investigators maintain that the testing documented not only the stability and strength of the assembly but also of the prosthesis-cement-bone interfaces. The tests also demonstrated satisfactory range of motion, kinematics, and deceleration cam mechanism function.[22] The early failure of the Herbert prosthesis led the investigators to perform fatigue investigations of the linkage and housing. Early results identified several areas of considerable surface strain where fatigue failure could occur. Multiple design revisions resulted in the thickening of all prosthetic surface intersections as well as reinforcing the anterior notch housing. At the conclusion of these mechanical investigations and subsequent design modifications, the institutional review board at the Uni-

versity of Michigan approved clinical use of the Spherocentric knee in 1973.[22]

Matthews et al. reported a midterm result of 58 of the first 81 Spherocentric knees in 1982.[22] The specific indications for using the Spherocentric knee were fixed varus or valgus greater than 20 degrees, flexion contracture greater than 30 degrees, instability greater than a 20-degree arc, and severe metaphyseal bone loss. Duration of follow-up averaged 48 months, with a range of 24 to 73 months. All implants were cemented in first-generation technique. No patellae were resurfaced. The majority of patients experienced markedly improved range of motion, stability, ambulatory capacity, and pain. In comparison with reports with other devices, the complication rate was quite low. The deep infection rate was 3.5% (3 of 84 knees). Only 7 knees (8.3%) required reoperation for infection, instability, or pain.[22] Early clinical enthusiasm was dampened when it was reported that 52% of radiographically followed patients displayed some radiolucency at the prosthesis-cement or cement-bone interface. Longer-term follow-up displayed only modest deterioration of the results, but was limited to only 21 patients.[23] Nevertheless, the basic principles for the design of modern linked prostheses and the methodology for investigating the devices, both in the laboratory and in the clinical setting, are grounded in the Spherocentric experience.

Attenborough

The Attenborough hinged knee (Figure 20-10) was introduced in 1974 and was one of the first prostheses to compromise between the highly constrained first-generation hinged knees and the unconstrained condylar prosthesis.[24] The Attenborough hinged knee was comprised of a

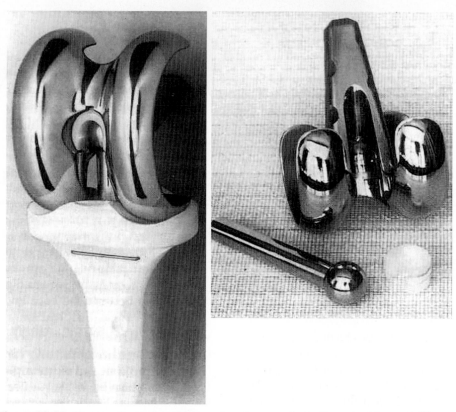

Figure 20-10. The Attenborough total knee arthroplasty prosthesis. (From Attenborough,[24] by permission of *J Bone Joint Surg Br.*)

polyethylene tibial component, which was cemented in place. The metal femoral component consisted of the femoral articular surface and a short stem, which was also cemented in place. The original knee prosthesis had a stabilizing rod, which was contained in the femoral component. This rod fit inside the tibial component and allowed some lateral and rotational laxity. In the newer modified models, the stabilizing rod is separate from the femoral component and is locked into the femoral component with a polyethylene circlip. This separation of the rod from the femoral component allowed for greater ease in insertion of the prosthesis and facilitated the removal of cement. The femoral-tibial articulation of this prosthesis is similar to the knees used today. The difference lies with the stabilizing rod. The stabilizing rod provides the linkage of the prosthesis but allows for some lateral and rotational laxity. When the lateral and rotational movements occur, the joint opens and tightens the soft tissues, which produce a gradual deceleration of movements instead of a sudden block to movement.[24] This was the conceptual advantage over other second-generation hinged knees that limited movement with a hard block, which may lead to early loosening.

Early clinical results were promising. Attenborough short-term results of 245 knees showed only 2 cases of tibial loosening.[24] Vanhegan also presented his short-term results with 100 knees at 2.5 years of follow-up. He found 85% good results with only 2 knees having loosened.[25] However, as with the early generation hinged knees, long-term results deteriorated. Kershaw et al. in 1988 reported on 132 arthroplasties with a 77-month average follow-up (49 to 120 months). He found a 30% loosening rate and a 19% wound healing complication rate. The survivorship analysis using revision as the end point showed survivorship to be 77% at both 6 and 10 years. However, if pain and radiographic loosening were used, then survivorship declined to 65% at 6 years and 52% at 10 years.[26]

Noiles

The Noiles total knee (Figure 20-11) was introduced in the late 1970s by Joint Medical Products (Stamford, CT).[27] The prosthesis consisted of a modified constrained hinge that allowed 20 degrees of varus/valgus as well as axial rotation. The cemented femur and uncemented tibial components were linked via a cemented poly sleeve and a hinge pin. Knee simulator data showed torque similar to that of an unconstrained design and less than that of a semiconstrained design total knee prosthesis.[27]

The clinical adaptation of the Noiles design was intended for patients with anticipated heavy use and severe varus/valgus instability as well as revision surgery.[27,28] The late 1970s and early 1980s clinical experience was very positive. However, poor results were reported by Shindell in 1986.[28] Twenty-three knees in 19 patients with an average age of 61 years were followed for up to 75 months. HSS scores improved from 41.3 to 76.8 at 6 months, but 10 knees failed at an average of 32 months. The majority of failures were in heavy patients (>200 lb) and in patients with large tibial metaphyses. A significant rate of subsidence of the tibial prostheses occurred (5.1 mm) even in well-functioning knees. Subsidence of greater than 10 mm was reported in rheumatoid patients.[28] Despite the clinical failure of the original Noiles hinge design, the device further advanced hinge technology by coupling decreased constraint with decreased mechanical failure of the link.

Kinematic

In 1978 the Kinematic Rotating Hinge device (Figure 20-12) was introduced for clinical use.[29] Like the Noiles and Spherocentric prostheses, the Kinematic Rotating Hinge prosthesis was designed to decrease the clinical and mechanical failure mechanisms of earlier designs. Several fundamental principles required for a well-functioning linked prosthesis were identified, and extensive mechanical and wear testing of the design was performed before clinical release.

The design team proposed 5 primary questions: (1) How is hyperextension limited and what is the range

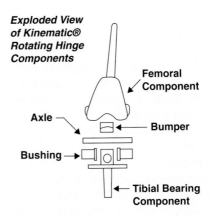

Figure 20-12. Exploded Kinematic Rotating Hinge prosthesis. Note the modular link, the metal on polyethylene articulating surfaces, and the polyethylene extension block. (From Walker, Emerson, and Potter,[30] by permission of *Orthop Clin North Am.*)

of flexion before impingement? (2) Is the prosthesis unrestricted in axial rotation? (3) How is varus-valgus alignment restricted? (4) Is there provision for patellar replacement/resurfacing? (5) How much bone is resected from the intercondylar area?[29] The resultant design was a cast cobalt chrome femoral component with condylar replacement and intramedullary stems for use with cement. Removable, condylar, polyethylene bushings prevent metal-on-metal contact between the femoral component and a snap-in axle that provides flexion and extension. A cobalt chrome tibial bearing component articulates between the femoral snap-in axle and an all-polyethylene tibial component. The all-polyethylene tibial component is cemented to the tibia and has a central cylinder to receive the rotational axle of the cobalt chrome tibial bearing component.[29]

The prosthetic linkage controls 2 of 3 degrees of linear freedom, while the soft tissue sleeve limits distraction.[29,30] The prosthesis also controls varus-valgus motion, while allowing flexion-extension and axial rotation. The limits of flexion are related more to soft tissue restraints than to prosthetic design. Extension is limited by the posterior soft tissues, and also by a polyethylene bumper on the tibial bearing component that engages the femoral axle at 3 degrees of hyperextension. Posterior placement of the axle in the condyles helps facilitate unlimited flexion and lock-out in hyperextension. Axial rotation of the prosthesis is limited to 12 degrees internal and external rotation by the incongruent curvatures of the all-polyethylene tibia and the base plate of the cobalt chrome tibial bearing component.

Wear analysis of the polyethylene bushings was performed through a 30-degree arc of motion in a simulator loaded to approximately 3 times standard body weight,

Figure 20-11. Schematic of exploded Noiles total knee arthroplasty prosthesis. Note the link modularity and metal on polyethylene articulating surfaces. (From Kester, Cook, Harding,[27] by permission of *Clin Orthop.*)

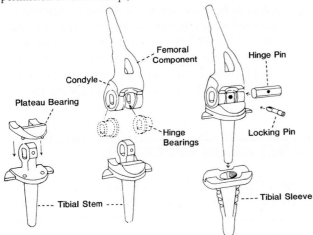

at 37 degrees C, with distilled water as a lubricant, for up to 5 million cycles.[30] Most flexion-extension rotation occurred between the axle and the polyethylene bushings, creating a maximum wear of 0.23 mm at 5 million cycles. No significant changes were noted in any other component. However, when an off-center load was applied in a similar experiment, permanent deformation of both the bushing and polyethylene tibial component were noted.[30] Despite the authors' claim that the deformation was mild in both components, the results indicate that reconstruction of a neutral mechanical axis of the lower extremity is crucial to the longevity of this design.

Finite element analysis of the relationship between the cobalt chrome tibial bearing component and both the condylar portion of the femoral component and the all-polyethylene tibial component concluded that the majority of weightbearing force in a normally aligned knee reconstruction passes from the tibia to the femur via the condyles.[30] The risk of fatigue fracture of the rotational axle is extremely low. Mechanical testing of the rotational axle confirmed the fatigue limit of the metal to be slightly higher than the expectant forces as calculated by finite element analysis.[30] These results also indicate that neutral axis reconstruction with the Kinematic Rotating Hinge prosthesis is critical to the longevity of the prosthesis. Excessive varus or valgus produces moments greater than those predicted and could result in fatigue failure of the polyethylene bushings, the all-polyethylene tibial component, or the rotational axis of the cobalt chrome tibial bearing component. Five of the first 200 devices implanted suffered fatigue fracture of the rotational axle at its junction with the base plate. Subsequently, the design was modified to thicken the rotational axle and improve the tolerance between the femoral condyles and the cobalt chrome tibial bearing component.[30] The Kinematic Rotational Hinge experience furthered the scientific approach to introducing a new prosthesis, and many of the design principles are preserved in newer design-linked prostheses.

The first clinical results with the Kinematic Rotating Hinge were published in 1982.[30] Twenty-two knees were followed for an average of 12 months with a range of 5 to 24 months. The indications for a constrained prosthesis were a combination of marked collateral ligament deficiency and bone loss, in which a condylar-type replacement was considered unsuitable. All but one case was a revision procedure. All patients without prior patellectomy underwent patella resurfacing. Half of the extensor mechanisms required lateral release for patellar stabilization. The short duration of follow-up in this series prevented the authors from reporting radiographic or clinical results of mechanical failure. However, 17 of 22 knees reported trivial or no pain, 16 of 22 patients had

the same or improved range of motion, there were no cases of postoperative sepsis, and no re-revisions were performed.[29]

Good early clinical results using the Kinematic Rotating Hinge prosthesis were also reported independently by Shaw and Rand.[29,31] Follow-up periods ranged from 25 to 79 months and averaged approximately 4.0 years. Satisfaction rates in the primary setting range from 80% to 90%. Satisfaction rates after revision surgery to the Kinematic Rotating Hinge were worse, however, ranging from 74% to 83%. Patellar instability, the most frequently reported complication by both investigators, was reported as high as 36%. More serious complications reported by Rand included sepsis in 3 cases and implant breakage in one. Of greatest concern was the report by both authors that, despite the short-term follow-up period, progressive radiolucent lines were present in as many as 25% of cases.[29,31,32]

Unlike the experience with many hinged devices, midterm follow-up with the Kinematic Rotating Hinge has recently been reported by Springer et al.[33] Sixty-nine knees were followed for an average of 75 months with a range of 24 to 199 months. The indications for implanting a linked device were (1) severe bone loss combined with ligamentous instability; (2) periprosthetic fracture; (3) severe collateral ligament instability; (4) congenital dislocation of the knee; and (5) reimplantation after sepsis. The average range of motion was from 1 degree shy of full extension to 94 degrees of flexion. At final follow-up, Knee Society Scores had improved an average of nearly 40 points. However, complications were frequent and often severe. Thirty-two percent of patients experienced at least one complication. Postoperative infection was greater than 14%, and component fatigue failure was 10%. Patellar pain was reported as severe in 13% of patients, the majority of whom had an unresurfaced patella. Radiographic analysis of the surviving components revealed that 13% of patients had definite loosening of either or both the femoral and tibial components.[33] Although unreported, failure for any reason can be interpreted as high as 40% at an average of approximately 6 years in this patient population. The authors concluded that linked prosthetic reconstruction with the Kinematic Rotating Hinge should be reserved for salvage situations.[33]

OVERVIEW OF FIRST- AND SECOND-GENERATION IMPLANTS

In 1986, the Swedish Orthopaedic Society published the survivorship analysis of over 8000 knee arthroplasties enrolled in the Swedish Knee Arthroplasty Project between 1975 and 1983.[34] Included in the report, subdivided by primary diagnosis of osteoarthritis and rheumatoid arthritis, was an independent survivorship analysis of 4 first-generation and 3 second-generation hinged knee arthroplasty designs. Arthroplasties were designated as failures if one or more prosthetic components had been added, removed, or replaced during the observation period. At 6 years, 140 first-generation hinges implanted for primary diagnosis of osteoarthritis had a survivorship of only 65%. One hundred two second-generation hinges implanted for the same diagnosis had a survivorship of 83% at the same follow-up duration. The majority of failures in both first- and second-generation designs were secondary to infection and mechanical loosening.[34] The Swedish experience clearly linked improved prosthetic design and surgical technique to improved prosthetic longevity. Nevertheless, the fundamental problems with linked prosthetic designs were also highlighted. Despite improved survivorship, unacceptable rates of loosening and major complications such as deep infection persisted. Survivorship of both first- and second-generation hinges was notably inferior to that of both unicompartmental and tricompartmental unlinked designs. In rheumatoid arthritis, survivorship was similar in all hinged designs, but inferior to the survivorship of unlinked tricompartmental arthroplasty.[34] This report accurately encapsulated the unsatisfactory clinical performance of hinge knee arthroplasty designs up to that point; however, it also provided promise that continued design evolution could improve longevity.

THIRD-GENERATION HINGES

Finn

The Finn rotating hinged knee (Biomet, Inc., Warsaw, IN) introduced in 1990, is a modular CoCr implant.[35,36] The prosthesis functions via an axle and yoke construct and approximates the anatomic profile of the knee. The link is not significantly weightbearing as contact between the femoral and tibial components is maintained throughout the range of motion. The design improves the distribution of weightbearing forces and patellofemoral kinematics by several specific design modifications. Anatomically sized femoral components have a deep patellar tracking groove and an anatomic axis of motion with a posterior center of rotation.

Preservation of the joint line is made possible through different sizing of the femoral component and selecting different thickness of the modular polyethylene bearing. Lastly, femoral and tibial geometry is congruent with a broad ultra-high molecular weight polyethylene (UHMWPE) surface contact throughout the range of motion. The net result is a prosthesis with improved stress

distribution, 135 degrees of flexion, 20 degrees of internal rotation, and 20 degrees of external rotation. The design further includes both modular cemented and uncemented femoral and tibial stem extensions, as well as distal femoral and proximal tibial replacement.[35,36]

The clinical results have been good in the short-term follow-up. In 1991 Finn reported no cases of failed fixation, instability, or patellofemoral maltracking in 23 knees at 9 months follow-up.[36] Later follow-up of 42 knees revealed a 25% incidence of overall complications in tumor reconstruction and suggested that mechanical failure was still an issue.[37] Westrich et al. in 2000 reported on 24 Finn prostheses with an average of 33 months of follow-up.[35] All the patients had significant improvement in the Knee Society Scores (average preoperative score 44, average postoperative 83). One patient (2 knees) had progressive femoral radiolucent lines no greater than 2 mm. Five patients had patellar subluxation but none were symptomatic.[35] Currently, there are no long-term series in the literature to report mechanical loosening rates with this implant. Of note, the Finn knee reports showed decreased rates of infection when compared with most first- and second-generation designs.[35–37] This was likely related to improvements in surgical technique.

The Finn knee designers' greatest contribution to the evolution of the hinge knee design was a formal kinematic analysis of gait and stair-stepping published in 1999.[38] Young (average 29.7 years) and older (average 56.2 years) patients with Finn rotating hinge knee prostheses were evaluated with regard to gait and stair stepping ability. Results were compared with both normal controls and patients with unlinked, posterior cruciate ligament (PCL)-retaining prostheses. The younger patients were as capable as younger controls and differed only in stride length and the external rotatory moment about the knee. Many of the younger patients had proximal tibia and soft tissue resected for tumor along with compromised extensor mechanisms reconstructed with rotation of the medial gastrocnemius. Decreased stride length was thought to be related to weakened calf musculature and push-off strength.[38]

Older patients were also noted to be equally as functional with regard to the activities of daily living tested in this study. The cadence and velocity of gait was similar to both the unlinked, PCL-retaining arthroplasty patients, and the controls. However, stride length was significantly short when compared with controls despite the lack of confounding soft tissue procedures. Older patients with Finn knee prostheses ambulated with an externally rotated, stiff-legged gait. The patients locked their knees in full extension at heel strike and maintained their knees in that position during early and midstance. Flexion of the torso placed the center of mass forward and reduced the demand on the extensor mechanism by creating an extension moment at the knee. Reliance on external moments to facilitate extension must increase prosthesis-cement and cement-bone stresses and may have a detrimental effect on prosthetic longevity. In contradistinction, rotatory moments on the knee were lessened. Without collateral ligaments, rotation of the prosthesis is checked predominantly by the lines of action of the knee flexors and extensors. The resultant moment in patients with the Finn prosthesis produced increased external rotation of the tibia during both stance phase and stair-stepping. Older patients with Finn rotating hinge knees were observed to externally rotate their torsos in the direction of the externally rotated foot during stair-stepping, thereby reducing normal internal rotatory forces about the knee. It was concluded that reduction in torque would reduce prosthesis-cement and cement-bone stresses and the potential for loosening.[38] This reduction would not be possible in first-generation, uniaxial hinge designs.

The kinematic data parallel the clinical experience of the Swedish Knee Arthroplasty Project.[34,38] Increased prosthesis-cement and cement-bone stresses associated with a stiff-legged gait result in early mechanical loosening when compared with unlinked prostheses. However, axial rotation, a second-generation design modification, decreases prosthesis-cement and cement-bone stresses, thereby improving longevity.

S-ROM

The S-ROM rotating hinged total knee (Figure 20-13) is a third-generation hinge that was developed from its precursor the Noiles hinged knee.[39] As discussed previously, the Noiles was an axle yoke system that allowed 20 degrees of rotation as well as flexion and extension. However, several problems with the Noiles such as failure at 32 months, single size, subsidence, and poly wear led to its abandonment.[27,28] The S-ROM is a modification of the Noiles that has addressed these problems. The prosthesis is CoCr, and the femoral component has a deepened groove for improved patellar tracking. The tibial component is broad with a polished finish. These femoral and tibial components are augmented with press-fit diaphyseal stems with slots or flutes. These are modular and have several sizes to obtain the best fit and fill and optimal load transmission. In addition to the stems, augments are available to restore the joint line. The polyethylene is congruent with the femoral component and allowed to rotate on the tibial component.[39,40]

The clinical results of this and other third-generation rotating hinged prostheses are encouraging. In a combined series of 2 surgeons, 30 knees with a mean follow-up of 49 months showed excellent results.[39] These midterm results were obtained using press-fit diaphyseal stems with metaphyseal filling sleeves and cemented components. The Knee Society Scores improved from 52 preoperatively to 134 postoperatively. The visual analog pain scales for walking showed significant improvement from 6.6 preoperative to 2.8 postoperative. The visual analog pain scales for stair climbing ability also improved from 7.6 preoperatively to 3.9 postoperatively. Finally, no mechanical failures of the implants have been seen in the midterm follow-up.[39]

Several other third-generation prostheses are commercially available. The MOST, the Kotz, the LINK, and others are modular prostheses with capabilities for managing severe bone loss. These systems have predominantly been applied after bone tumor resection about the knee,

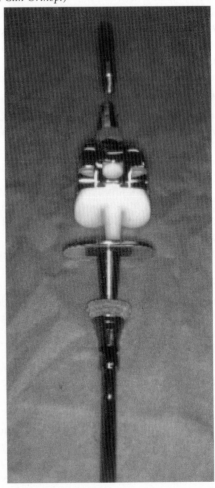

Figure 20-13. Exploded S-ROM modular, mobile bearing hinge knee prosthesis. Note modular stem extensions and modular metaphyseal filling components. (From Jones, Barrack, Skedros[39] by permission of *Clin Orthop.*)

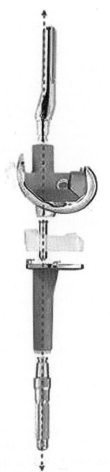

Figure 20-14. NexGen RHK, exploded view depicting axial association of parts. (Images copyright Zimmer, Inc. Used by permission only.)

and little is known about survivorship. Data in the revision arthroplasty setting are also lacking. However, each design is an axle yoke system with polyethylene bearing surfaces that transfer the majority of weightbearing force through the femoral condyles. It is reasonable to expect clinical performance to parallel that of other third-generation prostheses.

NexGen RHK

The Zimmer (Warsaw, IN) NexGen Rotating Hinge Knee is a CoCr resurfacing prosthesis, is the latest of the modern hinged devices, and may represent a new generation of prostheses.[41] The prosthesis, like most modern unlinked revision prostheses, is designed as a resurfacing prosthesis. A slightly larger, intercondylar box cut accommodates the link, and flexibility is achieved through standard revision stem and augment modularity.[41]

This hinged device is not linked in the same manner as traditional hinges. The hinge consists of a CoCr hinge

post that is preassembled to the intercondylar box of the femoral component. Metal-on-metal contact is prevented by a polyethylene box liner and bushing (Figure 20-14). A hinge pin secures the mechanism. After the components have been implanted, a CoCr hinge post extension is threaded into the preassembled hinge post and inserted into a polyethylene bushing located inside the tibial base plate stem. Like the Finn knee, the link is unloaded, and the majority of weightbearing forces (95%) are transmitted from the tibia to the femur via a highly conforming polyethylene bearing. The device allows 25 degrees of internal and external rotation about the post extension, but prevents dislocation with a jump distance of 4 cm. Flexion and extension are permitted from 0 to 120 degrees with 2 modes of dampening the terminal extension load.[41] Like many of the third-generation prostheses, peer-reviewed outcomes in revision knee arthroplasty are not available with the NexGen RHK.

INDICATIONS FOR HINGED IMPLANTS

A review of the literature indicates that hinged prostheses represent fewer than 1% of all knee arthroplasties performed in the United States.[32] In our practice as well, linked prostheses are infrequently required. Most are performed in association with large bone deficits encountered during revision arthroplasty or after tumor resection. However, as the number and complexity of revision surgeries increase, we anticipate the increased need for hinged total knee arthroplasty.

We believe that uniaxial hinge prostheses have no role in modern arthroplasty. Instead, all linked reconstructions should be performed with a prosthesis that allows some degree of axial rotation and varus-valgus motion. It is also preferable for the condylar reconstruction to dissipate forces through load sharing. In this manner, the axle and link are protected from fatigue fracture as the weightbearing forces are partially dissipated through host bone. Decreased constraint and condylar load sharing also decrease stresses at the prosthesis-cement and prosthesis-bone interfaces, and potentially increase prosthesis longevity.

The absolute indications for rotating hinge reconstruction in our practice are (1) femoral and/or tibial tumor resections that sacrifice the origins or insertions of the collateral ligaments; (2) gross ligamentous incompetence defined as the clinical absence of all 4 major knee ligaments; and (3) severe bone loss from osteolysis, sepsis debridement, or component removal that has eliminated the origin or insertion of the collateral ligaments.[42-44]

TABLE 20.1. AORI Femoral Bone Loss Classification.

AORI Femur Grade	Deficit	MCL/LCL	Bone Reconstruction
F1	Intact Metaphyseal Bone	Intact	Cement or Particulate Graft
F2a	Metaphyseal Loss Single Condyle	Intact	Cement or Metal Augment
F2b	Metaphyseal Loss Both Condyles	Intact	Cement, Metal Augment or Structural Graft
F3	Deficient Metaphysis	Compromised	Structural Allograft or Segmental Replacement

In revision knee arthroplasty we grade bone loss intraoperatively, after primary component removal, using the AORI classification (Tables 20.1 and 20.2). Bone loss is graded separately for the femur and tibia on a progressive scale from 1 to 3.[45] The implication is that grade F3 and T3 bone loss is frequently associated with compromised collateral ligaments. Hinged total knee arthroplasty substitutes for the collateral ligaments and often is the optimal reconstruction choice for grade F3 and T3 bone loss.

Relative indications for rotating hinge reconstruction in our practice include (1) severe valgus or varus deformity combined with severe flexion contracture that necessitates complete release of both collaterals; (2) severe uncorrectable flexion-extension gap imbalance that may result in cam dissociation of an unlinked design; (3) primary or revision arthroplasty in patients with neuromuscular diseases such as polio; (4) compromised extensor mechanism; and (5) severe recurvatum.[42–44] The author's algorithm for selecting an appropriate prosthesis with regard to ligament competence and bone loss is represented by Figure 20-15.

Technique

Surgical exposure of the knee and subsequent removal of implants is difficult in revision surgery. Several modifications to the standard medial parapatellar approach have been suggested to improve exposure in difficult cases. These include the quadriceps snip, V-Y quadricepsplasty, quadriceps turndown, tibial tubercle osteotomy, and medial epicondylar osteotomy, which are discussed in Chapter 6. Our preferred technique is the quadriceps snip because the technique is simple to perform, provides excellent improvement in exposure, and may be performed without alteration in postoperative therapy protocols. The tibial tubercle osteotomy may be combined with the quadriceps snip to provide increased exposure; however, postoperative protocols must be altered to include cast or brace immobilization in extension for several weeks followed by passive range of motion. Active extension is delayed 4 to 6 weeks and full weightbearing is delayed 6 weeks when a tibial tubercle osteotomy is needed.

Once the knee has been exposed, the soft tissue envelope is assessed. The medial and lateral gutters, the suprapatellar pouch, and potential space between the patellar tendon and the anterior tibia proximal to the tubercle are reestablished through scar excision. Medial and lateral collateral ligament competence can now be assessed through palpation and manual testing. Full extension and several positions of flexion should be assessed because contracted tissues such as the posterior capsule may

TABLE 20.2. AORI Tibial Bone Loss Classification.

AORI Tibial Grade	Deficit	MCL/LCL	Bone Reconstruction
T1	Intact Metaphyseal Bone	Intact	Cement or Particulate Graft
T2a	Metaphyseal Loss Med **or** Lat Plateau	Intact	Cement or Metal Augment
T2b	Metaphyseal Loss Med **and** Lat Plateau	Intact	Cement, Metal Augment or Structural Graft
T3*	Deficient Metaphysis	Compromised	Structural Allograft or Segmental Replacement

*Possible extensor mechanism compromise.

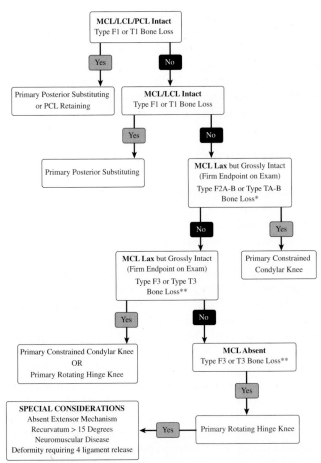

Figure 20-15. Algorithm for ligament competence and bone loss. *Bone loss made up with augments and cement; stem tibia and/or femur. **Bone loss cannot be made up by augments and cement; must use structural graft or segment replacement.

provide apparent stability in extension despite incompetent collateral ligaments.

The components to be revised are next assessed for positioning prior to removal. Frequently, component malposition and/or improper sizing can be determined as the source of patellar maltracking/dislocation, stiffness, and instability. These clues can be used to help guide the proper reconstruction. After component removal with thin osteotomes and/or a Gigli saw, bone loss is assessed and graded using the AORI classification (Tables 20.1 and 20.2). Rotating hinge reconstruction is performed only when less constraining prostheses are unlikely to provide adequate stability, or severe bone loss (F3 and/or T3) exists.

The first step is to provide the ultimate reconstruction with a stable tibial platform and a correct joint line. Minimal proximal tibia is osteotomized perpendicular to its anatomic axis, and the platform is leveled or raised by

block or segmental augmentation as necessary. Preoperative planning and even contralateral radiographs are helpful in reestablishing the joint line. Frequently used landmarks for reestablishing the joint line when working on the tibia are the inferior pole of the patella and the head of the fibula. Elevating the joint line may create patellar baja, cause anterior impingement of the extensor mechanism in flexion, alter the kinetics of the patellofemoral joint, and limit the range of motion. Most current hinged devices combat this issue by placing a cutout in the anterior polyethylene and providing the ability to manipulate the joint line through the use of various sized modular wedge and segment options. The tibia is next machined to accept appropriate stem sizes and then oriented in rotation based on the position of the tibial tubercle. If the tubercle is absent we base rotation off an extramedullary guide rod positioned parallel to the lateral tibial crest and located distally just lateral to the anterior aspect of the medial malleolus. Most rotating hinge prostheses do not require a posterior tibial slope (no rollback in linked prosthesis), and it is usually recommended that the proximal tibia be cut perpendicular to the long axis. The perpendicular cut also helps prevent flexion instability and prosthesis dissociation.

The femur is first reconstructed with respect to rotation. Three degrees of external rotation of the femoral component is optimal for proper patellar tracking. The easiest landmark to assess rotation is the epicondylar axis. If the epicondyles are absent, then Whiteside's line can be used. Posterior referencing is often less useful in the assessment of femoral rotation because in the revision setting the condyles are deficient. The posterior condyles are helpful, however, in assessing the position of the implant that is to be revised. If the primary component appears internally rotated, then one must be prepared to perform a new anterior reference cut in the proper rotation. Once rotation is established, the femur is sized in the AP plane and cut to fit a trial component. Revision knee systems provide 5-degree and/or 7-degree valgus femoral stems, and the distal femoral resection must be made appropriately. Bone deficiency and the need for augmentation are easily assessed by examining the unsupported portions of the femoral trial. Great care is taken at this point to establish the proper joint line from the femoral side. Distal augments or segments should be trialed until the medial joint line is 25 to 30mm distal to the medial epicondyle and 20 to 25mm distal to the lateral epicondyle. This joint line should match the joint line established via tibial reconstruction, including 10 to 16mm of polyethylene tibial insert. If the epicondyles are absent (F3 bone loss), then the femoral reconstruction is simply brought down to the joint line established by tibial reconstruction. Keep in mind that the joint line may be elevated pre-revision due to femoral collapse and the routine use of *plus cuts* on the distal femur during primary arthroplasty. This slight elevation of the joint line on the femoral side is commonly required during revision reconstruction to ensure full extension. Once the joint line is confirmed, the femur is machined for the appropriate size augments and stem.

Balance of the flexion and extension gap at the appropriate joint line is easily accomplished with modern instrumentation and modular hinge designs. The trial reduction should be balanced much the same as a primary arthroplasty. Care must be taken to eliminate gross flexion instability, as this may lead to dissociation of the hinge post from the tibial polyethylene bearing surface in some *unlinked* rotating hinge prostheses. The modern hinge device typically provides a 3- to 4-cm *jump distance*. Soft tissue releases are frequently needed to balance the flexion and extension gaps, but most work should be done on the bony side by a combination of resection and augmentation. Range of motion should be from full extension to beyond 90 degrees flexion. Mild joint line elevation with respect to femoral positioning is best tolerated when trial reduction does not achieve full extension.

The trial reduction is then inspected with regard to patellofemoral function. Mild patella baja associated with patellar tendon fibrosis and contracture is well tolerated if the joint line has been properly restored. If the extensor mechanism impinges on the anterior tibial reconstruction despite an appropriately recessed polyethylene design, then mild joint line lowering with respect to the tibial reconstruction is appropriate. Care should also be taken to ensure that the femoral trial component is not oversized. The AP size increase of the femoral component varies per design, but is approximately 4 mm per size. Downsizing the femoral component decreases extensor mechanism tension during flexion. Tibial and femoral component rotation should be rechecked and corrected if patellofemoral tracking is poor. Lateral releases are required more commonly in the revision setting than in the primary setting, but the underlying causes for maltracking are the same. Component position should be addressed before performing a lateral release. We routinely release the tourniquet before performing a lateral release to prevent tethering of the quadriceps musculature and to help in maintaining strict hemostasis. Persistent genicular bleeding after lateral retinacular release may result in postoperative hemarthrosis, stiffness, and wound compromise.

Once satisfactory trial reconstruction is achieved, the bony surfaces are prepared for cementing. The authors routinely cement the tibial and femoral components and stems. We commonly use cement restrictors to limit the extent of cementing, but do not routinely pressurize the medullary spaces. Concern exists in both linked and unlinked reconstructions regarding the longevity of *hybrid* techniques, in which the components are cemented and the stems are not. In the future, newer cementless techniques and design modifications may become available and obviate the need for cement.

CONCLUSION

In conclusion, hinged total knee arthroplasty has undergone a unique design evolution, from single-size, uniaxial devices with poor fixation methods to current designs with multiple sizes, modularity, multiple modes of fixation, and decreasing constraint. The evolution parallels the scientific evolution of orthopedics and knee surgery in general. Increasing laboratory testing and engineering have been part of each new advance. Clinical reports and kinematic testing support the notion that these design modifications can affect prosthetic longevity and improve outcomes. Nevertheless, no hinged prosthesis has midterm clinical results comparable with those of unlinked designs. Long-term data have not been reported with any linked device. As such, hinged prostheses should be reserved for specific indications. Despite design advances and future promise, hinged devices serve predominantly as a salvage option in cases of tumor reconstruction, severe bone loss, severe ligamentous instability, severe deformity, and extensor mechanism dysfunction.

Example Case

A 45-year-old woman has an infected total knee arthroplasty and history of patellar tendon avulsion (Figure 20-16A). Components were removed and radical debridement undertaken. The tibia was reconstructed originally with an antibiotic-impregnated cement tibial spacer and recementing of the autoclaved original femoral component with antibiotic impregnated cement (Figure 20-16B, C). Repeat debridement was undertaken before permanent reconstruction. After 6 weeks of intravenous antibiotic and 3 months of oral antibiotic, the knee was aspirated and documented free of infection. At the time of reconstruction, the extensor mechanism was compromised, the medial collateral ligament (MCL) was absent, and the bone stock was graded as F3 and T2. Reconstruction with a rotating hinge prosthesis was undertaken with reconstruction of the extensor mechanism (Figure 20-16D, E). Nearly 2 years postoperatively, the patient ambulates without assistive device, has flexion to 95 degrees, and has only a 5-degree extensor lag (Figure 20-16F).

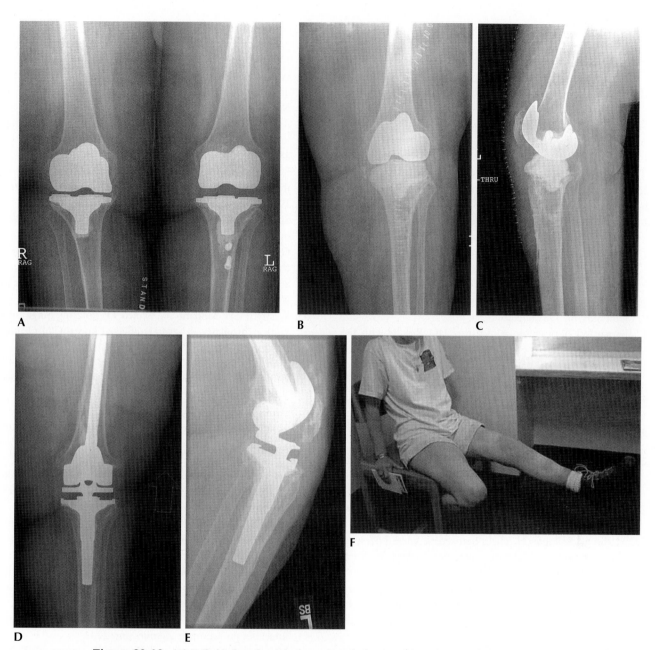

Figure 20-16. (A) Failed infected arthroplasty. (B and C) AP and lateral views of the first stage of revision. (D and E) AP and lateral views of rotating hinge prosthetic implant reconstruction. (F) Two-year postoperative range of motion.

REFERENCES

1. Jones GB. Total knee replacement—the Walldius hinge. *Clin Orthop.* 1973;94:50–57.

2. Habermann ET, Deutsch SD, Rovere GD. Knee arthroplasty with the use of the Walldius total knee prosthesis. *Clin Orthop.* 1973;94:72–84.

3. Jackson JP, Elson RA. Evaluation of the Walldius and other prostheses for knee arthroplasty. *Clin Orthop.* 1973;94:104–114.

4. Freeman PA. Walldius arthroplasty: a review of 80 cases. *Clin Orthop.* 1973;94:85–91.

5. Bain AM. Replacement of the knee joint with the Walldius prosthesis using cement fixation. *Clin Orthop.* 1973;94:65–71.

6. Wilson FC, Fajgenbaum DM, Venters GC. Results of knee replacement with the Walldius and geometric prostheses. *J Bone Joint Surg Am.* 1980;62A:497–503.

7. Hui FC, Fitzgerald RH. Hinged total knee arthroplasty. *J Bone Joint Surg Am.* 1980;62A:513–519.

8. Arden GP. Total knee replacement. *Clin Orthop.* 1973;94:92–103.

9. Shiers LGP. Arthroplasty of the knee. preliminary report on a new method. *J Bone Joint Surg Br.* 1954;36B:553.

10. Shiers LGP. Hinge arthroplasty for arthritis. *Rheumatism.* 1961;17:54–60.

11. Phillips RS. Shiers' alloplasty of the knee. *Clin Orthop.* 1973;94:122–127.

12. Brady TA, Garber JN. Knee joint replacement using Shiers knee hinge. *J Bone Joint Surg Am.* 1974;56A:1610–1614.

13. Lettin AWF, Deliss LJ, Blackburne JS. The Stanmore hinged knee arthroplasty. *J Bone Joint Surg Br.* 1978;60B:327–332.

14. Karpinski MRK, Grimer RJ. Hinged knee replacement in revision arthroplasty. *Clin Orthop.* 1987;220:185–191.

15. Jones EC, Insall JN, Inglis AE. Guepar knee arthroplasty results and late complications. *Clin Orthop.* 1979;140:145–152.

16. LeNobel J, Patterson FP. Guepar total knee prosthesis. *J Bone Joint Surg Br.* 1981;63B:257–260.

17. Bargar WL, Cracchiolo A, Amstutz HC. Results with the constrained total knee prosthesis in treating severely disabled patients and patients with failed total knee replacements. *J Bone Joint Surg Am.* 1980;62A:504–512.

18. Barrack RL. Evolution of the rotating hinge for complex total knee arthroplasty. *Clin Orthop.* 2001;392:292–299.

19. Sheehan JM. Arthroplasty of the knee. *J Bone Joint Surg Br.* 1978;60B:333–338.

20. Rickhuss PK, Gray AJ, Rowley DI. A 5- 10-year follow-up of the Sheehan total knee endoprosthesis in Tayside. *J R Coll Surg Ed.* 1994;39(5):326–328.

21. Murray DG, Wilde AH, Werner F. Herbert total knee prosthesis. *JBone Joint Surg Am.* 1977;59A:1026–1032.

22. Mathews LS, Kaufer H. The spherocentric knee: a perspective on seven years of clinical experience. *Orthop Clin North Am.* 1982;13(1):173–186.

23. Mathews LS, Goldstein SA, Kolowich PA. Spherocentric arthroplasty of the knee. *Clin Orthop.* 1986;205:58–66.

24. Attenborough CG. The Attenborough total knee replacement. *J Bone Joint Surg Br.* 1978;60B:320–326.

25. Vanhegan JAD, Dabrowski W, Arden GP. A review of 100 Attenborough stabilized gliding knee prostheses. *J Bone Joint Surg Br.* 1979;61B:445–450.

26. Kershaw CJ, Themen AEG. The Attenborough knee: a four- to ten-year review. *J Bone Joint Surg Br.* 1988;70B:89–93.

27. Kester MA, Cook SD, Harding AF. An evaluation of the mechanical failure modalities of a rotating hinge prosthesis. *Clin Orthop.* 1988;228:156–163.

28. Shindell R, Neumann R, Connolly JF. Evaluation of the Noiles hinged knee prosthesis. *J Bone Joint Surg Am.* 1986;68A:579–585.

29. Shaw JA, Balcom W, Greer RB. Total knee arthroplasty using the kinematic rotating hinge prosthesis. *Orthopedics.* 1989;12(5):647–654.

30. Walker PS, Emerson R, Potter T. The kinematic rotating hinge: biomechanics and clinical application. *Orthop Clin North Am.* 1982;13(1):187–199.

31. Rand JA, Chao EYS, Stauffer RN. Kinematic rotating-hinge total knee arthroplasty. *J Bone Joint Surg Am.* 1987;69A:489–497.

32. Kabo MJ, Yang RS, Dorey FJ. In vivo rotational stability of the kinematic rotating hinge knee prosthesis. *Clin Orthop.* 1997;336:166–176.

33. Springer BD, Hanssen AD, Sim FH. The kinematic rotating hinge prosthesis for complex knee arthroplasty. *Clin Orthop.* 2001;392:283–291.

34. Knutson KAJ, Lindstrand A, Lindgren L. Survival of knee arthroplasties: a nation-wide multicenter investigation of 8000 cases. *J Bone Joint Surg Br.* 1986;68B:795–803.

35. Westrich GH, Mollano AV, Sculco TP. Rotating hinge total knee arthroplasty in severely affected knees. *Clin Orthop.* 2000;379:195–208.

36. Finn HA, Kniel JS, Kane LA. Constrained endoprosthetic replacement of the knee: a new design. *J Bone Joint Surg Br.* 1991;(Suppl 2):177–178.

37. Finn HA, Golden D, Kneisi JA. The Finn knee; rotating hinge replacement of the knee. complications of limb salvage, prevention, management and outcome. *Montreal Int Soc Limb Salvage.* 1991;413–415.

38. Draganich LF, Whitehurst JB, Chou LS. The effects of the rotating-hinge total knee replacement on gait and stair stepping. *J Arthroplasty.* 1999;14(6):743–755.

39. Jones RE, Barrack RL, Skedros J. Modular, mobile-bearing hinge total knee arthroplasty. *Clin Orthop.* 2001;392:306–314.

40. Barrack RL, Lyons TR, Ingraham RQ. The use of a modular rotating hinge component in salvage revision total knee arthroplasty. *J Arthroplasty.* 2000;15(7):858–866.

41. 97-5880-03 10ML. The next generation of rotating hinge knee: design rationale. *Zimmer, Inc.* 2002.

42. Murray DG. Editorial: in defense of becoming unhinged. *J Bone Joint Surg Am.* 1980;62A:495–496.

43. Cuckler JM. Revision total knee arthroplasty: how much constraint is necessary? *Orhtopedics.* 1995;18(9):932–936.

44. Scuderi GR. Revision total nnee arthroplasty: how much constraint is enough? *Clin Orthop.* 2001;392:300–305.

45. Engh GA, Rorabeck CH. *Revision Total Knee Arthroplasty.* 1st ed. Baltimore: Williams & Wilkins; 1997.

CHAPTER 21

Total Knee Arthroplasty After Fractures About the Knee

Russell E. Windsor and William L. Walter

Gonarthrosis in a patient who has had a fracture about the knee may result from direct injury to the articular surface at the time of fracture or it may result secondarily from altered mechanics across the knee with associated ligament injuries and bony deformities. It may be incidental to the fracture that has occurred in the metaphyseal or diaphyseal region of the knee. Also, secondary arthritic deterioration may develop from hardware penetrating into the joint.

Total knee arthroplasty in these patients presents an array of technical challenges to the surgeon. Damage to the soft tissue envelope of the knee makes exposure more difficult and may lead to healing problems and stiffness due to the associated scarring that may develop from the fracture itself or from the extent of surgery required to initially fix the fracture.[1] There is a greater risk of infection due to soft tissue envelope compromise and possible bacterial colonization of bone or hardware.[1,2] Bone loss, bone deformity, and fracture nonunion can present problems that may require augments, long-stemmed implants, or even an osteotomy to solve.[3] Furthermore, issues relating to the patella present their own challenges.[1] Finally, soft tissue balancing of the knee can be difficult particularly if the collateral ligaments have been damaged.

Although primary total knee replacement is not infrequently performed for post-traumatic osteoarthritis secondary to fracture, the technical challenges these clinical cases offer demand techniques that are more frequently seen during revision total knee replacement. The only significant difference between primary total knee replacement for arthritis involving an intra-articular or extra-articular fracture and revision surgery is that the surgeon may have more bone stock at his or her disposal when performing the reconstruction. Only in severe intra-articular tibial plateau or femoral condylar fractures could there be extenuating circumstances in which there is extraordinary bone loss secondary to the severity of the fracture (Figure 21-1).

PREOPERATIVE CONSIDERATIONS

Infection Risk

Knee arthroplasty after fracture about the knee has been shown to carry a higher risk of infection.[1,2,4] This may be due to a damaged soft tissue envelope resulting from the original injury and/or open reduction and internal fixation exposure or to colonization of hardware, especially in the case of external fixators. The preoperative workup should include laboratory tests for markers of infection (complete blood count, C-reactive protein, and erythrocyte sedimentation rate). An aspiration of the knee should be obtained and the specimen sent for Gram's stain, culture, and sensitivities.[5] During the total knee replacement operation itself, intraoperative Gram's stain and culture may also be useful. If there is a high index of suspicion of infection at the time of surgery it may be appropriate to perform a staged primary total knee replacement with the first stage consisting of a thorough debridement of the knee, including making the definitive bone cuts for the arthroplasty. The implantation of the prosthesis is delayed until the presence of infection in the knee tissue is resolved. During the first stage, the initial distal, anterior, and posterior femoral bone resections are performed. The proximal tibial resection and posterior patellar resection is also done and an antibiotic-impregnated acrylic spacer block is inserted. This procedure basically serves as a very aggressive debridement since the articular surfaces are resected at this stage. Finishing resections such as femoral chamfers and tibial stem preparation are done during the second stage when the prostheses themselves are implanted with antibiotic

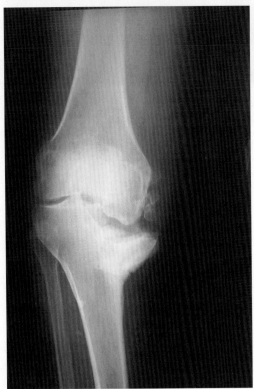

FIGURE 21-1. Anteroposterior radiograph showing a medial tibial plateau fracture with severe depression of the medial tibial condyle.

impregnated cement. Considerable success has been achieved in treating patients at high risk in this way. Implantation of the knee prostheses may be done as early as 1 week after this first stage if the intraoperative culture results are negative. However, if they are positive, implantation is delayed for 6 weeks or more while the infection is treated with an appropriate course of parenteral or oral antibiotics. This scenario is similar to the two-stage treatment of an infected total knee replacement. Antibiotic impregnated cement should be used during the second stage even if there was no evidence found of an active infection.

Imaging

In addition to a routine series of radiographs of the knee it may be necessary to obtain additional imaging such as a full-length standing anteroposterior radiograph or CT scan to clearly define any deformity resulting from the fracture.[3] A Technetium-diphosphonate bone scan or gallium scan may be useful for localizing infection if there is a high suspicion for its presence. These scans are particularly suggested in cases in which numerous operative procedures were performed or cases in which the patient had a prolonged, complicated course of treatment.

The full-length standing radiographs are important for preoperative planning to determine the possible need for corrective osteotomy.[3] This is particularly important if there is a significant malunion present that may affect the overall alignment of the knee. Malunion may make it difficult or impossible to use intramedullary instrumentation to gain appropriate alignment of the distal femoral or proximal tibial resection. Hence, extramedullary alignment guides should be used to obtain a correctly aligned resection.

A good rule for handling malunion situations is to mark out a line on the standing radiograph of the planned resection that would provide the correct mechanical axis. If there is the risk of violating the collateral ligament insertions on the femur, then a corrective osteotomy should be contemplated. If osteotomy is required, it is usually performed at the site of the original malunion. Otherwise, a swan-neck or curved bow deformity would be obtained because of the malunion site and the osteotomy site working together to create this anatomic relationship.

EXPOSURE

Soft Tissue Envelope

The soft tissue envelope may be compromised either as a result of the initial injury or as a result of subsequent surgeries. An effort should be made to incorporate old incisions if possible. In the case of multiple incisions, the most lateral incision that is practical should be used.[1] If there are old incisions that cannot practically be used, then it may be necessary to adjust the incision medially or laterally to increase the width of the skin bridge. Hockey stick incisions and transverse incisions may present a particular concern. In general, an incision can be crossed at right angles but should not be crossed obliquely. Incisions older than 10 years can probably be ignored. If there are particular concerns about the soft tissue envelope, the surgeon may perform the skin incision only and delay the definitive procedure. The healing of this incision can be monitored and if necessary the definitive procedure may be performed with the cover of a vascularized flap.[1,6]

A *delay* procedure only may be performed to determine the healing potential of the wound. During this procedure, the incision and underlying soft tissue dissection is performed and the wound is closed. Healing is observed for a 2-week period to determine the presence of eschar formation and to permit neovascularization of the soft tissue flaps. If skin necrosis develops, then separate soft tissue coverage grafts would be needed prior to the knee replacement implantation stage. A gastrocnemius muscle flap or vascularized free myocutaneous flap may be used in this situation to obtain healthy soft tissue coverage.[2]

In situations in which the skin is adherent to the underlying extensor mechanism, tissue expanders may be inserted to stretch the skin and create neovascularized environment before the primary total knee replacement. As in revision situations, it may be necessary to extend the original incision proximally and distally to more clearly define the subcutaneous tissue planes. This enables the surgeon to find the proper depth of the plane between the extensor mechanism and subcutaneous adipose tissue or scar.

Scar tissue and bone deformity or overgrowth may make exposure of the knee quite difficult. The surgeon may need to consider techniques such as a rectus snip, lateral retinacular release, or tibial tubercle osteotomy to facilitate exposure.[4,7] The rectus snip is generally the preferred choice due to its relative simplicity and ability to be extended. It is performed by extending proximally and laterally the standard medial arthrotomy that is performed during most primary replacement surgeries. Early lateral retinacular release is performed when there is difficulty with exposure and eversion of the patella or in cases in which there is considerable scarring from a previous lateral incision or adherent scar along the lateral femoral gutter. Tibial tubercle osteotomy is used when patellar eversion is still not possible even with the use of the quadriceps snip. This technique is particularly recommended if a previous tibial tubercle osteotomy was used during the initial approach for open reduction and internal fixation of a tibial plateau fracture.

Since there is frequently scar tissue present from previous open reduction procedures, it may be necessary to recreate the medial and lateral gutters. With this technique, the scar tissue adhesions that have formed between the quadriceps mechanism and femur may be fully excised. In rare situations, skeletonization of the distal femur may be required if there is substantial preoperative ankylosis. In these latter situations, the surgeon should be prepared to use prostheses with further built-in constraint, such as a constrained condylar knee, or total condylar III implant. In extraordinary cases of severe distal femoral malunion or severe proximal tibial condyle disruption and bone loss, constrained rotating hinge designs may be required.

REMOVING HARDWARE

Removal of hardware is not mandatory unless the presence of the hardware interferes with instrumentation, placement, or function of the arthroplasty. A longer inci-

sion and greater exposure are usually required to remove hardware. It is only necessary to use the original medial or lateral incision if it is clear that the implant is not reachable by the standard midline incision that will be used during the replacement. Often, buttress plates affixed to the lateral tibial plateau may be simply removed by entering the anterolateral muscle compartment through and extended midline incision. The soft tissue envelope should be assessed preoperatively to determine the likelihood of success. Obese patients may have enough adipose tissue coverage to permit easy access to the lateral side of the joint by further lateral dissection through the midline incision. A separate incision may be necessary if instrumentation can not be easily applied to the implants through the midline incision. Use of a single midline incision simplifies the exposure and decreases the risk of skin flap necrosis that may arise as a result of the presence of two freshly made incisions (Figure 21-2).

FIGURE 21-2. Medial and lateral plates may be removed from the midline incision used during the total knee replacement. Also, these plates may be removed as a separate procedure.

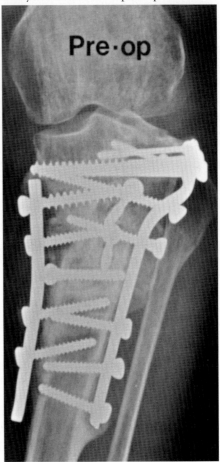

Nevertheless, as a general rule, all hardware should be removed unless this procedure unnecessarily places the operative environment in danger of necrosis or additional bone loss by difficult extraction techniques. If there is a suspicion of infection, the hardware may be removed during a separate stage and a sample of deep tissue can be obtained and sent for frozen section, routine pathology, culture, and sensitivity. A separate removal stage is generally reserved for large implants that may extend far away from the knee joint itself.

Proximal intramedullary femoral nails that extend to the distal metaphysis would interfere with the use of intramedullary alignment instrumentation. In this case, extramedullary alignment instruments should be considered. The nail should only be removed if there is little risk of disrupting the proximal aspect of the femur.

BONE LOSS

Contained defects of the tibial plateau or femoral condyles can be filled with morsellized bone graft that can usually be obtained from the resected bone.[1] However, it may be necessary to add a stem to the component to add stability to the construct if there is still proximal discontinuity that mandates additional fixation.[8] If there is an uncontained tibial or femoral defect, then augments and a stems should be added to the component. Frequently, it may be necessary to combine grafting with the use of metal augmentation.

Larger defects may require the use of a distal femoral or proximal tibial replacement that is used for the treatment of tumor excisions in this area. Bulk allografts may be also used in these situations and the surgeon must weigh the risk and benefits of allograft incorporation, stability, and long-term survivorship. This decision-making process is somewhat age-dependent, as allograft usage would be considered in the younger patient with better bone stock and large constrained, distal femoral or proximal tibial replacements are better suited for the older patient with more compromised bone stock.

BONE DEFORMITY

Malunion or nonunion may result in deformity of either the tibia or the femur. This may be in the coronal plane (varus/valgus), sagittal plane (flexion/extension), the axial plane (rotation), or any combination of these. If the deformity is not corrected, the altered mechanics that may have caused the arthritis could lead to early failure of the device.[9,10]

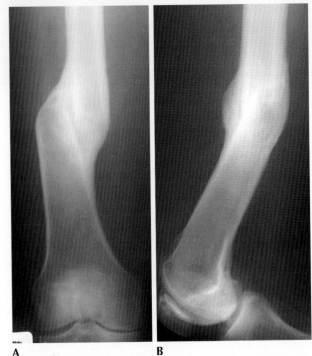

A   **B**

FIGURE 21-3. (A and B) Anteroposterior and lateral x-ray of a midshaft femoral malunion. This patient underwent corrective osteotomy as a separate procedure, prior to the performance of a total knee replacement.

Intra-articular deformity (deformity within the collateral ligaments) may be corrected with the bone cuts or may require augments; however, extra-articular deformity (deformity proximal to the femoral origin of the collateral ligaments or distal to the tibial insertion) may need to be corrected by osteotomy[3,10] (Figure 21-3).

NONUNION

Open reduction and internal fixation of nonunited fragments with screws or plate and screws may be possible at the time of arthroplasty.[1] If implant stability is compromised, a stem may be added to a femoral or tibial component. Long stemmed prosthesis may be appropriate to span a transverse nonunion. Bone graft, bone graft substitutes, and adjuvants can also be considered.

For proximal tibial nonunions or femoral condylar nonunions, the initial resection of bone may be significant enough that the nonunited segment is almost completely excised. In these cases, simple metal augments may be used. The resected bone, however, serves as an excellent source for autogenous graft material and is packed around a persistent non-union site. The combination of stem extensions, fixation of the nonunited fracture frag-

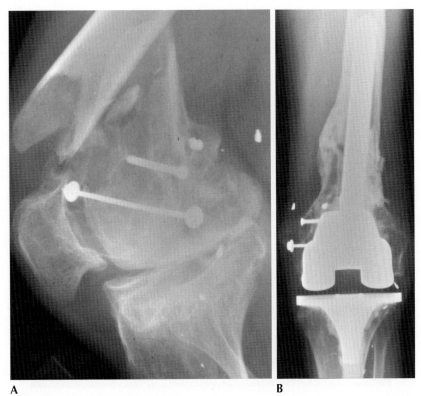

FIGURE 21-4. (A and B) Preoperative and postoperative x-ray of a supracondylar femur fracture. The resected one was used as autograft. An intramedullary stem extension was utilized to obtain control of the fracture.

ments with a cemented or porous implant and autologous bone graft is quite successful in bringing about union of the fracture site and handling of the arthritic condition (Figure 21-4).

Protected weightbearing may be necessary based on the overall stability of the reconstruction. However, in most cases, the postoperative rehabilitation course progresses uneventfully.

ACUTE FRACTURE

In the majority of cases a fracture about the knee should be treated by open reduction and internal fixation as appropriate. Arthroplasty is then performed later if and when arthritis has developed. However, if there is poor prospect for normal joint function (in the case of preexisting arthritis or significant chondral injury), particularly in an elderly or frail patient, arthroplasty may be appropriate at the time of the acute fracture.[11,12]

Certainly, open reduction and internal fixation should be considered first, as every attempt should be made to preserve bone stock. If post-traumatic arthritis occurs after the fracture has healed, total knee replacement can be performed in the area where the fracture has united. Nevertheless, in the elderly, fracture treatment may dictate partial or nonweightbearing, or prolonged bed rest that may pose the threat of venous thromboembolic disease or pulmonary embolism. In this case, it may be more prudent to consider primary knee replacement, especially when treating intra-articular fractures. The benefits include quick rehabilitation and early mobilization without the need for prolonged protected weight bearing. In general, all attempts should be made to preserve the natural knee anatomy. However, there may be extenuating circumstances when total knee replacement is the more prudent option.

PATELLA CONSIDERATIONS

Care should be taken to avoid rupture of patella tendon at the time of surgery by using techniques previously mentioned to facilitate the exposure without putting undue tension on the patella tendon.[1] If the exposure is difficult, it may be necessary to secure the patella tendon to the tibial tubercle with a bone pin. There is a higher risk of delayed rupture of the extensor mechanism in this

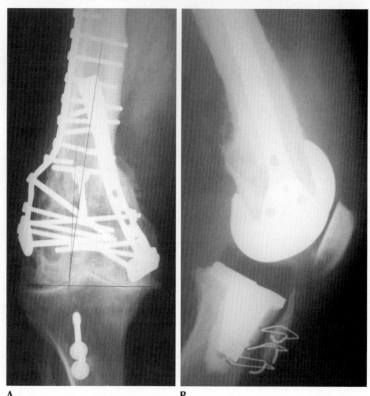

A   **B**

FIGURE 21-5. (A and B) Preoperative and postoperative radiograph of a knee with a complex femoral fracture that was initially exposed using a tibial tubercle osteotomy. A non-union developed and two attempts at bone grafting and fixation of the tibial tubercle were required before healing occurred. Bone graft adjuvants were required. The large size of the tibial tubercle osteotomy permitted ultimate fixation and healing to occur.

patient group that may occur during extensor mechanism eversion and flexion of the knee, particularly in patients who have diabetes or are taking oral steroids.[1,2]

Fractures of the proximal tibia can result in scarring of the patella tendon and patella baja. Mild cases may require fashioning of a recess in the anterior portion of the tibial polyethylene but more severe cases may require tibial tubercle osteotomy or even an extensor mechanism allograft.

In cases in which a tibial tubercle osteotomy was performed to expose a tibial fracture for reduction and internal fixation, the tibial tubercle may progress to nonunion (Figure 21-5). In addition to fixation with screws, this may require bone grafting and bone graft adjuvants and perhaps also reinforcement with a cable or wires. It may be necessary to splint the limb in extension postoperatively and may compromise overall rehabilitation of the arthroplasty.

Patella fracture if unhealed and not amenable to fixation may be treated by simple debridement of prominent bone or by complete patellectomy keeping in mind that extensor strength will be compromised.

SOFT TISSUE BALANCING

Stiffness

Preoperative range of motion may be less than normal in which case the surgeon should expect poorer postoperative range of motion, particularly in the case of distal femoral fracture. Some cases require manipulation of the knee in the first 6 to 12 weeks postoperatively.[1] Extensor mechanism scarring is difficult to release. Extensor mechanism lengthening is not recommended as secondary quadriceps mechanism weakness may develop despite the possibility of improved flexion. Scar tissue may be excised in the medial and lateral gutters. But, flexion may only be marginally increased if interstitial scarring of the quadriceps muscle is present. The vastus intermedius may be lifted off and dissected free from the anterior aspect of the femur.

Stiffness is less of a secondary problem after tibial plateau or shaft fractures. The stiffness that is created is generally intra-articular rather than extra-articular, which is the case in supracondylar femur or femoral shaft fractures.

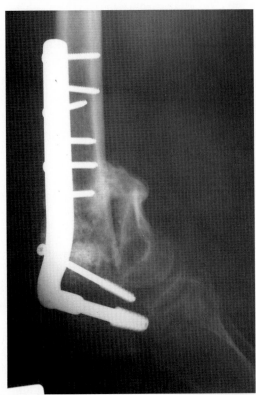

FIGURE 21-6. Radiographs of a patient with a severely comminuted distal femur fracture and non-union. The distal femoral fragment is underneath the posterior aspect of the proximal fragment and it is flexed. The supracondylar screw pulled through the distal fragment as well. A rotating hinge was required due to severe bone loss, deformity and lack of knee ligament stability.

Ligament Balancing

If extra-articular deformity is corrected by intra-articular compensatory angular resection, balancing may not be possible. These particular deformities may be more appropriately treated by an osteotomy. Extensive soft tissue release may be necessary at the time of surgery either to correct deformity or for stiffness. Substantial soft tissue release may compromise stability of the knee. Also, ligament injuries, which may result from the original trauma or are secondary to the subsequent abnormal mechanics, may also compromise knee stability. A more constrained device, in conjunction with stems to strengthen fixation may be required. In the most significant cases of severe bone loss and soft tissue scarring, rotating hinged prostheses may be required (Figure 21-6).

REFERENCES

1. Saleh KJ, Sherman P, Katkin P, Windsor R, Haas S, Laskin R, Sculco T. Total knee arthroplasty after open reduction and internal fixation of fractures of the tibial plateau: a minimum five-year follow-up study. *J Bone Joint Surg Am.* 2001;83-A(8):1144–1148.
2. Lonner JH, Pedlow FX, Siliski JM. Total knee arthroplasty for post-traumatic arthrosis. *J Arthroplasty.* 1999;14(8): 969–975.
3. Lonner JH, Siliski JM, Lotke PA. Simultaneous femoral osteotomy and total knee arthroplasty for treatment of osteoarthritis associated with severe extra-articular deformity. *J Bone Joint Surg Am.* 2000;82(3):342–348.
4. Jain R. Complications of total knee arthroplasty after open reduction and internal fixation of fractures of the tibial plateau. *J Bone Joint Surg Am.* 2002;84-A(3):497–500.
5. Duff GP, Lachiewicz PF, Kelley SS. Aspiration of the knee joint before revision arthroplasty. *Clin Orthop.* 1996;(331): 132–139.
6. Gerwin M, Rothaus KO, Windsor RE, Brause BD, Insall JN. Gastrocnemius muscle flap coverage of exposed or infected knee prostheses. *Clin Orthop.* 1993;286:64–70.
7. Whiteside LA. Surgical exposure in revision total knee arthroplasty. *Instr Course Lect.* 1997;46:221–225.
8. Windsor R, Bono J. Management of bone loss in total knee arthroplasty. In: Callaghan J, Dennis D, Paprosky W, Rosenberg A, eds. *Orthopaedic Knowledge Update: Hip and Knee Reconstruction.* Rosemont, IL: American Academy of Orthopaedic Surgeons; 1995:277–282.
9. Nelson CL, Saleh KJ, Kassim RA, Windsor R, Haas S, Laskin R, Sculco T. Total knee arthroplasty after varus osteotomy of the distal part of the femur. *J Bone Joint Surg Am.* 2003; 85-A(6):1062–1065.
10. Wolff AM, Hungerford DS, Pepe CL. The effect of extraarticular varus and valgus deformity on total knee arthroplasty. *Clin Orthop.* 1991;(271):35–51.
11. Wilkes RA, Thomas WG, Ruddle A. Fracture and nonunion of the proximal tibia below an osteoarthritic knee: treatment by long stemmed total knee replacement. *J Trauma.* 1994;36(3):356–357.
12. Wolf LR, Rothman RH, Hozack WJ, Balderston RA, Booth RE Jr. Primary total knee arthroplasty for displaced, acute intraarticular knee fractures. a report of four cases. *Clin Orthop.* 1992;(276):229–236.

CHAPTER 22

Insert Exchange

Rahul V. Deshmukh and Richard D. Scott

Modularity in tibial components for total knee arthroplasty (TKA) is controversial. Advantages of insert modularity include component inventory management and the potential for late insert exchange to treat instability or polyethylene wear. In addition, *prophylactic* insert exchange to an improved polyethylene can be accomplished at the time of arthrotomy for a reason unrelated to the tibial component. Disadvantages of modular tibial inserts include outright failure of the locking mechanism or the potential for insert-tray movement leading to backside wear and potential synovitis or osteolysis.[1-7]

Among the many advances in Total Knee Prosthetic design in the past 30 years has been the incorporation of metal backing and modularity as standard attributes of present-day total knee systems. Metal backing was added to tibial components to improve load transfer across the proximal tibia based on the finite element analysis of Bartel and others.[8] Its continued routine use, however, remains controversial. In 1991, Apel et al.[9] presented a series of total knee arthroplasties comparing 62 patients with all-polyethylene tibial components with 69 patients with metal-backed tibial components. They reported no significant difference at 6-year follow-up. In fact, they maintained that the incorporation of metal-backing posed the risk of decreased polyethylene thickness and that an all-polyethylene component of 8 to 10 mm thickness will have greater durability than a metal-backed component due to more favorable surface wear.

In contrast, later series with longer follow-up document the importance of metal-backing the tibial component. Colizza et al. published a 1995 review[10] of posterior stabilized TKA that documented 96% survival for the metal-backed tibial component vs. 87% for the all-polyethylene tibial components (P = 0.02). In a later study in 1997 with a larger database and longer follow-up, Font-Rodriguez et al.[5] performed a review of 2629 cemented

primary TKR with follow-up ranging from 14 to 22 years that documented 90% to 94% (0.38% to 0.46%/yr) survival for all-polyethylene tibial components vs. 98% (0.14%/yr) survival for metal-backed tibial components. In an evaluation of 2001 implants using the AGC Knee, Ritter and colleagues[11] in 1995 demonstrated a 98% 10-year survival rate with their flat on flat, compression molded, nonmodular metal-backed tibial components. A subsequent study in 1999[12] evaluating the midterm (4.19-year follow-up) results of 538 knees using an all-polyethylene tibia in the same design reported 50 tibial component revisions, 45 knees with medial plateau collapse, and 155 knees with more than 1 mm of medial plateau radiolucency. In a landmark study of 9200 TKA performed at the Mayo Clinic, Rand and Illstrup[13] identified several factors predictive of increased implant survival. On multivariate analysis, there were 4 independent factors that each lowered the risk of failure, namely primary TKA, diagnosis of rheumatoid arthritis, age > 60, and a metal-backed tibial component. If all 4 factors were present, patients had a 97% 10-year survival. Interestingly, a recent follow-up study by Rand et al. clarified some further points.[14] A review of 11 606 primary total knees demonstrated that on multivariate analysis, the ideal total knee replacement would be a cemented posterior-cruciate retaining prosthesis with a nonmodular metal-backed tibial component and an all-polyethylene component in a woman, older than 70 years, with inflammatory arthritis. On univariate analysis, these authors found a significant difference in survivorship between those prostheses with a nonmodular metal-backed tibial component (92%) and those with a modular metal-backed tibial component (90%). There was no significant difference between implants with either metal-backed design and those with the all-polyethylene tibial component. Although there is some controversy, the preponderance of data suggests therefore that metal backing of the tibial component is indeed of benefit in improving the survival of TKA.

With metal backing of the tibial component, 3 other advances were made possible in TKA: cementless fixation, mobile bearing designs, and modularity. Modular systems allow greater intraoperative flexibility (to address issues of clearing cement, trialing, fracture, or osteotomy), size interchangeability between polyethylene insert and femoral component, and ease of stocking/availability. Modularity also serves to address the issues of bone loss, poor bone quality, polyethylene wear, and instability. In addition, "prophylactic" insert exchange to an improved polyethylene can be accomplished at the time of arthrotomy for a reason unrelated to the tibial component. Brooks et al., through measuring tray-bone deflections, found that the best support for the tibial tray with a wedge-shaped defect was with modular metal wedges or custom implants.[15] Disadvantages of modularity include corrosion or fretting at the metal interfaces, potential failure of the polyethylene locking mechanism, and, perhaps most contentious, insert-tray movement leading to backside wear and potential synovitis or osteolysis.[1–7]

Modularity was originally predicted to be most useful in the event of progressive polyethylene wear to facilitate exchange of the liner without necessitating removal of the components. Insert exchange has also been advocated in the treatment of instability in total knee replacement. There are 4 major studies that address these issues. Bert et al.[1] published a multicenter retrospective review in 1998 looking at 62 revision TKA performed as a result of modular tibial insert failure. Their findings were striking in that 55 cases (88.7%) had such scoring and/or damage to the femoral and/or tibial components that one or both components had to be revised. The authors conclude that this series "clearly does not support the premise that polyethylene exchange is common at the time of revision surgery for tibial polyethylene insert failure." They further suggest that a simple liner exchange will only be possible with the benefit of close evaluation to detect progressive wear before damage occurs to the tibial and femoral components. In 2000, Engh et al.[4] published a very informative evaluation of the results of isolated exchange of modular polyethylene liners, following 48 liner-exchanged knees for an average of 7.4 years. Of those 48 exchanges, 22 were for severe polyethylene wear and 6 of those 22 (27%) failed at an average of less than 5 years. The authors maintain that polyethylene wear is influenced by both implant-related factors (insert thickness, type of locking mechanism, and the design and finish of the bearing surfaces) and patient-related factors (age, weight, height, activity level, length of time with implant in situ, and component alignment). Isolated insert exchange can improve the polyethylene factors so that the surgeon implants a thicker or even angled polyethylene; machined or compression-molded polyethylene rather than heat pressed; or polyethylene sterilized without the use of gamma irradiation in air. In the end, however, the surgeon must assess whether the main problem is isolated to the liner or if it is more involved. Indeed, Engh et al. maintain that if there is (1) severe delamination, (2) grade 3 or 4 undersurface wear and/or damage to the tibial baseplate, (3) full-thickness wear-through, or (4) severe wear within 10 years of the primary procedure, then an isolated insert exchange should *not* be performed. Rather, attention should be turned to the reasons for the accelerated wear. Most recently in 2002, Babis et al.[16,17] published their findings on a review of 56 isolated modular tibial insert exchanges on a variety of prosthetic designs. Inclusion criteria were limited to patients with a worn insert or instability and any patient undergoing insert exchange in the setting of component loosening, infection, stiffness, component malposition, or extensor mechanism problems was excluded. They reported an overall 25% re-revision rate after a mean of 3 years (range, 0.5 to 6.8 years) and determined that cumulative overall survival was 63.5% at 5.5 years. They also noted a trend that early initial failure portends a poorer outcome of an isolated insert exchange (p < 0.09). In looking at the subgroups of instability and wear, 12 (44%) of 27 knees undergoing exchange for instability failed at a mean of 3 years with a cumulative survival rate of 54.4%, noting that patients with global instability had a worse survival rate than those with isolated varus-valgus instability (p < 0.035). The authors report that 33% of knees (8 of 24) undergoing exchange for insert wear failed at a mean of 4 years with a cumulative survival rate of 71.6% at 5.5 years. Finally, Brooks et al.[18] in 2002 examined outcomes of polyethylene liner exchange to treat instability in a series of 14 knees at a mean follow-up of 56 months. Although the authors found 71% success with their procedure, they describe some important caveats in treating the 3 types of instability, which they define. Type I instability with competent but unbalanced ligaments is well treated with isolated liner exchange and ligament release. Types II and III instability with ligamentous incompetence or flexion/extension mismatch more often require femoral component revision followed by polyethylene exchange and potential tibial tray retention.

Backside wear (mode 4 wear)[6] is another area of recent controversy with modular knee systems. A review published by Ezzet et al.[19] in 1995 on the effect of component fixation method on osteolysis in TKA showed that the interface between the screw head and polyethylene liner is an important source of wear debris. These authors further postulate that the screw hole not only serves as a conduit for the transmission of wear debris to the metaphysis, but also is a source of metal-on-metal fretting with the screw head itself. They conclude with a "caution against the routine use of screws in any fixation scheme." Wasielewski et al.[20] in 1997, identified backside wear as a major source of polyethylene debris contributing to osteolysis. The authors reviewed 62 cementless TKA for an average of 5 years and determined that osteolytic lesions of the tibial metaphysis found directly below tibial tray screw holes link backside wear as a significant source of the polyethylene debris. Although the bulk of debris created in TKA is from larger particles generated in surface wear, the abrasive wear occurring at the insert-base plate junction can create the submicron particles implicated in osteolytic reactions.[19,20] Indeed, these authors demonstrate a statistically significant relationship between severe (grade 4) backside wear and tibial osteolysis (P = 0.001), whereas the association between severe articular wear and tibial osteolysis was not significant (P = 0.09). Moreover, no association was found between osteolysis formation and implant type, patient weight, implant loosening, or insert thickness. This study as well as an insert micromotion study published by Parks et al.[21] in 1998 have documented the importance of the modular interface as a significant source of the submicron debris associated with osteolysis. Parks et al. caution against the use of highly constrained components as this transfers increased load to the modular interface just as highly constrained components have been shown to transfer

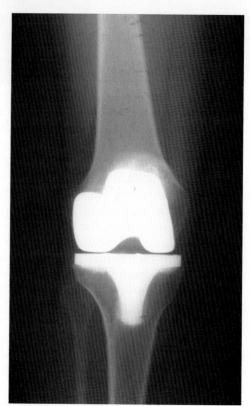

FIGURE 22-1. JRA patient presenting 10 years postop with painful TKR, synovitis, and evidence of polyethylene wear on AP x-ray.

TABLE 22.1. Reasons for Reoperation in 2000 Total Knee Arthroplasties.

- 13 metastatic infection
- 8 insert wear with synovitis
- 8 insert wear with osteolysis
- 6 asymptomatic insert wear
- 6 metal-backed patellae
- 6 instability (3 traumatic, 3 atraumatic)
- 4 broken femoral components
- 4 unresurfaced patellae
- 4 recurrent rheumatoid arthritis
- 4 recurrent hemarthroses
- 4 stiffness requiring arthroscopic debridement
- 3 loose cementless tibial components
- 2 ganglion cysts
- 1 loose cementless femur
- 1 loose hybrid tibia
- 1 loose cemented tibia
- 1 fractured proximal tibia

76 Total Reoperations
45 involving insert exchanges
0 failures of locking mechanism

increased load to the implant-bone interface in nonmodular systems. Both studies stress the need to minimize abrasive sources at the modular interface such as prominent screw heads, screw holes, or interposed cement or tissue. They also recommend that implant design should be modified to polish the tibial tray and improve the insert locking mechanism. Both studies must be interpreted for now as prosthesis specific and not necessarily generic to the modularity issue.

These studies raise the significant question of whether modularity is truly beneficial for patients or simply places them at greater risk for osteolysis and implant failure. In a recent study by the authors, an attempt was made to answer this question. In a series of 2000 consecutive PCL-retaining TKA from a single surgeon, 76 revisions were performed, 45 involving insert exchanges (Table 22.1). Twenty-eight insert exchanges were advantageous to either treat wear (18 cases) (Figure 22-1, 22-2, and 22-3), instability (6 cases), or allow isolated femoral revision with retention of the tibial tray (4 cases). Seventeen incidental insert exchanges allowed minimally worn inserts to be replaced with improved polyethylene at arthrotomy

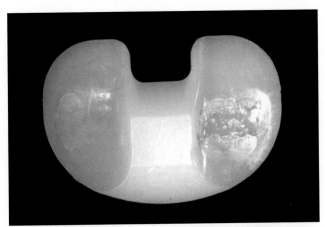

FIGURE 22-2. Retrieved polyethylene liner (treated by gamma irradiation in air) demonstrating surface delamination (mode 1 wear).

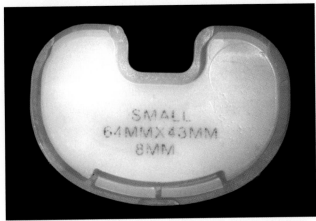

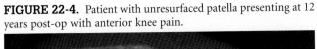

FIGURE 22-3. Undersurface of retrieved liner demonstrating minimal backside (mode 4) wear.

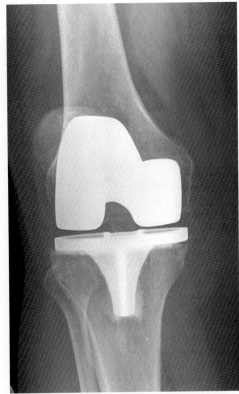

FIGURE 22-5. Preoperative films suggest well-preserved polyethylene liner.

performed for another cause (Figures 22-4 through 22-7). The 18 exchanges performed for polyethylene wear enjoy a 100% survival rate whereas of the 6 patients undergoing exchange for laxity, 2 of them (33%) underwent re-operation. While average 3- to 5-year follow-up results from both Engh and Babis suggest that isolated tibial insert exchange is not a viable option for polyethylene wear, with 27% and 33% re-revision rates, respectively, data from this current series suggest otherwise, with

FIGURE 22-4. Patient with unresurfaced patella presenting at 12 years post-op with anterior knee pain.

FIGURE 22-6. At time of arthrotomy for patellar resurfacing, evidence of oxidation and delamination is seen.

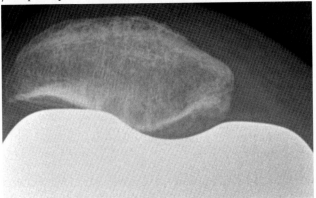

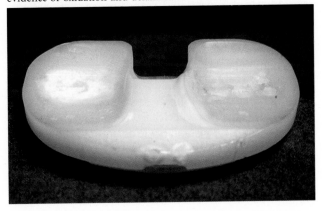

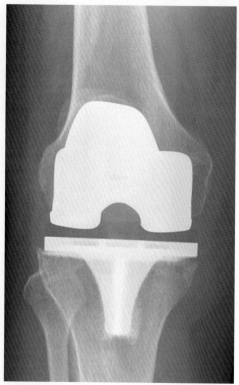

FIGURE 22-7. After patellar resurfacing and incidental liner exchange, patient is doing well 1 year postoperatively.

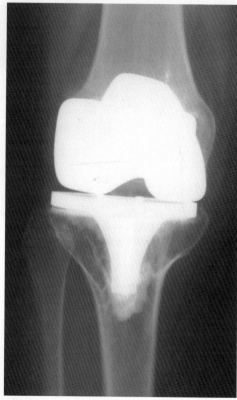

FIGURE 22-8. Asymptomatic patient presenting at 8 years postoperatively with varus deformity and polyethylene wear.

no re-revisions at average 6-year follow-up reported in the subset of patients undergoing insert exchange for wear. Among the factors making this series distinct are usage of a single implant design and limitation to a single surgeon. Although difficult to validate, such differences in outcome between these series may be a function of implant quality, patient selection, and surgical technique.

Of these 45 insert exchanges, 6 were performed for instability and of these, 2 underwent re-exchange for repeat traumatic instability. Although the numbers are small, this 33% failure rate at average 6-year follow-up is in keeping with rates reported by Babis et al. of a 44% re-revision rate at a mean of 3 years. One of these patients had a prior patellectomy with quadriceps insufficiency. She was stabilized successfully at her second revision by conversion to a posterior stabilized femoral component and stabilized insert with retention once again of the tibial tray. The second patient was discovered to have a thoracic syringomyelia and her subsequent neurologic deterioration confined her to a wheelchair. These data suggest that insert exchange for instability yields unpredictable results and that the onus is on the surgeon to consider the type and cause of instability before considering isolated insert exchange. While a thicker insert may tighten the collateral ligaments and enhance stability of the knee joint, it

cannot compensate for insufficiency of the collateral ligaments, unequal flexion and extension gaps, or insufficiency in extensor mechanism or motor control.

Apart from addressing wear, another advantage of modular insert exchange seen in our series was the ability to correct or improve limb alignment with the use of an angled bearing. Shaw first reported this concept in 1992.[7] Angled bearings of 3, 5, and 5 degrees, respectively, were used among our 45 insert exchanges. Two of these improved the alignment of knees in residual varus with asymptomatic medial polyethylene wear (Figures 22-8, 22-9, and 22-10). At 9 and 11 years post-revision, both

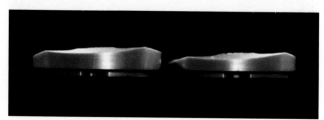

FIGURE 22-9. Custom angled bearings.

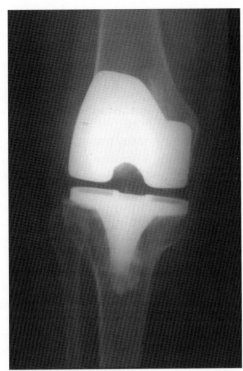

FIGURE 22-10. Eight years postoperatively with restored alignment and improved joint space.

maintain their polyethylene joint space. One angled bearing was used incidentally 11 years after the index surgery at the time of secondary patellar resurfacing to improve the cosmetic appearance of a knee with residual valgus alignment.

Angled bearings may be indicated to treat minor limb malalignment with and without instability. An appropriate case might be a patient with medial polyethylene wear at 10 years after initial surgery whose limb alignment shows a neutral anatomic axis or roughly 5 to 6 degrees of mechanical axis varus. With an angled bearing, the malalignment can be corrected merely by exchanging the insert. Another example might be a patient with a total knee placed in too much valgus with residual lateral laxity. An angled bearing can correct the cosmetic deformity and stabilize the lateral side at the same time.

Preoperative planning for these cases involves independent measurement on long films of the mechanical axis of the femoral and tibial components. The angle of the custom bearing is the complement of the sum of these 2 values. For example, if the femoral component mechanical axis is 2 degrees of varus and the tibial axis is 5 degrees of varus, the insert should be angled into 7 degrees of valgus.

Since these angled bearings are custom made, they can be expensive. The surgeon should attempt to make accurate preoperative measurements so that one or at most 2 potential inserts are fabricated. Trial inserts are helpful, but they, too, are expensive. The best way to size the thickness of the angled insert is to base measurements off of the more lax side as measured on an AP varus and valgus stress roentgenograms.

SUMMARY

Insert exchanges in this series were utilized in 45 of 2000 knees or 2.2% of cases at average 9-year follow-up. Although this number is small, it does represent 59% of the 76 reoperations performed in this series. Evaluation of follow-up data for patients undergoing exchange for polyethylene wear demonstrates 100% survival at average 6-year follow-up. In contrast to other data in the literature, data from this series suggest that insert exchange for polyethylene wear can be a reasonable treatment option and that patients do well if the procedure is performed for the correct indications. Exchange for instability appears to be an unpredictable prospect, with 2 of 6 failing in this series and 44% failure in the study by Babis et al. Overall, modularity would appear to have significant benefit during re-operation with this specific knee system whose tibial tray has remained unchanged for the 19 years since its introduction. These data do not condemn, however, the use of nonmodular, all-polyethylene tibial components since 98% of cases at 9 years did not require modularity, especially the elderly. The average age of the entire series of 2000 knees was 68 years at initial surgery, whereas the average age of the patient taking advantage of an insert exchange was 58 years. In addition, only one octogenarian in the entire series had an insert exchange, and this was the patient with a syringomyelia whose exchange, in fact, was of no benefit. Perhaps as experience and follow-up evolves, reliable age criteria can be developed for the arthroplasty surgeon to choose between modular and nonmodular designs.

Insert exchange may be considered to treat problems of progressive polyethylene wear with or without synovitis, progressive osteolysis, or incidentally at the time of surgery for another reason such as metastatic infection. Insert exchange for instability yields unpredictable results and the onus is on the surgeon to consider the type and cause of instability prior to considering isolated insert exchange. Custom angled bearings may occasionally play a role in these cases. As mentioned previously, while a thicker insert may tighten the collateral ligaments and enhance stability of the knee joint, it cannot compensate for insufficiency of the collateral ligaments, unequal flexion and extension gaps, or insufficiency in extensor mechanism or motor control. As seen in the literature, if there is (1) severe delamination, (2) grade 3 or 4 undersurface wear and/or damage to the tibial base plate, (3) full-thickness wear through, or (4) severe wear within 10 years of the primary procedure, then an isolated insert exchange should *not* be performed. Rather, attention should be turned to the reasons for the accelerated wear.

REFERENCES

1. Bert J, Reuben J, Kelly F, Gross M, Elting J. The incidence of modular tibial polyethylene insert exchange in total knee arthroplasty when polyethylene failure occurs. *J Arthroplasty.* 1998;13(6):609–614.

2. Brassard M, Insall J, Scuderi G, Colizza W. Does modularity affect clinical success? a comparison with a minimum 10-year follow-up. *Clin Orthop.* 2001;388:26–32.

3. Engh G, Dwyer K, Hanes C. Polyethylene wear of metal-backed tibial components in total unicompartmental knee prostheses. *J Bone Joint Surg.* 1992;74B:9–17.

4. Engh G, Koralewicz L, Pereles T. Clinical results of modular polyethylene insert exchange with retention of total knee arthroplasty components. *J Bone Joint Surg.* 2000;82A: 516–523.

5. Font-Rodriguez D, Scuderi G, Insall J. Survivorship of cemented total knee arthroplasty. *Clin Orthop.* 1997;345: 79–86.

6. Jacobs J, Shanbhag A, Glant T, Black J, Galante J. Wear debris in total joint replacements. *J Am Acad Orthop Surg.* 1994;2:212–220.

7. Shaw J. Angled bearing inserts in total knee arthroplasty. *J Arthroplasty.* 1992;7:211–216.

8. Bartel DL, Burstein AH, Santavicca EA, Insall JN. Performance of the tibial component in total knee replacement—conventional and revision designs. *J Bone Joint Surg.* 1982; 64A:1026–1033.

9. Apel D, Tozzi J, Dorr L. Clinical comparison of all-polyethylene and metal-backed tibial components in total knee arthroplasty. *Clin Orthop.* 1991;273:243–252.

10. Colizza W, Insall J, Scuderi G. The posterior stabilized total knee prosthesis. *J Bone Joint Surg.* 1995;77A:1713–1720.

11. Farris PM, Ritter MA, Keating EM, Meding JB. Midterm follow-up of all-poly tibial component flat-on-flat design. *J Arthroplasty.* 1999;14:245.

12. Ritter M, Worland R, Saliski J, Helphenstine J, Edmonson K, Keating M, Faris P, Meading J. Flat-on-flat, nonconstrained, compression molded polyethylene total knee replacement. *Clin Orthop.* 1995;321:79–85.

13. Rand J, Illstrup D. Survivorship analysis of total knee arthroplasty. *J Bone Joint Surg.* 1991;73A:397–409.

14. Rand J, Trousdale R, Ilstrup D, Harmsen W. Factors affecting the durability of primary total knee prostheses. *J Bone Joint Surg.* 2003;85A:259–265.

15. Brooks PJ, Walker PS, Scott RD. Tibial component fixation in deficient tibial bone stock. *Clin Orthop.* 1984;184: 302–309.

16. Babis GC, Trousdale RT, Morrey BF. The Effectiveness of isolated tibial insert exchange in revision total knee arthroplasty. *J Bone Joint Surg.* 2002;84A:64–68.

17. Babis GC, Trousdale RT, Pagnano MW, Morrey BF. Poor outcomes of isolated tibial insert exchange and arthrolysis for the management of stiffness following total knee arthroplasty. *J Bone Joint Surg.* 2001;83A:1534–1536.

18. Brooks DH, Fehring TK, Griffin WL, Mason JB, McCoy TH. Polyethylene exchange only for prosthetic knee instability. *Clin Orthop.* 2002;405:182–188.

19. Ezzet K, Garcia R, Barrack R. Effect of component fixation method on osteolysis in total knee arthroplasty. *Clin Orthop.* 1995;321:86–91.

20. Wasielewski R, Parks N, Williams I, Surprenant H, Collier J, Engh G. Tibial insert undersurface as a contributing source of polyethylene wear debris. *Clin Orthop.* 1997;345: 53–59.

21. Parks N, Engh G, Topoleski T, Emperado J. Modular tibial insert micromotion. *Clin Orthop.* 1998;356:10–15.

CHAPTER 23

Management of the Stiff Total Knee Arthroplasty

Van P. Stamos and James V. Bono

The ultimate goal of total knee arthroplasty is to achieve a stable, painless knee with an excellent range of motion allowing for maximum function. A normal knee should have a range of motion from 0 to approximately 140 degrees, although functional demands for most activities of daily living such as walking, sitting, driving, and climbing stairs can be easily accomplished with motion from 10 to 95 degrees. The uncomplicated total knee arthroplasty usually results in a range of motion of 0 to 5 degrees to 115 to 120 degrees, which, although not as full as a normal knee, allows greater motion than is needed for basic function.[1,2] Recalling this basic information is critical when evaluating a knee with a limited range of motion.

Stiffness following total knee arthroplasty can be extremely disappointing to both patient and surgeon. It can also be one of the most difficult complications to remedy. When faced with a stiff knee, the surgeon must remember that the best predictors of postoperative motion are preoperative motion and the passive motion achieved at surgery with the patella reduced and the joint capsule closed.[2–7] This fact is particularly important when evaluating a patient who has been operated by another surgeon; if only 60 degrees of flexion was achieved at surgery and the patient has 60 degrees 2 weeks postoperatively, he is doing quite well. However, if 125 degrees of flexion was achieved at surgery and 2 weeks later the patient has only 60 degrees of flexion, he is doing quite poorly. The treating surgeon must consider the passive range of motion at the time of surgery when assessing the stiff knee; one should not be influenced by arbitrarily defined numbers.

Knee stiffness can be the result of myriad causes, with some being more easily remedied than others. It is imperative that the surgeon fully evaluate the stiff knee and properly identify the cause so that appropriate treatment can be administered. Differentiating the stiff painful knee from the stiff painless knee can be particularly helpful.

CAUSES

Infection

Infection following total knee arthroplasty may present in many ways. Fortunately, it is the rare patient who presents with systemic signs of sepsis such as fever, chills, and/or shock. Far more common is the patient who is slow to progress following total knee arthroplasty despite aggressive physical therapy and other modalities. Flexion goals are not met, and the knee is insidiously painful and stiff. Constitutional symptoms as well as local wound problems are often absent, leaving pain and stiffness as the only signs of infection. It is therefore imperative that sepsis be excluded when presented with the stiff knee. The evaluation and treatment of infected total knee arthroplasties is fully discussed in Chapter 5, Skin Exposure Issues.

Associated Conditions

Knee stiffness may not be directly attributable to the knee itself. Disorders of the hip and spine may present as pain in the knee. Evaluation of both areas should be performed when assessing the stiff knee to exclude hip or spine pathology.[8] A flexion contracture of the hip may contribute to a flexion contracture of the knee. Ideally, hip abnormalities should be corrected before addressing disorders of the knee.

A wide array of nerve or muscular disorders must also be considered when evaluating the stiff knee. Diseases of the central nervous system that result in spasticity markedly affect motion and impede physical therapy. As revision surgery is rarely helpful in this patient group, they must be identified to prevent the surgeon from proceeding with surgery that will almost certainly not achieve its intended goals.

Reflex Sympathetic Dystrophy

Reflex sympathetic dystrophy is a particularly troublesome disorder that results in knee pain and stiffness. It is often difficult to diagnose and may be extremely difficult to treat. Any additional insult such as trauma or surgery to a limb exhibiting this condition usually aggravates symptoms. Therefore, it is critical that the surgeon identify this disorder before any surgical intervention.

Because reflex sympathetic dystrophy is commonly described as a disorder of the upper extremity, lower extremity involvement is often overlooked. The incidence following total knee arthroplasty has been reported as 0.8%,[9] so the surgeon must have a high index of suspicion to make the appropriate diagnosis. Diagnostic tests are seldom useful; the diagnosis is made on clinical grounds. Pain out of proportion to objective findings on physical examination is the classic sign, but the patient usually also exhibits delayed functional recovery, vasomotor disturbances, and trophic changes.[9–11] Physical examination may reveal skin hypersensitivity, decreased temperature, edema, and hyperhydrosis. In late stages, atrophy of the skin may be present. Limitation of motion affects flexion more commonly than extension, and the patellofemoral joint is often quite sensitive.

Treatment should be instituted immediately once the diagnosis is made. If symptoms have been present for less than 6 weeks, nonsteroidal anti-inflammatory medication and physical therapy for range of motion and desensitization are the mainstays of treatment.[10] The patient should be encouraged to bear weight and use the limb as much as possible. If the duration of symptoms has been greater than 6 weeks, lumbar sympathetic block may be required. Blockade of the sympathetic nervous system to the lower extremities is both therapeutic and diagnostic. It should alleviate symptoms, at least initially. When it does not, the diagnosis of reflex sympathetic dystrophy becomes suspect. Usually, several sequential blocks are required to provide lasting relief. Critical to success is the institution of aggressive physical therapy immediately following blockade. Some authors have reported success rates of as high as 80% with this regimen.[12] The key factors for a positive outcome are early recognition, aggressive treatment, and the avoidance of additional surgery or trauma to the extremity.[10]

Heterotopic Ossification

Occasionally, heterotopic ossification can be identified following total knee arthroplasty (Figure 23-1). Most

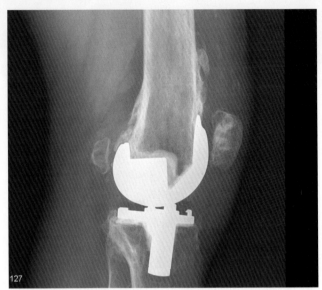

FIGURE 23-1. Heterotopic ossification is seen in the extensor mechanism and can limit flexion of the knee. Limited surgical dissection in the supra-patellar pouch may potentially avoid this complication.

commonly it is seen in the quadriceps muscle or anterior supracondylar region of the femur but other locations have also been reported. Historically, its incidence following knee arthroplasty was considered low.[13] It was also considered a rare cause of knee stiffness. Two separate case reports describe patients who developed severe myositis ossificans following knee replacement with porous ingrowth prostheses.[14,15] In one, the diagnosis of hypertrophic osteoarthritis was thought to be a predisposing factor when combined with extensive surgical exposure of the distal femur at the time of surgery and postoperative manipulation of the knee. In addition, the authors noted difficulty managing the dosage of coumadin in the postoperative period in this patient.

However, a more recent retrospective review of 98 primary knee arthroplasties in 70 patients demonstrated an incidence of heterotopic ossification of 26%.[16] The authors identified significantly elevated lumbar spine mineral bone density in those patients who developed heterotopic ossification as compared with a matched control group of patients who did not develop ectopic bone. Based on these findings they identified increased lumbar spine bone mineral density as an indicator of patients at risk for the development of postoperative heterotopic ossification.

Treatment consists of excision of ectopic bone followed by prevention of recurrence with either radiotherapy or pharmacologic means. The response to this treatment in not entirely predictable so it should be reserved for cases in which there is severe limitation of motion and extensive heterotopic ossification.

Arthrofibrosis

Arthrofibrosis is probably the most common cause of knee stiffness in patients with mechanically sound reconstructions.[4,17] These patients develop adhesions or dense scar within the joint or extensor mechanism that either act to tether or mechanically impede full joint motion. Fibrous nodules may also form on the undersurface of the quadriceps tendon leading to patellar clunk syndrome, particularly in posterior stabilized designs. Although this syndrome responds well to arthroscopic resection of the fibrous nodules, it is not commonly associated with diminished range of motion.[18] Attempts to identify predisposing factors for the development of arthrofibrosis have been largely unsuccessful. Thus, preventive measures are limited. A prolonged period of immobilization is certainly a causative factor. Currently, most joint surgeons implement aggressive rehabilitation in the postoperative period in an attempt to decrease the incidence of this complication. At many institutions this often includes the use of continuous passive motion, the efficacy of which is uncertain. Several studies have concluded that continuous passive motion has no effect on range of motion when measured at three months and one year.[5,7,19] These studies do, however, demonstrate significantly greater flexion in the early postoperative period for patients who were treated with continuous passive motion.

Posterior Cruciate Ligament Tightness

In patients with stiffness following implantation of posterior cruciate retaining devices, several authors have suggested tightness or contracture of the posterior cruciate ligament as the etiology.[17,20,21] Significant improvement in range of motion following open or arthroscopic release of the posterior cruciate ligament was achieved in the majority of these patients.

Technical Considerations

The etiology of stiffness following knee arthroplasty is often technique related, which often can be elucidated on radiography or by physical examination. These patients can be distinguished from patients with arthrofibrosis by comparing their postoperative motion with that achieved at surgery. Limitation of motion, if technique related, will be present at the time of surgery. Prior to attributing these imperfections to surgical error, one must consider a few points. While it should be the goal of every surgeon to implant prosthetic components in anatomic position and perfect alignment to allow full range of motion, this is not achievable in all cases due to variations in anatomy and technical limitations available. Because there are limits to

the sizes and configurations of implants used and the variations in anatomy are infinite, compromises are often necessary after considering the alternatives.

Five broad categories of technical imperfections can lead to knee stiffness. These are retained bone or osteophytes of the posterior femoral condyles, malalignment, imbalance of the extension gap and flexion gap, improperly sized components, and improper reconstruction of the patellofemoral joint.

At the time of primary knee arthroplasty, bone or osteophytes along the posterior femoral condyles and femur should be removed, if possible. This is best accomplished in the following fashion: With a trial femoral component in position, a curved osteotome is used to resect any excess posterior bone. The trial component is used as a template so the surgeon can precisely remove the correct amount of bone and often includes the removal of a small portion of normal posterior femoral condyle. If resection of posterior bone is incomplete, the remaining bone can impinge on the posterior edge of the tibial component or tibia, resulting in a mechanical impediment to full flexion. Residual posterior bone can be identified on a lateral radiograph and should be looked for when a patient presents with a stiff knee (Figure 23-2).

Restoration of proper mechanical alignment is critical to ensure both proper function and longevity of a knee

FIGURE 23-2. Incomplete resection of posterior osteophyte. The remaining bone can impinge on the posterior edge of the tibial resulting in a mechanical impediment to full flexion, and can tent the posterior capsule resulting in incomplete extension.

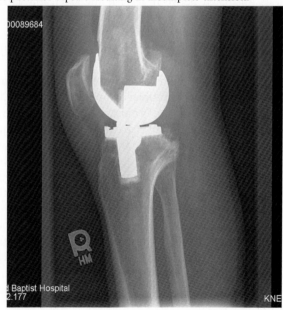

implant.[22] This includes alignment in sagittal, coronal, and rotational planes. Significant malalignment in any of these planes can result in decreased range of motion. Standing 3 foot anteroposterior and lateral radiographs are most helpful in assessing alignment and should be obtained for any patient in whom revision surgery is being considered. In the coronal plane, it is not uncommon to see errors of up to 3 degrees on either the femoral or tibial component.[1] It would be highly unusual for this amount of malalignment to result in motion limitation.[1,22] However, when measurements exceed 5 degrees, the likelihood of resultant loss of motion increases dramatically. In the sagittal plane, excessive flexion or extension of the femoral component can lead to limitation of motion, but the degree of error must be quite large and is rarely seen as the cause. This is not the case with the tibial component, in which a relatively small degree of malalignment in this plane can significantly affect motion. The slope of the tibial prosthesis relative to the long axis of the tibia should be carefully evaluated. Excessive posterior slope may result in lack of full extension and instability in flexion. Anterior slope (i.e., hyperextension of the tibial component) is likely to lead to recurvatum deformity and lack of full flexion. Of course, the amount of posterior slope designed into the particular component implanted must be taken into account when evaluating the radiograph. When possible, comparison of the patient's preoperative anatomic tibial slope to that achieved postoperatively can be enlightening.

Improper balance of the extension and flexion gaps can clearly lead to stiffness following knee arthroplasty. This includes both asymmetry of the individual gap as well as mismatch between gaps. If the extension gap is tight relative to an appropriate flexion gap, lack of full extension is the result. Conversely, if the flexion gap is tight relative to an appropriate extension gap, limited flexion is observed.

Incorrect sizing of the implant affects knee motion. For both the femoral and tibial components, appropriate anteroposterior dimension is most important for restoration of knee mechanics. Oversizing of the femoral component results in tightening of the collateral ligaments in flexion. The resultant flexion/extension gap mismatch leads to incomplete flexion. Undersizing of the tibial tray, when combined with excessive anterior placement on the tibia, also affects motion. In this situation, the uncovered posterior cortex of the tibia leads to a mechanical block from contact between the posterior femur and tibia as the knee is flexed. Finally, oversizing of the composite thickness of the tibial component and liner results in a knee that is globally too tight, limiting both flexion and extension.

Complications associated with reconstruction of the patellofemoral joint can result in decreased flexion.[18,23] Maltracking or tilting of the patella can have an effect on motion by both mechanical and pain-mediated pathways. Patients with these findings often demonstrate an unwillingness to fully flex their knees. If the reconstructed patella is too thick, increased forces across the patellofemoral joint may impede flexion.

Identification of technical imperfections when presented with the stiff knee is relatively straightforward. The difficulty lies in whether those findings are the actual cause of stiffness. The surgeon must remember that technical imperfections can be identified in many well-functioning total knee replacements.

Miscellaneous

Anecdotal cases of loose bodies within the joint have been described. In one case report, an intraarticular fragment of methylmethacrylate was identified.[24] Knee motion was restored after arthrotomy and removal of the offending loose body. Fracture of the polyethylene should also be considered when determining the cause of knee stiffness.

TREATMENT

General

Treatment should be directed at the causative factor. The previous section addressed the treatment of infection, reflex sympathetic dystrophy, and heterotopic ossification. The remainder of this section discusses treatments for stiffness related to arthrofibrosis, posterior cruciate ligament tightness, or technical errors. Included are some associated with significant complications of which the surgeon and patient must be aware before embarking on these courses of action. Manipulation and arthroscopy are directed toward the treatment of arthrofibrosis. These modalities should be reserved for patients who originally had adequate motion but have lost it over time. The patient who never had adequate motion is unlikely to benefit from arthroscopy or manipulation.

Manipulation

Although controversy exists regarding its use and effectiveness, manipulation of the stiff total knee arthroplasty can be a useful treatment if used appropriately. Timing is probably the most critical element if manipulation is to be successful. The surgeon must remember that manipulation is theoretically designed to produce disruption of immature, early adhesions. It is not designed to disrupt solidly formed adhesions or to stretch tendon or muscle. Therefore, its effectiveness is markedly diminished beyond 6 weeks postoperatively when adhesions are nearing maturity. Beyond this time, the increased risk of complications such as femur fracture, patellar fracture, or rupture of the extensor mechanism should discourage the surgeon from performing a manipulation. The most effective time to perform a manipulation is within 6 weeks of surgery, so patients need to be identified and treated early if one is to be successful.

The current prevailing opinion of most joint replacement surgeons is that manipulation does not affect ultimate range of motion after knee arthroplasty. This conclusion is based on studies that compared patients who underwent manipulation under anesthesia with those who did not.[13,17] These investigations found the ultimate motion at one year after surgery to be the same in these two groups. On the surface, one might then conclude that manipulation has no influence on ultimate motion. However, because of inherent bias, these 2 groups are not matched, making such a conclusion suspect. The patients who underwent manipulation were chosen because they were slow to progress as compared with the unmanipulated group. Ultimately, motion was comparable in both groups. Manipulation allowed the slower patients to, in effect, catch up to the other, rapidly progressing patients. Based on studies to date, it is extremely difficult to determine the true long-term influence of manipulation. Regardless of the actual influence on ultimate range of motion, one cannot deny the very positive benefits, particularly psychological, of a successful manipulation on the patient, therapist, and surgeon.

In order to be effective, manipulation, like any procedure, needs to be performed correctly. General or regional anesthesia is mandatory to provide adequate muscle relaxation and control of pain, thereby decreasing the risk of fracture or extensor mechanism rupture. Once the patient is under anesthesia, passive range of motion should be measured with the patient supine. Extension is assessed by supporting the heel with the hip slightly flexed. The amount of extension is recorded. Flexion is measured by supporting the lower extremity from the thigh with the hip flexed to 90 degrees. The knee is allowed to bend passively to maximum flexion with gravity. Once the arc of motion has been determined, manipulation is performed. With the patient's leg supported by both hands around the calf and the ankle in the surgeon's axilla, a gentle steady flexion force is applied. As the adhesions are torn, the surgeon will feel a sensation of crepitus and flexion of the knee will gradually increase. Alternatively, the leg may be allowed to freely fall from full extension into flexion. This maneuver is repeated several times; the weight of the limb itself is used to disrupt adhesions. With the knee in extension, an attempt at mobilization of the patella should be performed by applying inferior and medially directed forces, which assist in lysis

of adhesions in the suprapatellar pouch. These maneuvers should be repeated until the motion attained at surgery is reproduced or no further progress is made. Postmanipulation motion is then measured in the fashion described previously. Continuous passive motion should be instituted immediately and set to the maximum extension and flexion achieved with manipulation. Following the procedure, adequate analgesia must be given so the patient does not experience pain and resist the motion that has been achieved. An epidural catheter maintained for 24 to 48 hours following the manipulation is often beneficial. An aggressive physical therapy program is then instituted to avoid losing the motion gained with manipulation.

Arthroscopy

Arthroscopic treatment of disorders of the knee is the most common procedure in orthopedic practice. Its use in the treatment of problematic knee arthroplasty, however, has historically been relatively uncommon.[25,26] As experience with this technique has increased, its utility and safety have grown.[27] When contemplating the use of arthroscopy for the stiff knee, the indications and prerequisites are similar to those for manipulation; that is, the motion of the knee is less than that attained at surgery, rehabilitation is slow to progress, and the etiology is thought to be arthrofibrosis or tightness of the posterior cruciate ligament. Arthroscopy, though, can be attempted after the 6-week postoperative time period in which manipulation is most effective. Because the adhesions are released directly, even mature secondary scar can be removed safely. Intuitively, one might think arthroscopic lysis of adhesions followed by aggressive therapy would be a highly effective treatment of arthrofibrosis. In reality this approach has yielded limited success.[27–30] The most promising results have been in patients treated for tethered patella syndrome, in which the fibrous bands of secondary scar are isolated to the patellofemoral joint. These patients have a reproducible pattern of symptoms characterized by painful patellar grinding and crunching when actively extending the knee and some limitation of motion. There is a consistent pattern of fibrous band formation with the most common occurring at the superior border of the patellar component.[31–33] Less common are bands that tether the patella or fat pad to the intercondylar notch region. In patients with these constellations, long-term results have been excellent following arthroscopic removal of these *tethering bands*.

In patients with cruciate-retaining designs, arthroscopic release of the posterior cruciate ligament has been shown to increase range of motion and result in increased patient satisfaction.[20]

One might also reasonably consider the use of the arthroscope for the removal of a foreign body that is impeding motion. Although no series have been reported, one would expect a positive outcome if used to treat the case described earlier of an intraarticular fragment of methylmethacrylate limiting joint motion.

Revision Surgery

Ultimately, the surgeon must address the stiff knee that is the result of technical imperfections. Attempts to improve motion in these patients require revision knee arthroplasty and the potential complications associated with such an undertaking. Therefore, before embarking on such a potentially hazardous course, the potential benefit must be clearly demonstrated. This benefit should be determined in the context of the functional range of knee motion described in the introductory section of this chapter and the true functional requirements of the patient. When contemplating revision surgery for knee stiffness, the surgeon and patient must have reasonable expectations and goals. The surgeon must have experience in revision surgery and have a clear surgical plan. The patient must understand that the ultimate outcome with revision surgery may not be improved and may in fact be worsened. Both must be prepared for complete revision of all components. As the saying goes: "Hope for the best, prepare for the worst."

Techniques used for revision of total knee replacements are described in detail in Chapter 6. What follows is merely an overview of revision surgery as it pertains to treatment of the stiff knee.

Revision of the stiff knee arthroplasty requires attention to detail that begins with the skin incision and surgical approach. Previous incisions should be used whenever possible. Because the skin is often contracted and tenuous in this group of patients, excision of hypertrophic scar is strongly discouraged as it may not allow a tension-free closure at the completion of the procedure. In addition, closure may require rotational flaps or grafts, so the surgeon must be prepared by using appropriate incisions and handling all tissues carefully. Nearly all cases require an extensile approach to avoid the disastrous complication of avulsion of the patellar tendon. Favored approaches include the quadriceps snip, V-Y quadriceps turndown, and tibial tubercle osteotomy, all of which are thoroughly described in Chapter 6.

Next, the suprapatellar pouch and medial and lateral gutters are examined. All scar and fibrous tissue in these areas is excised, and the undersurface of the quadriceps tendon is debrided. The knee is then flexed, and the components are examined for evidence of loosening or abnormal polyethylene wear. Patellar tracking and function of the extensor mechanism are assessed. If the patella has been resurfaced, the composite thickness should be measured with a caliper. Measurements greater than 26 mm in men and 24 mm in women may indicate inadequate resection at time of patellar reconstruction.[23] As described earlier in this chapter, the resultant overly thick patella can be a cause of limited flexion. Range of motion is then assessed once thorough debridement of scar and mobilization of the extensor mechanism are complete. Occasionally, adequate motion will have been restored. More commonly, however, further evaluation is required.

Overall static alignment and symmetry of the extension and flexion gaps are then assessed. If abnormalities are observed, one must determine if correction can be achieved with exchange of the polyethylene and soft tissue releases. Custom designed angled bearing inserts have been described for use in these situations.[34] This is described in more detail in Chapter 22. If present, the modular tibial insert is then removed, and attention is directed posteriorly. Dense scar and residual bone along the posterior femur are excised. Adequacy of removal is assessed by finger palpation. Subsequently, range of motion is checked after replacement of the tibial insert. If it is considered inadequate, revision of the femoral and/or tibial components is performed if a technical imperfection has been identified.

Flexion of the knee is evaluated both with the patella everted and with the patella reduced. Diminished flexion with the patella reduced compared with the patella everted indicates extrinsic tightness of the extensor mechanism due to scarring and fibrosis. In this setting, lenghtening of the quadriceps mechanism may be accomplished by creating several relaxing incisions in the tendon with a No. 11 knife blade.

Prior to closure, patellar tracking is reevaluated carefully. Lateral release and/or revision of the patellar component to decrease its thickness may be required. The surgical wound is then closed using meticulous surgical technique and cautious handling of the tissues.

CONCLUSION

The knee that is stiff following total knee arthroplasty presents a difficult problem to the surgeon.[35–38] Prior to embarking on a treatment regimen that may include revision surgery, which is fraught with complications, one must be certain the benefits to the individual patient outweigh the risks. Knee motion from 10 to 95 degrees may be perfectly adequate for some and unacceptable for others. Similarly, the cause of limitation of knee motion and corrective treatment with acceptable risk must be identified. Revision surgery should be pursued only after these factors are considered.

REFERENCES

1. Krackow KA. Postoperative period. In: Krackow KA, ed. *The Technique of Total Knee Arthroplasty.* St. Louis: C.V. Mosby; 1990:385–424.

2. Kim JM, Moon MS. Squatting following total knee arthroplasty. *Clin Orthop.* 1995;313:177–186.

3. Fox JL, Poss R. The role of manipulation following total knee replacement. *J Bone Joint Surg.* 1981;63-A:357–362.

4. Harvey IA, Barry K, Kirby SP, et al. Factors affecting the range of movement of total knee arthroplasty. *J Bone Joint Surg.* 1993;75-B:950–955.

5. Maloney WJ, Schurman DJ, Hangen D, et al. The influence of continuous passive motion on outcome in total knee arthroplasty. *Clin Orthop.* 1990;256:162–166.

6. Menke W, Schmitz B, Salm S. Range of motion after total condylar knee arthroplasty. *Arch Orthop Trauma Surg.* 1992; 11:280–281.

7. Wasilewski SA, Woods LC, Torgerson WR, et al. Value of continuous passive motion in total knee arthroplasty. *Orthopedics.* 1990;13:291–296.

8. Vince KG, Eissmann E. Stiff total knee arthroplasty. In: Fu FH, et al., eds. *Knee Surgery.* Baltimore: Williams and Wilkins; 1994:1529–1538.

9. Katz MM, Hungerford DS. Reflex sympathetic dystrophy affecting the knee. *J Bone Joint Surg.* 1987;69-B:797–801.

10. Cooper DE, DeLee JC. Reflex sympathetic dystrophy of the knee. *J Am Acad Orthop Surg.* 1994;2:79–86.

11. Katz MM, Hungerford DS, Krackow KA. Reflex sympathetic dystrophy as a cause of poor results after total knee arthroplasty. *J Arthroplasty.* 1986;2:117–122.

12. Ogilvie-Harris DJ, Roscoe M. Reflex sympathetic dystrophy of the knee. *J Bone Joint Surg.* 1987;69-B:804–809.

13. Daluga D, Lombardi AV, Mallory TH, et al. Knee manipulation following total knee arthroplasty: analysis of prognostic variables. *J Arthroplasty.* 1991;6:119–128.

14. McClelland SJ, Rudolf LM. Myositis ossificans following porous-ingrowth TK replacement. *Orthop Rev.* 1986;15: 223–227.

15. Freedman EL, Freedman DM. Heterotopic ossification following total knee arthroplasty requiring surgical excision. *Am J Orthop.* 1996;25(8):559–561.

16. Furia JP, Pellegrini VD. Heterotopic ossification following primary total knee arthroplasty. *J Arthroplasty.* 1995;10: 413–419.

17. Maloney WJ. The stiff total knee arthroplasty: evaluation and management. *J Arthroplasty.* 2002;17(4 Suppl 1):71–73.

18. Johanson NA. The stiff total knee replacement: causes, treatment, and prevention. *Instr Course Lect.* 1997;46: 191–195.

19. Ververeli PA, Sutton DC, Hearn SL, et al. Continuous passive motion after total knee arthroplasty. analysis of cost and benefits. *Clin Orthop.* 1995;321:208–215.

20. Williams RJ, Westrich GH, Siegel J, Windsor RE. Arthroscopic release of the posterior cruciate ligament for stiff total knee arthroplasty. *Clin Orthop.* 1996;331:185–191.

21. Christensen CP, Crawford JJ, Olin MD, Vail TP. Revision of the stiff total knee arthroplasty. *J Arthroplasty.* 2002;17: 409–415.

22. Hungerford DS. Alignment in total knee replacement. *Instr Course Lect.* 1995;44:455–468.

23. Barnes CL, Scott RD. Patellofemoral complications of total knee replacement. *Instr Course Lect.* 1993;42:303–307.

24. Robins PR. Internal derangement of the knee caused by a loose fragment of methylmethacrylate following total knee arthroplasty. a case report. *Clin Orthop.* 1977;4:208–210.

25. Johnson DR, Friedman RJ, McGinty JB, et al. The role of arthroscopy in the problem total knee replacement. *Arthroscopy.* 1990;6:30–32.

26. Lintner DM, Bocell JR, Tullos HS. Arthroscopic treatment of intraarticular fibrous bands after total knee arthroplasty. a follow-up note. *Clin Orthop.* 1994;309:230–233.

27. Diduch DR, Scuderi GR, Scott WN, Insall JN, Kelly MA. The efficacy of arthroscopy following total knee replacement. *Arthroscopy.* 1997;13(2):166–171.

28. Bocell JR, Thorpe CD, Tullos HS. Arthroscopic treatment of symptomatic total knee arthroplasty. *Clin Orthop.* 1991; 271:125–134.

29. Campbell ED. Arthroscopy in total knee replacements. *Arthroscopy.* 1987;3:31–35.

30. Sprague NF, O'Connor RL, Fox JF. Arthroscopic treatment of postoperative knee fibroarthrosis. *Clin Orthop.* 1982;166: 165–172.

31. Thorpe CD, Bocell JR, Tullos HS. Intra-articular fibrous bands. patellar complications after total knee replacement. *J Bone Joint Surg.* 1990;72-A:811–814.

32. Beight JL, Yao B, Hozack WJ, et al. The patellar "clunk" syndrome after posterior stabilized knee arthroplasty. *Clin Orthop.* 1994;299:139–142.

33. Vernace JV, Rothman RH, Booth RE. Arthroscopic management of the patellar clunk syndrome following posterior stabilized total knee arthroplasty. *J Arthroplasty.* 1989;4: 179–182.

34. Shaw JA. Angled bearing inserts in total knee arthroplasty. a brief technical note. *J Arthroplasty.* 1992;7:211–216.

35. Scuderi GR, Tria AJ. *Surgical Techniques in Total Knee Arthroplasty.* New York: Springer-Verlag; 2002.

36. Nichols DW, Dorr LD. Revision surgery for stiff total knee arthroplasty. *J Arthroplasty.* 1990;5:573–577.

37. Vince KG. Revision knee arthroplasty. In: Chapman MW, Madison M, eds. *Operative Orthopaedics.* Philadelphia: J.B. Lippincott Company; 1993:1988–2010.

38. Blesier RB, Matthews LS. Complications of prosthetic knee arthroplasty. In: Epps CH, ed. *Complications in Orthopaedic Surgery.* Philadelphia: Lippincott, Williams and Wilkins; 1994:1075–1086.

CHAPTER 24

Aseptic Synovitis

Wolfgang Fitz and Richard D. Scott

Aseptic effusions are occasionally seen after total knee arthroplasty, but their source is not well understood. Effusions immediately following total knee arthroplasty (TKA) gradually disappear several weeks or a few months after surgery, and even though frequent, they raise no significant clinical concern. A new onset of an effusion beyond the postoperative period of 1 year or more is infrequent and raises clinical concern.

Some minimal effusions occur gradually, most of the time without other symptoms, and may not even be noticed by the patient. The time between surgery and the onset of an effusion varies, and problems related to polyethylene wear increase with time. Several technical issues that require consideration may play a role in accelerated polyethylene wear: the quality of polyethylene; the sterilization method;[1–4] its shelf-life;[5] the use of extruded versus press-molded polyethylene;[6] its thickness; third body wear; mechanical problems that may lead to increased wear, such as backside wear; and designs that are too conforming, among others. Misalignment of components and tissue balancing play important roles and have to be considered as contributors to excessive wear. Therefore, the joint aspirate should be examined in addition to the normal work-up with polarized light microscopy for polyethylene wear debris.[7]

However, catastrophic failures due to poor polyethylene quality, poor implant designs, or poor surgical techniques usually represent no diagnostic but rather a surgical challenge.

Some effusions have an acute onset with or without a history of trauma. Some are accompanied by pain and some by a change in stability or alignment. The combination of effusion with pain and a change in alignment is related to the loosening of the implant and is easy to diagnose. So far, no specific markers have been described for specific diagnosis, such as inflammation, metallosis, particulate cement debris, or hypersensitivity allergic reactions.

Joint fluid cell analysis is based on joints without implants, based on the guidelines published by the American College of Rheumatology[8–10] (Table 24.1). It is considered to be normal with a white blood cell count (WBC) of less than 200/mL, and less than 25% polymorphonuclear leukoctyes (PML).[11] Osteoarthritic patients (noninflammatory, group I) may have a WBC of <2000/ml with <25% PML to be considered as normal, whereas inflammatory arthritis (group II), such as rheumatoid, gouty, or pseudogouty arthritis, can have WBC ranging between 2000 and 50000/mL with >50% PML, whereas the criteria for septic synovial fluid would be WBC >50000/ml with >75% of PML. The amount of WBC in inflammatory arthritis is not associated with accelerated bone degradation in normal joints.[12] It has been shown that these guidelines apply for failed aseptic TKA, too.[11]

The most important differential diagnosis of an effusion is infection, which must be ruled out in every case. Aspiration of these joints provides easy access for further diagnostic studies and should be combined with basic blood workup and other diagnostic workups. The most important differential diagnoses include gout and pseudogout. A significant challenge in TKA is the diagnosis of a low-grade infection, in which aspirates remain aseptic.

LOW-GRADE INFECTION

The combination of pain and aseptic effusion should raise suspicion of an infection, which is sometimes difficult to diagnose. Whereas the diagnosis of an acute infection is relatively easy, based on the acute onset of effusion, redness, swelling, systemic infectious symptoms (see

TABLE 24.1. Standard Workup for Aseptic Synovitis Includes Serum Tests, Analysis of Synovial Fluid, and Radiography.

Blood test
    Erythrocyte sedimentation rates
    White blood cell counts
    C-reactive protein levels
Synovial fluid analysis
    Aerobic and anaerobic cultures
    Fungus cultures
    Gram's staining
    Leukocyte counting
    Glucose and protein level
    Crystals
    Polarized light microscopy for polyethylene wear debris
Radiographic analysis
    Radiography
    Scintigraphy
    Gallium
    Indium
    Technetium

Chapter 16 for discussion) a low-grade infection may not present with classical symptoms but rather with aseptic effusion and different levels of pain. Laboratory studies, including complete blood cell count, sedimentation rate, and C-reactive protein are useful in evaluating a suspected infected total knee replacement.[13,14] Synovial fluid cultures and white blood cell counts, including its differential are commonly performed. The literature has demonstrated reliable specificity (80%–100%), but a variable sensitivity of 0% to 90% for aspirations in total hip arthroplasty.[15–19] The use of white blood cell counts and its differential was found to be helpful in a series of 79 failed TKR [11]. Only eight knees showed a white blood cell count >2000. The authors concluded that patients with a primary diagnosis of osteoarthritis and a WBC <2000/mL and a differential of <50% PMLs of the synovial fluid had a greater than 98% negative predictive value for excluding infection.[11]

The standard test for the detection of bacteria is arthrocentesis, followed by a Gram's stain testing and culture, which actually fail to detect infection in 15% or even up to 50% of such cases. The percentage of false-negative test results from standard microbiologic assays may be reduced significantly by the use of the polymerase chain reaction (PCR).[20] PCR testing results of 32 preoperative aspirates were all positive, whereas standard microbiologic culturing assays performed preoperative and intraoperative were positive in only 15 samples. PCR testing yielded no false-positive results in 21 negative control specimens obtained from aseptic joints. PCR may help to identify bacteria even under antibiotic therapy in the detection of both live and dead bacteria as recently shown,[21] but its clinical use is still very limited.

In addition to aspirate analyses, the serum level of WBC, the determination of C-reactive protein levels, and bone scans, among other analyses, may not significantly improve the sensitivity of a suspected infected TKR.[11] However, the combination of all these measures have not been studied yet.

A low-grade infection may be present with an aseptic effusion. Microbial colonies produce a carbohydrate-rich biofilm that encases the bacteria on the surface of the biomaterial, dispersing over the surface and between the implant-bone interface. The infectious process with clinical symptoms and positive aspirates does not start before the bacteria leave the surface of the biomaterial and invade surrounding tissue, specifically bone tissue, thereby provoking local osteomyelitis. Sooner or later the bacteria come into contact with the synovial fluid; the aspirate may become positive at this point. However, it may take months or even years before the infection becomes manifest. During this phase, the synovial fluid may remain free of bacteria and testing may produce false-negative test results.

The contamination of the culture media, also may lead to a false-positive diagnosis. Culture of both tissue and synovial fluid may help reduce false-positive results. Repetitive aspirations every 2 to 4 weeks without the administration of antibiotics are recommended, but it remains unclear when arthroscopic or open-tissue sampling should be performed.

GOUTY SYNOVITIS

One of the most important differential diagnoses of an acute infected TKA is gouty or pseudogouty synovitis, since its treatment for this diagnosis may result in the unnecessary removal of the implants. Its presentation may be undistinguishable from an acute infected TKR with erythema, pain, redness, effusion, elevated erythrocyte sedimentation rate (ESR), and fever. The crystals, which are either intracellular or extracellular, are usually visible with light microscopy under polarized light. Histological examination of synovial tissue may be necessary to confirm the correct diagnosis under polarized light [22]. Both conditions reveal a high WBC count ranging from 50000 to 100000/mL in septic synovitis and from 20000 to 80000/mL in gouty arthritis.[10] In the differential WBC count for septic synovitis, the percentage of polymorphonuclear (PML) cells ranges from 75% to 100% and is usually greater that 90%,[10] whereas the percentage in gouty synovitis is usually slightly lower: 60% to 90%. A careful clinical evaluation, including a medical history of previous gouty episodes, serum levels of uric acid, assessment of the total WBC count and the PML cell count, and the presence or absence of monosodium urate crystals under light microscopy may provide the correct diagnosis.

The clinical presentation of pseudogouty synovitis after TKA has been described as similar to that of septic synovitis. In a series of 50 patients with a pseudogout attack, 14 patients were initially suspected or misdiagnosed as having septic arthritis.[23] Only 1 of the 50 patients showed no calcium pyrophosphate dihydrate crystals (CPPD) in the synovial fluid, and arthroscopic biopsy helped establish the diagnosis. Clinically, the 2 most important clues in the differentiation to septic arthritis are the presence of intracellular CPPD crystals in synovial aspirates and the involvement of more than one joint.[23] The absence of crystals does not exclude gouty and pseudogouty synovitis and septic arthritis. Gout or pseudogout can occur simultaneously with septic synovitis.

POLYETHYLENE WEAR

The initial clinical symptom of failure of a total knee replacement due to wear is a painless effusion. The occurrence of additional pain was considered to be the criterion for operative intervention[24] and may suggest a loosening of any of the components.

Failure of the patellofemoral compartment may result in patellofemoral pain with crepitus, caused by a nonreplaced patella, wear failure, or loosening or fracture of the patella (or a combination of each). Clinically, a flexion contracture with an associated weakness of the vastus medialis muscle should raise attention to the patellofemoral compartment. The combination of a tight lateral retinaculum, a malpositioned femoral (internal rotation, too much valgus, medial positioning), malpositioned tibial (internal rotation and medial positioning), and/or a patellar component malpositioning (lateral) may lead to an increased lateral force vector on the patella. This may in combination lead to early failure of the patellofemoral compartment. Some studies show an advantage of a conforming patellofemoral groove and a 3-peg oval patellar component design.[25–27] A single-peg patellar design caused a high prevalence of patellar fracture in one series.[27]

At least 3 components of synovial fluid can contribute to periprosthetic bone resorption and aseptic loosening: wear particles, soluble factors, and the physical effect of synovial fluid pressure.[28] Wear particles are released into the joint fluid and are dispersed throughout the joint space. They cause a cellular response in the synovial tissue, resulting in release of inflammatory enzymes and in inflammatory synovitis.[29,30] The single cell layer of the synovial membrane consists of two types of synoviocytes.[31] Synovial macrophages (type A) remove cellular and particulate debris from the synovial fluid, whereas synovial fibroblasts (type B) repair the damage of the synovial membrane. The activated synovial macrophages produce a variety of inflammatory cytokines, such as interleukin (IL-1β, IL-6), tumor necrosis factor (TNF), interferon, and prostaglandin (PGE$_2$). IL-1β has been shown to increase osteoclastic activity. In a study comparing 7 severely osteoarthritic knees with 20 failed total knee replacements, the levels of IL-1β and tartrate-resistant acid phosphatase were elevated in the latter group, suggesting that wear particulates caused significant elevations in these cytokines.[32]

Various amounts and sizes of wear particles, mostly polyethylene particles, are generated during the normal function of a total knee replacement. The amount of particles generated increases with malalignment and excessive activity and is influenced by the quality of the polyethylene[2,4] and implant-specific design issues. It is unclear if the shape, size, or relative number of wear particles influence the amount of osteolysis. One study reported a mean particle size of polyethylene debris in failed total knee replacement between 200 and 300 nm and observed the volume fraction differed by a factor of 2 in osteolytic and nonosteolytic cases.[30] Wolfarth et al. reported submicron-sized debris in failed total knee replacement either in the synovial fluid or in tissue samples surrounding TKA with osteolysis. Others examined the synovial fluid for particles larger than 5 μm in diameter and found three fractions in failed total knee replacement: 94% consisted of globular particles with a mean diameter of 10 μm, 4% of long fibrous particles with a mean surface area of 1164 μm, and large rhomboidal particles with a mean surface area of 557 μm regardless of the wear pattern.[33] No submicron particles were analyzed. Larger polyethylene particles were found in failed TKR with gross polyethylene wear,[29] supporting the recommendation to analyze the joint fluid aspirate for polyethylene wear particles.[7]

The clinical triad of effusion, pain, and progressive change in the coronal alignment of the knee is characteristic of accelerated polyethylene wear[34] and presents no diagnostic problem for the orthopedic surgeon. The diagnosis is made with regular radiographs comparing immediate postoperative with recent films for the detection of component changes. A septic workup with bone scan and knee aspiration for WBC count, differential, and cultures is recommended and provides the diagnosis of a failed total knee arthroplasty.

The combination of effusion with or without pain is much more problematic, since the incidence of a painful total knee replacement is actually higher than we assume.

In a prospective study for the evaluation of pain before and after total knee replacement, after the exclusion of patients with chronic pain, the pain decreased 50% every 3 months postoperatively. At 12 months a surprisingly high 10% of patients reported significant pain.[35] Therefore, a careful and thoughtful assessment of a painful effusion is recommended.

Early failure of polyethylene in total knee replacement is rare today, but care should be taken in regard of third-body wear. With new interest in mobile-bearing designs, the mechanism of abrasive wear should be reconsidered to improve surgical techniques, since the bearing surfaces are enlarged. Abrasive wear is caused through third-body wear from fretting, bone chips, loose grafts, and loose or broken pieces of bone cement. Therefore, the elimination of these particles during surgery is important to improve long-term results in younger and more active patients. In 13 consecutive patients despite a careful implantation and a meticulous cementing technique, the removal of a large amount of debris required intense irrigation with at least several liters of fluid.[36]

Some mobile-bearing TKRs have less constrained motion at the tibial counterface, which may lead to further increase of wear.[37] Scratching and surface roughening through bone cement may lead to accelerated wear. Figure 24-1 shows a moderately painful total knee

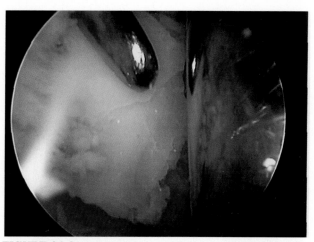

FIGURE 24-2. Arthroscopic removal of residual bone cement in the posterolateral corner with complete pain relief postoperative and subsidence of the knee effusion.

replacement with a small effusion and a radiopaque body in the posterolateral corner 2 years postoperatively. After arthroscopic removal of the cement, the patient had complete pain relief and a subsidence of the knee effusion (Figure 24-2). Figure 24-3 shows a maltracking patella with painful effusion 18 months after surgery. Accelerated early polyethylene wear is also seen with malalignment: Too much posterior slope in the sagittal plane led to early wear (Figure 24-4) in a posterior stabilized total knee replacement through impingement of the tibial post in the femoral box (Figure 24-5), causing villous hypertrophic synovitis (Figure 24-6).

Adhesive wear can occur rapidly with thin or altered polyethylene. Thicker polyethylene inserts and improved sterilization processes in ETO and neutral gases have

FIGURE 24-1. Residual bone cement in the posterolateral corner of a posterior stabilized modular TKR with mild effusion and continuous pain postoperatively.

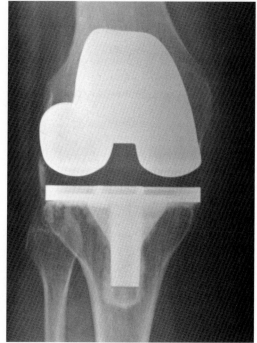

FIGURE 24-3. Patella maltracking with painful effusion 18 months after surgery.

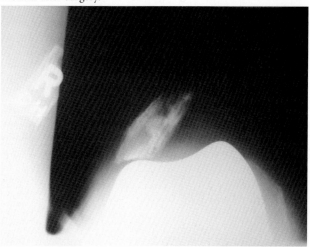

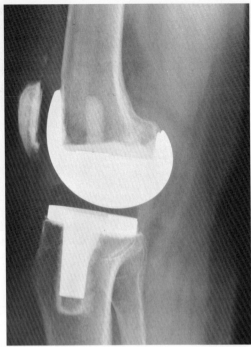

FIGURE 24-4. Posterior slope of 12 degrees in a posterior stabilized TKR with post-cam impingement.

improved adhesive wear.[1,2,5] More recent studies demonstrate reduced radiolucent lines and less revisions with a compression-molded monoblock versus ram-extruded modular tibia in TKR with intermediate to long-term follow-up.[6] Figures 24-7 and 24-8 show a nonconforming posterior cruciate retaining total knee replacement 7 years postoperative in an active 55-year-old patient with periprosthetic osteolyis.

FIGURE 24-5. Impingement of the tibial post in the femoral box *(arrow)* 2 years postoperative with mild effusion.

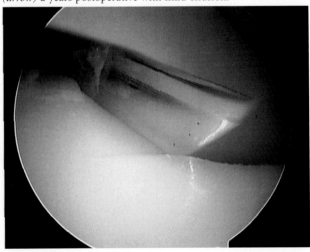

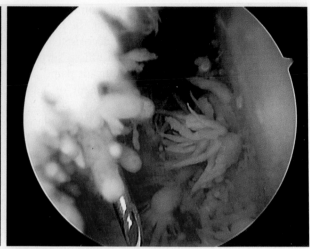

FIGURE 24-6. Villous hypertrophy secondary to early wear of post-cam impingement in a posterior stabilized TKR 2 years postoperatively.

More conforming tibial inserts may lead to increased micromotion between the insert and the tibial component of modular design, causing significant backside wear, and we may see more wear-related problems in these patients. We also have to be aware of the fact that certain production years of polyethylene may play an important factor. We observe currently more wear-related problems in total knee replacements implanted after 1996. The con-

FIGURE 24-7. Radiograph 7 years postoperative with mild medial wear and extensive osteolysis *(arrows).*

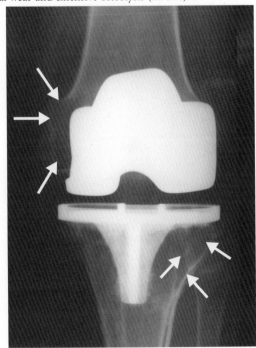

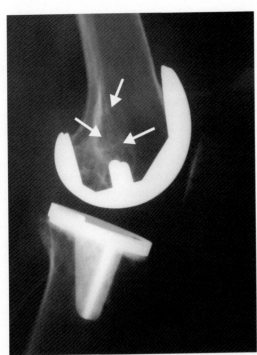

FIGURE 24-8. Lateral view of the same knee with osteolytic lesion (*arrows*) proximal to the femoral pegs.

comitant change to more conforming designs may present an additional disadvantage.

Aseptic synovitis secondary to polyethylene wear debris is the first symptom and should raise the surgeon's attention to various prosthetic, design, and surgical details to react promptly. These patients should be followed up closely, with regular follow-up visits before catastrophic failure of these total knee replacements occur.

SPONTANEOUS HEMARTHROSIS

Spontaneous hemarthrosis after knee arthroplasty is uncommon, and the incidence of hemarthrosis was found to be 0.5%.[38] Entrapment of synovial tissue between the components is postulated to be the etiology for recurrent bleeds. Spontaneous hemarthrosis after total knee replacement has been described in patients following total knee arthroplasty with proliferative synovitis,[38–40] hemophilia,[41] pigmented villonodular synovitis,[42,43] erosion of the lateral genicular artery,[44] and use of warfarin,[40,45] enoxaparin, and fondaparinux.[46] Furthermore, there is a group of idiopathic spontaneous hemarthrosis without any obvious finding, challenging its etiology.

REFERENCES

1. Collier JP, Sutula LC, Currier BH, et al. Overview of poly-ethylene as a bearing material: comparison of sterilization methods. *Clin Orthop.* 1996;333:76–86.
2. Collier JP, Sperling DK, Currier JH, et al. Impact of gamma sterilization on clinical performance of polyethylene in the knee. *J Arthroplasty.* 1996;11(4):377–389.
3. Sutula LC, Collier JP, Saum KA, et al. The Otto Aufranc Award. Impact of gamma sterilization on clinical performance of polyethylene in the hip. *Clin Orthop.* 1995;319: 28–40.
4. Nusbaum HJ, Rose RM. The effects of radiation sterilization on the properties of ultrahigh molecular weight polyethylene. *J Biomed Mater Res.* 1979;13(4): 557–576.
5. Bohl JR, Bohl WR, Postk PD, et al. The Coventry Award. the effects of shelf life on clinical outcome for gamma sterilized polyethylene tibial components. *Clin Orthop.* 1999;367: 28–38.
6. Weber AB, Worland RL, Keenan J, et al. A study of poly-ethylene and modularity issues in >1000 posterior cruciate-retaining knees at 5 to 11 years. *J Arthroplasty.* 2002;17(8):987–991.
7. Coutts RD, Engh GA, Mayor MB, et al. The painful total knee replacement and the influence of component design. *Contemp Orthop.* 1994;28(6):523–536, 541–545.
8. Gatter RA. *A Practical Handbook of Joint Fluid Analysis.* Philadelphia: Lea & Febiger; 1984.
9. Koopman WJ. *Arthritis and Allied Conditions: A Textbook of Rheumatology.* Baltimore: Williams & Wilkins; 1994.
10. Schumacher HR. *Primer on the Rheumatic Diseases.* 9th ed. Atlanta: Arthritis Foundation; 1988.
11. Kersey R, Benjamin J, Marson B. White blood cell counts and differential in synovial fluid of aseptically failed total knee arthroplasty. *J Arthroplasty.* 2000;15(3):301–304.
12. Aman S, Risteli J, Luukkainen R, et al. The value of synovial fluid analysis in the assessment of knee joint destruction in arthritis in a three year follow up study. *Ann Rheum Dis.* 1999;58(9):559–562.
13. Cuckler JM, Star AM, Alavi A, et al. Diagnosis and management of the infected total joint arthroplasty. *Orthop Clin North Am.* 1991;22(3):523–530.
14. Windsor RE, Bono JV. Infected total knee replacements. *J Am Acad Orthop Surg.* 1994;2(1):44–53.
15. Barrack RL, Harris WH. The value of aspiration of the hip joint before revision total hip arthroplasty. *J Bone Joint Surg Am.* 1993;75(1):66–76.
16. Lyons CW, Berquist TH, Lyons JC, et al. Evaluation of radiographic findings in painful hip arthroplasties. *Clin Orthop.* 1985;195:239–251.
17. Magnuson JE, Brown ML, Hauser MF, et al. In-111-labeled leukocyte scintigraphy in suspected orthopedic prosthesis

infection: comparison with other imaging modalities. *Radiology.* 1988;168(1):235–239.

18. O'Neill DA, and Harris WH. Failed total hip replacement: assessment by plain radiographs, arthrograms, and aspiration of the hip joint. *J Bone Joint Surg Am.* 1984;66(4): 540–546.

19. Gould ES, Potter HG, Bober SE. Role of routine percutaneous hip aspirations prior to prosthesis revision. *Skeletal Radiol.* 1990;19(6):427–430.

20. Mariani BD, Martin DS, Levine MJ, et al. The Coventry Award. Polymerase chain reaction detection of bacterial infection in total knee arthroplasty. *Clin Orthop.* 1996;331: 11–22.

21. Yin C, Jiranek W, Cardea J. Effect of Antibiotics on the diagnosis of joint infection: PCR versus culture. 47th Annual Meeting, Orthopaedic Research Society. San Francisco, Feb 25–28. 2001.

22. Williamson SC, Roger DJ, Petrera P, et al. Acute gouty arthropathy after total knee arthroplasty. a case report. *J Bone Joint Surg Am.* 1994;76(1):126–128.

23. Masuda I, Ishikawa K. Clinical features of pseudogout attack. a survey of 50 cases. *Clin Orthop.* 1988;229:173–181.

24. Tsao A, Mintz L, McRae CR, et al. Failure of the porous-coated anatomic prosthesis in total knee arthroplasty due to severe polyethylene wear. *J Bone Joint Surg Am.* 1993; 75(1):19–26.

25. Schai PA, Thornhill TS, Scott RD. Total knee arthroplasty with the PFC system. results at a minimum of ten years and survivorship analysis. *J Bone Joint Surg Br.* 1998;80(5): 850–858.

26. Ewald FC, Wright RJ, Poss R, et al. Kinematic total knee arthroplasty: a 10- to 14-year prospective follow-up review. *J Arthroplasty.* 1999;14(4):473–480.

27. Stern SH, Insall JN. Posterior stabilized prosthesis. results after follow-up of nine to twelve years. *J Bone Joint Surg Am.* 1992;74(7):980–986.

28. Schmalzried TP, Callaghan JJ. Wear in total hip and knee replacements. *J Bone Joint Surg Am.* 1999;81(1):115–136.

29. Bosco J, Benjamin J, Wallace D. Quantitative and qualitative analysis of polyethylene wear particles in synovial fluid of patients with total knee arthroplasty. a preliminary report. *Clin Orthop.* 1994;309:11–19.

30. Hahn DW, Wolfarth DL, Parks NL. Characterization of submicron polyethylene wear debris from synovial-fluid samples of revised knee replacements using a light-scattering technique. *J Biomed Mater Res.* 1996;31(3): 355–363.

31. Fox RI, Kang H. Structure and function of synoviocytes. In: McCarty DJ, Koopman, WJ, eds. *Arthritis and Allied Conditions.* Philadelphia: Lea & Febiger; 1993:263–278.

32. Kovacik MW, Gradisar IA Jr, Haprian JJ, et al. Osteolytic indicators found in total knee arthroplasty synovial fluid aspirates. *Clin Orthop.* 2000;379:186–194.

33. Peterson C, Benjamin JB, Sziveck JA, et al. Polyethylene particle morphology in synovial fluid of failed knee arthroplasty. *Clin Orthop.* 1999;359:167–175.

34. Jones SM, Pinder IM, Moran CG, et al. Polyethylene wear in uncemented knee replacements. *J Bone Joint Surg Br.* 1992;74(1):18–22.

35. Brander VA, Stulberg SD, Adams A. Chitranjan Ranawat Award: Predicting Those at Risk for Greater Total Knee Replacement Pain: A Prospective, Observational Study. The Knee Society Combined Specialty Day Meeting, New Orleans, Feb 8, 2003.

36. Helmers S, Sharkey PF, McGuigan FX. Efficacy of irrigation for removal of particulate debris after cemented total knee arthroplasty. *J Arthroplasty.* 1999;14(5):549–552.

37. Jones VC, Williams IR, Auger DD, et al. Quantification of third body damage to the tibial counterface in mobile bearing knees. *Proc Inst Mech Eng (H).* 2001;215(2): 171–179.

38. Worland RL, Jessup DE. Recurrent hemarthrosis after total knee arthroplasty. *J Arthroplasty.* 1996;11(8):977–978.

39. Oishi CS, Elliott ML, Colwell CW Jr. Recurrent hemarthrosis following a total knee arthroplasty. *J Arthroplasty.* 1995; 10(Suppl):S56–58.

40. Kindsfater K, Scott R. Recurrent hemarthrosis after total knee arthroplasty. *J Arthroplasty.* 1995;10(Suppl):S52–S55.

41. Magone JB, Dennis DA, Weis LD. Total knee arthroplasty in chronic hemophilic arthropathy. *Orthopedics.* 1986;9(5): 653–657.

42. Ballard WT, Clark CR, Callaghan JJ. Recurrent spontaneous hemarthrosis nine years after a total knee arthroplasty. A presentation with pigmented villonodular synovitis. *J Bone Joint Surg Am.* 1993;75(5):764–767.

43. Meyers BW, Masi AT, Feigenbaum SL. Pigmented villonodular synovitis and tenosynovitis: a clinical epidemiologic study of 166 cases and literature review. *Medicine.* 1980;59: 223–238.

44. Cunningham RB, Mariani EM. Spontaneous hemarthrosis 6 years after total knee arthroplasty. *J Arthroplasty.* 2001; 16(1):133–135.

45. Wild JH, Zvaifler NJ. Hemarthrosis associated with sodium warfarin therapy. *Arthritis Rheum.* 1976;19(1):98–102.

46. Bauer KA, Eriksson BI, Lassen MR, et al. Fondaparinux compared with enoxaparin for the prevention of venous thromboembolism after elective major knee surgery. *N Engl J Med.* 2001;345(18):1305–1310.

CHAPTER 25

Prodromes of Failure After Revision Total Knee Arthroplasty

Jess H. Lonner

Nearly 250000 primary total knee arthroplasties are performed annually, and it is estimated that this number may nearly double to 454000 by the year 2030.[1] While the long-term success and survivorship of primary total knee arthroplasties exceed 90% into the second decade,[2–4] there is an inevitable risk of failure and a need for subsequent revision. Despite the low percentage of failure, there is a large volume of revision total knee arthroplasties performed for aseptic failure since such a great number of primary knee arthroplasties are implanted annually. In 1999, it was estimated that 22000 revision knee arthroplasties were performed in the United States,[5] representing a 13% increase in the number of revision TKAs performed in the United States 4 years earlier.[6] The percentage growth in volume of revision TKAs may be even more dramatic in other regions, such as the Province of Ontario, Canada, which experienced an annual increase from 1989 to 1994 of 19.3% (compared with 14.1% for primary total knee arthroplasties).[7] And these numbers will likely continue to grow, particularly as total knee arthroplasties and unicompartmental arthroplasties are offered to the younger and more active sector of our population.

RESULTS AFTER REVISION TOTAL KNEE ARTHROPLASTY

Functional improvement after a well-performed revision total knee arthroplasty, at least in the short-term, can be expected. A meta-analysis of 37 studies found that while the results of revision TKA were clearly inferior to those of primary total knee replacement, significant improvements in the mean Knee Society Function Scores and Clinical Scores can be expected, improving from 30.4 points to 57.4 points (p < 0.0001) and from 32.8 points to 74.9 points (p < 0.0001), respectively.[8] Unfortunately, despite these functional improvements, revision total knee arthroplasties will statistically fail more frequently and earlier than primary TKAs, regardless of contemporary advancements in implant design, stems and augments, surgical technique, and quality and sterilization techniques of the polyethylene. Clearly, a great deal of variability exists in the success and survivorship of revision arthroplasty, complication rates, and patient satisfaction. The majority of reports have been relatively short-term with satisfactory results ranging from 46% to 84% at 3.5 to 5.0 years.[9–12]

The results of revision arthroplasty are impacted by the quality of bone stock, integrity of the collateral ligaments, function of the extensor mechanism, surgical proficiency, and implant selection.[9] Often, it is the former (i.e., quality of bone support) that deteriorates progressively in the failing revision arthroplasty, as a result of component motion and subsidence. This problem is compounded in the presence of osteolysis from particulate debris that is generated from polyethylene wear, metallosis, or other sources. Once a revision total knee arthroplasty has failed, the complexity, need for bone graft or augments, degree of implant constraint, and the eventual success of further revision procedures can be affected by the timeliness of detection of that failure and subsequent intervention.

SURVEILLANCE AFTER REVISION TOTAL KNEE ARTHROPLASTY

These points highlight the need for routine surveillance after revision total knee arthroplasty and early intervention once failure is detected. Looking at contemporary series, primary knee replacement failure modes include polyethylene wear (25%), loosening (24%), instability (21%), infection (17.5%), arthrofibrosis (14.6%), malalignment or malpositioning (11.8%), extensor mechanism deficiency (6.6%), avascular necrosis of the patella (4.2%), and periprosthetic fracture (2.8%).[13] Documented failure mechanisms after revision total knee arthroplasties include failure of fixation, subsidence, instability, loosening, fracture, and extensor mechanism dysfunction.[14] Again, clearly the most common reasons for failure after revision knee arthroplasty are related to the failure of structural support, which can compromise further revisional surgery if treatment is delayed. The need for reoperation after revision arthroplasty is approximately 15%, of which nearly 44% may require 2 or more additional surgeries.[15]

Routine Follow-Up

As in failures of primary knee replacements, identifying the mode of failure of the revision total knee arthroplasty is important to ensure that the intricacies of the problem are addressed at the time of subsequent re-operations. Further, routine surveillance is critical for even the well-functioning revision total knee arthroplasty to identify mechanical failures early, before the cascade of bone loss and component subsidence. Early diagnosis of and intervention for the failed revision TKA enhance the facility with which further revision knee replacement can be performed and potentially optimize the results of treatment. Despite the importance of routine surveillance, practically speaking it may be difficult to follow routinely all patients over an extended period of time because of a variety of barriers, some of which are self-imposed, but others that have either a geographic, economic, or procedural basis.[16–21] The obstacles to routine assessment are occasionally physician-imposed, in that we arbitrarily assign follow-up intervals. These intervals may be too infrequent to capture a failing arthroplasty early in the process.[16] Alternatively, patients who live far away from the treating surgeon may opt not to return for periodic assessment, or they may choose to follow up with a more locally accessible orthopedist. This problem may be hastened if regional centers are developed to care for patients with failed total knee replacements. Some patients may simply opt to discontinue routine follow-up visits because of their inconvenience. In one study, 45% of patients preferred not to return to the orthopedic office for an evaluation because of concerns regarding lost wages and expenditure of time.[22] Capitated care is another potential obstacle to routine surveillance after revision total joint replacement. While the trend common to the early and mid-1990s is less prevalent now, in which maintenance care, even after surgical interventions, was often relegated to the primary care physician, the future structure of health care delivery in the United States is uncertain. It is clear, though, that on some level our ability to routinely follow patients after revision total knee replacement surgery is being impacted. In light of these obstacles, an alternative method of surveillance of patients after revision total knee arthroplasty may be practical if it is proven effective at identifying those patients at risk for or actively undergoing implant failure. Surveillance should not be delayed, since more than 50% of revision surgeries may be necessary within the first 2 years after arthroplasty.[13]

Mail Questionnaires and Follow-Up Radiography

The use of mail questionnaires has been proposed to circumvent or complement direct patient follow-up, and this may in fact be an effective vehicle for following patients after revision arthroplasty. Several studies have detailed a variety of prodromal symptoms and signs that are most commonly associated with mechanical failure after total knee arthroplasty, and these signals of failure may be identified by mail questionnaires or telephone conversations.[16,23,24] The presence of these prodromal symptoms or signs that develop in the setting of implant *failure* should prompt radiographs and further direct hands-on evaluation. In a series of failed total knee arthroplasties with polyethylene wear, Tsao et al. noted the presence of pain in 75%, effusion in 63%, clicking in 28%, and stiffness in 6%.[23] A series by Knight et al. found that swelling was evident in 89%, stiffness in 72%, pain in 67%, clicking in 38%, and instability in 22%.[24] Comparable symptoms of mechanical failures after total knee arthroplasty were reported in a series by Lonner et al., including pain (84%), swelling (76%), progressive coronal plane deformity (19%), instability (17%), stiffness (17%), new onset of clicking or grinding (7%), catching (4%), and patellar pain, subluxation, or clicking (4%).[16] In the latter series, the average duration of symptoms before presentation was 13 months (range, 1 week to 5 years), suggesting that an annual symptom-based questionnaire (Table 25.1) and series of weightbearing radiographs of the knee can be an effective means of alternative surveillance after knee arthroplasty.[16] In that series, particularly in the absence of clinical symptoms, standing radiographs were considered an important supplement to the questionnaires for identifying failures. The dilemma with this means of surveillance (i.e., remote reporting of symptoms) is that it would not be pertinent for those patients who never recovered from the initial postoperative pain, stiffness, or swelling that usually resolves within the first year after revision surgery, or those with other uncommon causes of early dysfunction, such as instability from imbalance or patellar dysfunction not addressed

TABLE 25.1. Sample Symptom-Based Questionnaire.

Over the last 12 months have you experienced the following new symptoms that you had not previously noted?

Symptom	Yes	No
1. Pain	—	—
2. Swelling	—	—
3. Instability	—	—
4. Stiffness	—	—
5. Clicking	—	—
6. Progressive deformity	—	—
7. Grinding	—	—
8. Catching	—	—
9. Redness	—	—
10. Drainage	—	—
11. Fevers	—	—

For each positive response, address the following:

Was it associated with an injury? _____

Was the onset of symptoms acute or insidious? _____

Is it present both with activity and at rest? _____

With what activities are the symptoms associated? _____

Has it resolved or is it continuing? _____

Adapted from Lonner, Siliski, Scott,[13] by permission of *J Arthrop.*

at the time of revision surgery, reflex sympathetic dystrophy, arthrofibrosis, or infection. This method of alternative surveillance does not distinguish between aseptic and septic failure; suspicion for infection should always be high, and subsequent evaluation should include an appropriate workup for infection.

The potential for response bias in the reporting of patient satisfaction, function, and knee scores when using mail or telephone surveys is a legitimate concern.[25–27] But while there are potential inaccuracies of the questionnaires that are used for assessing clinical outcome and patient satisfaction, as well as a variety of other objective measurements, questionnaires can be a valuable vehicle for identifying symptoms of failure of knee arthroplasties that have previously been functioning well.[16] While these clues to failure should theoretically be easily gleaned from a questionnaire, there is an element of diminished efficacy of mail surveys. One recent survey of 472 surviving patients after total knee arthroplasty found that the response to questionnaires tends to diminish with time from the index surgery, such that the response rate to a standard questionnaire fell from 75% at 2 years to 54% at 10 years (p = 0.0016).[28] In that series, "nonresponders" tended to be those with inferior results; however, the study did not identify whether those who had new signs of problems were more or less likely to respond to the questionnaire than those who were faring well or those who had never done well after surgery.[28]

CONCLUSION

The potential value of mail surveys coupled with standing radiographs for identifying symptoms of mechanical failure cannot be overstated. A number of patients whose implants are failing may deny knee symptoms that are reflective of implant failure and this can only be reconciled by obtaining concurrent weightbearing radiographs of the knee. Complementing the questionnaire with standing radiographs will effectively identify the *occult* failures.[16] The administration of periodic questionnaires and standing radiographs every 12 to 24 months can be an effective method of surveillance after revision total knee arthroplasty, particularly when there are obstacles to direct annual follow-up. The possibility that the presence of acute pain or swelling can be indicative of deep infection should not be overlooked, and patients with new symptoms should always be scrutinized and evaluated for sepsis.

REFERENCES

1. Future demands for orthopaedic skill to soar. *AAOS Bull.* 1999;47:14.
2. Rodrigez JA, Bahende H, Ranawat CS. Total condylar knee replacement. a 20-year follow up study. *Clin Orthop.* 2001; 388:10–17.

3. Ritter MA, Herbst SA, Keating EM, Faris PM, Meding JB. Long-term survival analysis of a posterior cruciate-retaining total condylar total knee arthroplasty. *Clin Orthop.* 1994;309:136–145.

4. Stern SH, Insall JN. Posterior stabilized prostheses. results after follow-up of nine to twelve years. *J Bone Joint Surg.* 1992;74A:980–986.

5. Ingenix-Data Analyst Group. Columbus, OH: Ingenix; 1999.

6. Mendenhall S. Get the low down on orthopaedic implants. *Mater Manage Health Care.* 1996;5:30–32.

7. Coyte PC, Young W, Williams JI. Devolution on hip and knee replacement surgery? *Can J Surg.* 1996;39:373–378.

8. Saleh KJ, Rand JA, McQueen DA. Current status of revision total knee arthroplasty: how do we assess results? *J Bone Joint Surg.* 2003;85A(Suppl):18–20.

9. Haas S, Insall J, Montgomery W, Windsor R. Revision total knee arthroplasty with use of modular components with stems inserted without cement. *J Bone Joint Surg.* 1995; 77A:1700–1707.

10. Elia EA, Lotke PA. Results of revision total knee arthroplasty associated with significant bone loss. *Clin Orthop.* 1991; 271:114.

11. Goldberg VM, Figgie MP, Figgie HE, et al. The results of revision total knee arthroplasty. *Clin Orthop.* 1988;226:86.

12. Jacobs MA, Hungerford DS, Krackow KA, et al. Revision total knee arthroplasty using the kinematic stabilizer prosthesis. *J Bone Joint Surg.* 1988;70A:491.

13. Sharkey PF, Hozack WJ, Rothman RH, et al. Why are total knee arthroplasties failing today? *Clin Orthop.* 2002;404: 7–13.

14. Rand JA, Peterson LF, Bryan RS, Ilstrup DM. Revision total knee arthroplasty. *Instr Course Lect.* 1986;35:305–318.

15. Sierra RJ, Pagnano MW, Trousdale RT. Reoperations after 3200 revision total knee replacements: rate, etiology, and lessons learned. Proceedings of the 70th Annual Meeting of the AAOS. New Orleans, February 2003;40.

16. Lonner JH, Siliski JM, Scott RD. Prodromes of failure in total knee arthroplasty. *J Arthroplasty.* 1999;14:488–492.

17. McGinty JB. What is the meaning of "centers of excellence?" (editorial) *Orthop Today.* 1996;4.

18. Gottlieb S, Einhorn TA. Current concepts review: managed care: form, function, and evolution. *J Bone Joint Surg Am.* 1997;79A:125–136.

19. Kerr EA, Mittman BS, Hays RD, Leake B, Brook RH. Quality assurance in capitated physician groups. where's the emphasis? *JAMA.* 1996;276:1236–1239.

20. Michaels DM, Stiefel JD, Vogt WF. Subcapitation arrangements for specialists. *Med Group Manage J.* 1995;42(3): 41–46.

21. Rosenstein AH. Capitation and orthopedic services. *J Healthcare Resource Manage.* 1996;14(4):27–29.

22. Sethurman V, McGuigan J, Hozack WJ, Sharkey PF, Rothman RH. Routine follow-up office visits after total joint replacement: do asymptomatic patients wish to comply? *J Arthroplasty.* 2000;15:183–186.

23. Tsao A, Mintz L, McRae C, Stulberg SD, Wright T. Failure of porous coated anatomic prosthesis in total knee arthroplasty due to severe polyethylene wear. *J Bone Joint Surg.* 1993;75A:19–26.

24. Knight JL, Gorai PA, Atwater RD, Grothaus L. Tibial polyethylene failure after primary Porous Coated Anatomic total knee arthroplasty. aids to diagnosis and revision. *J Arthroplasty.* 1995;10:748–757.

25. Robertsson O, Dunbar MJ. Patient satisfaction compared with general health and disease-specific questionnaires in knee arthroplasty. *J Arthroplasty.* 2001;16:476–482.

26. Battish R, Lonner JH, Lotke PA. Efficacy of mail surveys for follow-up of total knee patients. Proceedings of the 68th Annual Meeting of the AAOS. San Francisco, February 2001.

27. McGrory BJ, Freiberg AA, Shinar AA, Harris WH. Correlation of measured range of motion following total hip arthroplasty and responses to a questionnaire. *J Arthroplasty.* 1996;11:565–571.

28. Kim J, Lonner JH, Lotke PA. Non-response bias in mail surveys for follow up after total knee arthroplasty. (unpublished data).

CHAPTER 26

Economics of Revision Total Knee Arthroplasty: Increasing Prevalence, Decreasing Reimbursement

Richard Iorio, William L. Healy, and Michael E. Ayers

The clinical success of total knee arthroplasty (TKA) is a testament to the collaboration of investigative orthopedic surgeons, biomechanical engineers, and the orthopedic joint implant industry during the late twentieth century. Primary TKA predictably relieves pain and improves function, and it is generally associated with patient satisfaction. However, while TKA is popular and successful, it is an expensive surgical procedure for healthcare payors. Due to expanded indications for TKA and the growth and aging of our population, the number of primary TKAs performed each year is increasing in the United States, and TKA will be a major healthcare expense in this country during the next decade.[1]

The increasing prevalence of TKA and the increased Medicare expenditure for TKA has contributed to the federal government's health care budget crisis. The centers for Medicare and Medicaid services (CMS, formerly HCFA) have implemented reductions in professional payment for all physician services, including primary and revision TKA. Medicare has also reduced payments to hospitals for revision TKA.[2]

The impact of reductions in payment for TKA is greater on revision TKA than on primary TKA. Revision TKA consumes more operative time, more physician work, and more hospital resources than primary TKA.[3] As the cost of hospital supplies increases, and reimbursement decreases, revision TKA can severely impact the bottom line of participating hospitals.[2] Revision TKA has been traditionally less profitable than primary TKA despite attempts at cost containment.[4] This chapter reviews the economic issues related to the cost of revision TKA and methods to improve the cost equation for hospitals that deliver revision TKA operations.

EPIDEMIOLOGY

In 2003, 43 million Americans suffer from arthritis, and by 2020 54 million people are projected to be affected by arthritis.[5] When patients develop arthritis of the knee, they experience pain, stiffness, and limitation of function. Total knee arthroplasty is a predictably successful treatment for arthritis of the knee, and the number of primary knee replacement operations in this country has steadily increased since the early 1980s. From approximately 40,000 operations in 1980 to 138,552 in 1990, to 308,250 in 2000, the growth of total knee arthroplasty is impressive (Table 26.1).[1,6] With a projected population of 351 million people by 2030, it is estimated that 474,319 total knee arthroplasty procedures will be performed annually in the United States at that time.[7]

Total knee arthroplasty can fail for many reasons: inadequate surgical technique, infection, bearing surface wear, osteolysis, loosening, implant breakage, fracture, and patient noncompliance. As a result of the increasing prevalence of primary total knee arthroplasty and the increasing longevity of the United States population, the prevalence of revision total knee arthroplasty is also increasing. In 1990, 11,369 revision knee replacement operations were performed in the United States;[6] by 1995, 19,138 revision TKA procedures were performed; and in the year 2000 that figure increased to 26,926.[1,8] It is estimated that by the year 2030, 41,432 revision total knee arthroplasty procedures will be performed in the United States (assuming the ratio of number of revision to primary total knee arthroplasty procedures equals 0.087 or 8.7%).[1,7]

TABLE 26.1. Prevalence of Primary and Revision Total Knee Arthroplasties in the United States, 1980 to 2030.

Year	No. of Primary Total Knee Arthroplasties	No. of Revision Total Knee Arthroplasties
1980	40 000	—
1990	138 552	11 369
2000	308 250	26 926
2030*	474 319	41 432

*Estimated numbers based on projected population data.

Data from References 1 and 6–8.

SURGEON REIMBURSEMENT

Professional reimbursement for orthopedic surgeons for revision total knee arthroplasty has decreased considerably since 1997. In 1997, the average Medicare reimbursement to orthopedic surgeons for revision total knee arthroplasty was $2,123. By 2002, professional payment dropped to $1,740. This represents a 26% decrease in professional reimbursement for revision TKA over 5 years. Professional payment for primary total knee arthroplasty also experienced a 26% decrease during this time period (from $1,816 to $1,514).[1,2]

Ritter et al. documented the inequity between the professional reimbursement for primary and revision total knee arthroplasty.[9] They studied the time required for primary and revision TKA, and they demonstrated that professional reimbursement for revision total knee arthroplasty is discounted 10% as a function of hourly payment when compared with primary total knee arthroplasty. They also raised the question of whether Medicare payment justifies the time spent and the risks assumed to perform revision total knee arthroplasty.

Barrack et al.[3] studied revision total and primary total knee arthroplasty in the context of surgeon work, input, and risk. Professional reimbursement was less per unit of surgeon work, and surgeons accepted greater risk with revision total knee arthroplasty. Increased surgeon work input in the operating room, and increased length of stay for patients in the hospital are measurable variables of increased physician work when compared with primary total knee arthroplasty. The immeasurable variables of intensity of care, preoperative evaluation, surgical planning, and preoperative and increased postoperative vigilance are unaccounted-for variables in the discrepancy between actual physician reimbursement for revision total knee arthroplasty and fair physician reimbursement for revision total knee arthroplasty.[3,9,10]

HOSPITAL COST AND REIMBURSEMENT

The most common method of hospital reimbursement for service is a single payment according to a payment schedule that is defined by a specific diagnosis or surgical case. Medicare pays for approximately two-thirds of knee replacement operations in this country. Eighty-six percent of Medicare cases are paid according to the diagnosis-related group (DRG) payment scale; the other 14% are reimbursed at a lower rate by managed Medicare programs. In fiscal year 2000, DRG 209 (major joint replacement) cost Medicare $3.2 billion.[1] As part of an effort to control Medicare health care expenditures, hospital Medicare payments for DRG 209 have been decreasing since 1998. The estimated average payment for 2002 was $9,057, a 1.8% decrease from the 2001 payment of $9,223.[1] The estimated average hospital cost for revision total knee arthroplasty is considerably higher than the DRG 209 reimbursement,[11–13] and revision TKA can cause considerable *red ink* on a hospital operating statement.

Revision total knee arthroplasty is associated with more operating room time, greater blood loss, a higher complication rate, and longer length of hospital stay than primary total knee arthroplasty.[3] Anesthesia costs and operating room costs have been reported as 12% higher for revision as compared with primary total knee arthroplasty.[12] The cost for inpatient nursing services and the hospital room were 31% higher for revision total knee arthroplasty.[12]

Revision total knee arthroplasty presents a difficult economic problem for hospitals. Revision total knee arthroplasty hospital costs exceed those of primary total knee arthroplasty hospital costs, yet Medicare hospital reimbursement for revision total knee arthroplasty does not compensate the hospital sufficiently for the additional expense.[10,12,13] It is unreasonable to expect hospitals to provide high-quality care to all patients who require revision total knee arthroplasty without sufficient reimbursement. Denying access to care is a concept that the American public has never embraced, and that we do not endorse. Unless reimbursement to hospitals is increased, budgetary restrictions on implants, operating room time, and criteria for admission and operating room use may be necessary.[14]

IMPLANT COSTS

Implant costs for total knee arthroplasty are an important component of the hospital costs of knee replacement. Healy and Finn[15] demonstrated that the hospital cost of total knee arthroplasty between 1983 and 1991 was controlled by utilization review, which effectively reduced the cost of a total knee arthroplasty operation for the hospital. However, the unit cost of the knee implants was not controlled during this period, and knee implant costs increased from 13% of the hospital cost of total knee arthroplasty in 1983 to 25% in 1991. The cost of knee implants in total knee arthroplasty has been increasing in absolute dollars since the 1980s.

Since 1991, orthopedic implant prices have increased 115%, while hospital payment increased 14% and physician payment decreased 40.3%.[16] The increase in manufacturer list prices for hip and knee implants increased 8.5% between 2001 and 2002, which was the second largest increase in implant price since 1992.[17] The average DRG 209 (major joint replacement) hospital payment decreased 1.8% in 2002, and the average physician payment for total knee arthroplasty decreased 9%.[1]

The cost of revision knee replacement implants can be considerably more than primary knee replacement implants without a meaningful increase in hospital reimbursement for the procedure.[4,11,17] In 2001 the average cost of primary knee implants in the Orthopaedic Research Network (a group of 27 hospitals that provided *Orthopaedic Network News* with detailed economic data concerning implant procedures) was $3,522 per procedure.[1] In sharp contrast, revision knee implant costs averaged $4,741 per procedure in the same hospitals.[1] However, there is wide variability in implant costs for revision TKA operations. Femoral and tibial components were required for 45% of the revision procedures.[1] Patella and tibial insert procedures accounted for 29% of revision operations with an average cost of only $980 per case.[1] Tibial revisions (11%) averaged $2,880 in implant costs and femoral revisions (6%) averaged $5,281 in implant costs.[1] The average cost of implants for a three-implant revision was $6,770 per procedure.[1] This cost to the hospital represents two-thirds of the Medicare DRG 209 hospital reimbursement.

Revision total knee arthroplasty frequently requires modular knee implant systems to treat difficult reconstructive problems. Femoral and tibial stems of various sizes, wedges and augments for the implants, and several degrees of constraint for ligamentous substitution are all necessary to ensure that the surgeon has the tools required for a successful reconstruction of a failed knee arthroplasty. In 2002, modular femoral stem extensions ranged in list price from $625 to $1,030 among major manufacturers.[18] Modular tibial stem extensions ranged in price from $413 to $850.[18] Wedges and augments ranged from $633 to $1,430.[18] Previously published (1994) list prices of major manufacturer femoral stems ($280 to $770),

tibial stems ($280 to $985), and wedges/augments ($200 to $950) were less than current listings.[19,20] Although the average selling price is less than the list price for hospitals with large total joint volumes, the trend toward higher costs for revision knee implants has been constant.

COST-CONTAINMENT MEASURES

The quality of health care in this country is perceived by Americans as the best in the world. However, many Americans believe the cost of health care is too high. Maintaining the quality of American health care, while controlling the cost, and without restricting access, is a fundamental paradox in health care economics in the new millennium.[10] Cost-containment measures are a hospital's only method of economic coping in an environment of decreasing reimbursement combined with rising material costs.

Healy and Finn[9] described the high cost of knee implants as a percentage of hospital reimbursement. These high implant costs offset utilization review programs, which reduce the volume of services and supplies associated with TKA. In the 1990s, Zuckerman et al.[21] instituted a surgeon education and institutional prosthesis utilization program that began a competitive bid system to reduce the cost of total joint implants. *The Journal of Bone and Joint Surgery* endorsed these cost-containment measures with the caveat that quality of care must remain the foremost consideration in any implant selection decision-making process.[22]

To further reduce TKA implant costs, an implant selection and cost-reduction program based on demand matching was developed at Lahey Clinic.[23] This program provides guidelines for knee implant selection that reduce the cost of knee implants for the hospital. Patients are assigned to demand categories based on 5 criteria: age, weight, surgeon-predicted postoperative-expected patient activity, general health, and bone stock. Implants are assigned to demand categories based on an implant's projected capacity to handle the patient's projected demand. This program was only applied to primary TKA operations. The use of all-polyethylene tibial components in lower demand categories provided most of the cost savings. A follow-up study evaluated the use of a clinical pathway and the knee implant standardization program as a control of resource utilization and hospital costs for TKA.[24] Short-term patient outcome was not affected, and hospital cost adjusted for medical inflation was reduced 19%.

To further reduce the cost of orthopedic knee implants, a Single Price/Case Price Purchasing Program was developed at Lahey Clinic.[25] The program was developed to eliminate potential conflicts between surgeons and hospital administrators regarding the selection and cost of implants for knee replacement operations. The vendor provided a single price for knee implants for every case without regard for which implant was used. The cost of knee implants was reduced 23% without changing vendors. The vendor was able to provide a price based on 3 years of historical utilization data.

Unfortunately, the cost of revision knee arthroplasty is more difficult to control than the cost of primary knee arthroplasty. Revision knee replacement operations are not suitable for a demand-matching system due to considerable variation in case severity and knee implant requirements. Stems are frequently needed on femoral implants, and femoral stems may have been underused in previous reports concerning primary knee implants used for revision knee replacement.[4] Although the use of all-polyethylene tibial components in primary TKA has been demonstrated to be cost effective and enduring, metal-backed tibial components remain the gold standard in revision TKA.[4,18,21] Recent reports concerning loosening and osteolysis secondary to backside wear and base plate locking mechanism deterioration have raised concerns about the long-term survivorship with metal-backed modular tibial components. The role of all-polyethylene tibial components in revision TKA remains to be defined.[26–28]

Retention of well-fixed knee implant components while revising failed components of a tricompartmental total knee arthroplasty can reduce implant cost for revision TKA. Obviously, by retaining well-fixed knee implant components, operative time and implant costs are saved. Unfortunately, routine retention of all well-fixed components may be unwise due to the multifactorial nature of total knee arthroplasty failure, which can include malrotation, instability, poor implant design, and patient noncompliance, which may compromise the retained components and lead to early revision total knee arthroplasty failure. A theoretical advantage of modular tibial implants is that well-fixed base plates can be retained and that unstable or worn modular inserts can be exchanged for new inserts. Unfortunately, isolated tibial insert exchange has a high failure rate. The cause of instability and polyethylene wear needs to be carefully examined before the modular insert is exchanged in isolation, even if the insert is specifically designed for the implant being revised.[29]

The retention of a well-positioned, stable, all-polyethylene patella component at the time of tibial-femoral revision arthroplasty can be successful, provided that the polyethylene is not oxidized. A mismatch of component manufacturers is acceptable with most modern designs, if the patella component articulates appropriately with the femoral implant.[30] Isolated revision of the patella component in revision total knee arthroplasty is a difficult clinical judgment. Isolated patellar revision with or without lateral retinacular release or other patella realignment procedures is associated with a high rate of reoperation. The variables of implant alignment and design need to be fully considered before isolated patellar revision is undertaken.[31]

CONCLUSIONS

As the prevalence of revision total knee arthroplasty increases, the potential for increased hospital financial losses increase. Cost containment for revision TKA can be achieved in 3 ways: (1) decreasing access to revision TKA; (2) improving efficiency of revision TKA such as at highly specialized centers; and/or (3) reducing the cost of knee implants for revision TKA. Revision total knee arthroplasty is an effective procedure for failed total knee arthroplasty based on global knee rating scales.[32] The literature also has shown that revision total knee arthroplasty provides substantial relief of pain and increased function.[14] However, there is a substantially higher rate of failure and infection when revision total knee arthroplasty is compared with primary total knee arthroplasty.[14] Cost reduction and quality are inextricably linked when the long-term implications of revision total knee arthroplasty surgery are examined.

For an operative intervention as complex as revision total knee arthroplasty, experience, efficiency, and skill are critical for the successful delivery of care. Lavernia and Guzman[33] studied the relationship of surgical volume on the short-term outcome of primary and revision arthroplasty of the hip and knee. In a review of both hospitals and surgeons, those with low volumes of patients (fewer than 10) had higher mortalities and increased length of stay compared with high-volume revision centers. Hospitals and surgeons can improve efficiency and outcome through a "practice makes perfect" scenario.[10,33]

The Knee Society and the North American Knee Arthroplasty Revision Study Group are currently performing a multicenter prospective study funded by the Orthopaedic Research and Education Foundation concerning revision total knee arthroplasty. A predictive severity index will be developed to aid in accurately categorizing revision total knee arthroplasty operations for both predictive outcome as well as reimbursement measures to more fairly reflect the wide spectrum of revision total knee arthroplasty operations. The ability of hospitals and physicians to be more accurately reimbursed for the work involved with these complex and demanding operative procedures is critical to maintaining access for the increasing cohort of patients who will require revision total knee arthroplasty now and in the future. As the American public continues to seek a reduction in the cost of health care, it is imperative that we, as orthopedic surgeons, stress the need for maintenance of quality to assure excellent outcomes for our patients.

REFERENCES

1. Mendenhall S. 2002 Hip and knee implant review. *Orthop Network News.* 2002;13(3):1–16.
2. Fine B. 2002 Medicare payments reduced. *AAOS Bull.* 2002; 50(1):26–29.
3. Barrack RL, Hoffman GJ, Tejeiro WV, Carpenter LJ Jr. Surgeon work input and risk in primary vs. revision total joint arthroplasty. *J Arthroplasty.* 1995;10:281–286.
4. Iorio R, Healy WL, Richards JA. Comparison of the hospital cost of primary revision total knee arthroplasty after cost containment. *Orthopaedics.* 1999;22:195–199.
5. Elders MJ. The increasing impact of arthritis on public health. *J Rheumatol.* 2000;60(suppl):6.
6. Mendenhall S. 1991 implant procedures increased 19%. *Orthop Network News.* 1992;3(4):1–11.
7. Frankowski JJ, Watkins-Castiello S. *Primary Total Knee and Hip Arthroplasty Projections for the U.S. Population to the year 2030.* Rosemont, IL: AAOS Dept of Research and Scientific Affairs; 2002:1–8.
8. Mendenhall S. 1996 Hip and knee implant review. *Orthop Network News.* 1996;7:1–7.
9. Ritter MA, Carr KD, Keating EM, Farris TM, Van Koff DO, Ireland PM. Revision total joint arthroplasty—does Medicare reimbursement justify time spent? *Orthopaedics.* 1996;19:137–140.
10. Iorio R, Healy WL. Cost equation in revision total knee arthroplasty. In: Engh GA, Rorabeck CH, eds. *Revision Total Knee Arthroplasty.* Philadelphia: Williams & Wilkins; 1996:183–194.
11. Najibi S, Iorio R, Surdam JW, Wang W, Appleby D, Healy WL. All polyethylene and metal-backed tibial components in total knee arthroplasty: a matched pair analysis of functional outcome. *J Arthroplasty.* 2003 (in press).
12. Meyers SJ, Reuben JD, Moye LA, Zang J. The actual inpatient cost of primary and revision total joint replacement. 65th AAOS Annual Meeting, 1994; New Orleans: 76.
13. Lavernia CJ, Drakeford MK, Tsao AK, Gittelsohn A, Krackow KA, Hungerford GS. Revision and primary hip and knee arthroplasty: a cost analysis. *Clin Orthop.* 1995; 311:136–141.
14. Saleh KJ, Rand JA, McQueen DA. Current status of revision total knee arthroplasty: how do we assess results? *J Bone Joint Surg.* 2003;85A(suppl):18–20.
15. Healy WL, Finn D. The hospital cost and the cost of the implant for total knee arthroplasty: a comparison between 1983 and 1991 for one hospital. *J Bone Joint Surg.* 1994;76A: 801–806.
16. Mendenhall S. Hip and knee implant prices rise 9.5%. *Orthop Network News.* 2003;14(1):1–16.
17. Mendenhall S. Hip and knee implant prices rise 8.5%. *Orthop Network News.* 2002;13(1):1–16.
18. Mendenhall S. 2002 Knee implant price comparison (special pull-out section). *Orthop Network News.* 2002; 13(3)(suppl).
19. Johnson & Johnson Orthopaedics. *Hospital Price List: Joint Reconstruction and Trauma Device Products.* Sept 26, 1994; 1–13.
20. Mendenhall S. 1993 hip and knee implant review. *Orthop Network News.* 1994;5(3):1–12.
21. Zuckerman JD, Kummer FJ, Frankel VH. The effectiveness of a hospital-based strategy to reduce the cost of total joint implants. *J Bone Joint Surg.* 1994;76A:807–811.
22. Clark CR. Cost containment: total joint implants (editorial). *J Bone Joint Surg.* 1994;76A:799–800.
23. Iorio R, Healy WL, Kirven FM, Patch DA, Pfeifer BA. Knee implant standardization: an implant selection and cost reduction program. *Am J Knee Surg.* 1998;11:73–79.
24. Healy WL, Iorio R, Ko J, Appleby D, Lemos DW. Impact of cost reduction programs on short-term patient outcome and hospital cost of total knee arthroplasty. *J Bone Joint Surg.* 2002;84A:348–353.
25. Healy WL, Iorio R, Lemos MJ, Patch DA, Pfeifer BA, Smiley PM, Wilk RM. Single price/case price purchasing in orthopaedic surgery. *J Bone Joint Surg.* 2000;82A:607–611.
26. Mikulak SA, Mahoney DM, Delarosa MA, Schmalzried TP. Loosening and osteolysis with a pressed fit condylar posterior cruciate substituting total knee replacement. *J Bone Joint Surg.* 2001;83A:398–403.
27. Engh GA, Lounici S, Rao AR, Collier NB. In vivo deterioration of tibial base plate locking mechanisms in contemporary modular total knee components. *J Bone Joint Surg.* 2001;83A:1660–1665.
28. O'Rourke MR, Callaghan JJ, Goetz DD, Sullivan PM, Johnston RC. Osteolysis associated with a cemented modular posterior cruciate substituting total knee design: 5- to 8-year follow-up. *J Bone Joint Surg.* 2002;84A: 1362–1371.
29. Babis GC, Trousdale RT, Morrey DF. The effectiveness of isolated tibial insert exchange in revision total knee arthroplasty. *J Bone Joint Surg.* 2002;84A:64–68.
30. Lonner JH, Mont MA, Sharkey PF, Siliski JM, Rajadhyaksha AD, Lotke PA. Fate of the unrevised all-polyethylene patella

component in revision total knee arthroplasty. *J Bone Joint Surg.* 2003;85A:56–59.

31. Leopold SS, Silverton CD, Barden RM, Rosenberg AG. Isolated revision of the patella component in total knee arthroplasty. *J Bone Joint Surg.* 2003;85A:41–47.

32. Saleh KJ, Dykes DC, Tweedi RL, Mohamed K, Ravichandran A, Saleh RM, Gioe TJ, Heck DA. Functional outcome after total knee arthroplasty revision: a meta-analysis. *J Arthroplasty.* 2002;17(8):967–977.

33. Lavernia CJ, Guzman JF. Relationship with surgical volume to short-term mortality, morbidity and hospital charges in arthroplasty. *J Arthroplasty.* 1995;10:133–140.

CHAPTER 27

Salvage Knee Surgery: Arthrodesis

James V. Bono and Steven R. Wardell

Primary arthrodesis or fusion of the knee is an uncommon procedure performed in the 21st century. It is rarely performed primarily for arthritis. The main role of knee arthrodesis is as a salvage procedure for unrevisable failed total knee arthroplasty (TKA).[1] Arthrodesis of the knee, in the face of grossly deficient bone stock and ligamentous instability, is difficult to achieve.[2–5] In limb salvage surgery for malignant and potentially malignant lesions about the knee, resection arthrodesis using an intramedullary rod and local bone graft has been reported as a successful primary procedure.[6] When performed as a primary procedure after trauma, arthritis, or instability, solid fusion may not always occur, with rates of union reported between 80% and 98% by various methods. Fibrous nonunion after attempted fusion frequently is painful,[3,7–10] and rigid internal fixation promotes bony union. Using strict patient selection criteria, knee arthrodesis should be reserved as a salvage procedure for severe infection, bone loss, or instability primarily following failed TKA.

INDICATIONS

Unilateral Posttraumatic Osteoarthritis in a Young Patient

In a healthy young male laborer with an isolated, severely damaged knee, an arthrodesis should be recommended.[11] A successful fusion is more durable over time than any other reconstructive option. However, arthrodesis is often refused by men and rejected unconditionally by women, which presents a dilemma for the surgeon. In the younger individual, a knee replacement is unlikely to endure a lifetime of hard use and will certainly require future revision. The patient's decision to undergo arthrodesis should be made carefully, since conversion of a knee arthrodesis to successful arthroplasty is not easily performed at a later date.[12] Fortunately, disabling unilateral, posttraumatic osteoarthritis in a young person is rare, and each case must be judged individually. Occasionally, joint debridement or realignment by osteotomy provides temporary symptomatic relief. Extensive preoperative discussion, including the risks, benefits, expectations, and alternatives to surgery help the patient decide whether to have surgery, postpone it, or avoid it altogether. Despite the long-term durability of fusion, the patient may still insist on TKA and the patient should understand that the success of arthrodesis following unsuccessful arthroplasty might be less predictable.

Multiple Operated Knee

Occasionally, there are patients who, despite or because of multiple operations, complain of a diffusely painful and usually unstable knee. The original insult may have been a ligament injury or patellar dislocation resulting in reflex sympathetic dystrophy with or without subsequent operative intervention. Underlying emotional and psychiatric problems may be present. These patients are challenging to treat, and additional knee surgery of any kind may be unwarranted and inadvisable secondary to its poor outcome. Management should consist of simple conservative care, bracing, physical therapy, evaluation by a pain service, and perhaps, psychiatric consultation. For a select few, arthrodesis may be the correct approach. In this situation, a preoperative trial of a cylinder cast is important to convey the functional limitations of knee arthrodesis to the patient.

Painful Ankylosis

Ankylosis of the knee is defined as a range of motion of no more than 10 to 20 degrees. Patients who develop stiffness from severe rheumatoid arthritis or osteoarthritis may be successfully treated by total knee arthroplasty[13] using quadriceps turn-down or tibial tubercle osteotomy techniques, *skeletonization* of the femur, and reestablishment of the medial and lateral gutters by scar excision. However, even in these cases, the likelihood of obtaining normal motion is small, with the final outcome often being less than 90 degrees of motion. In the ankylosed knee following sepsis or remote trauma, an arthroplasty may be either contraindicated or likely to produce a suboptimal result, particularly in terms of functional motion. Therefore, a painful ankylosis of the knee may benefit from an arthrodesis.

Paralytic Conditions

Currently, poliomyelitis is rare in the United States and Western Europe, where vaccination is widespread. Muscle weakness can usually be managed successfully by bracing, as these patients often have little pain. However, when associated with genu recurvatum, bracing is difficult and may not be successful. In this setting, arthroplasty is technically demanding.[14] In paralytic conditions, arthrodesis adequately addresses the quadriceps weakness and angular deformity.

Neuropathic Charcot Joint

Arthrodesis of a neuropathic knee joint has resulted in limited success and frequent nonunion. Thorough debridement of all bone detritus and complete synovectomy have been demonstrated to increase the rate of bony union.[15] Drennan reported 10 cases of arthrodesis of a Charcot knee in 9 patients.[15] The best results were obtained after complete removal of the thickened, edematous synovium in these knees. When the Charcot knee is painless, bracing and conservative management is the treatment of choice. However, some Charcot knees are painful and should be carefully selected for knee arthroplasty or arthrodesis. Variable results of TKA in Charcot joints have been reported.[16,17] However, if TKA is performed, bone defects should be treated by implants with metal augments rather than by bone grafting, and constrained posterior stabilized knee replacement designs are recommended.

Malignant and Potentially Malignant Knee Lesions

Certain potentially malignant and low-grade malignant tumors about the knee, such as aggressive giant cell tumor, chondrosarcoma, recurrent chondroblastoma, and carefully selected higher-grade malignant lesions may be satisfactorily controlled by adequate local resection of the lesion. Reconstruction of the defect created by such resection may be accomplished by (A) extremity shortening and arthrodesis; (B) arthrodesis with large intercalary bone grafts to preserve length; (C) arthroplasty with custom-made prosthetic replacements; and (D) allotransplantation of joints.[18–29] Local resection and arthrodesis for tumors about the knee was first described in 1907 by Lexer and others.[19,21,25,29,30] Success in controlling the tumor was frequently complicated by infection, nonunion, and late fatigue fracture. Enneking reported 20 patients with malignant or potentially malignant tumors (osteogenic sarcoma, giant cell tumor, synovial cell sarcoma, chondrosarcoma, and chondroblastoma) in the proximal tibia or distal femur.[6] These patients were treated by local resection and arthrodesis using a customized fluted intramedullary rod and autogenous segmental cortical grafts obtained from the same extremity.

Failed Total Knee Arthroplasty

Currently, the most frequent indication for knee fusion, as well as the most difficult circumstance in which to achieve union, is the failed TKA. Mechanical failure of an arthroplasty can nearly always be better managed by revision. Two-stage reimplantation may be the best choice when the failure is caused by sepsis. However, some cases of failed TKA with bone loss and infection can only be managed by resection arthroplasty and staged arthrodesis.

Arthrodesis as a salvage procedure for a failed septic knee replacement is indicated in the following circumstances: (A) persistent infection recalcitrant to repeated debridement and antibiotic regimen; (B) disruption of the extensor mechanism; (C) an infectious organism that is only sensitive to severely toxic antibiotic agents, such as *Candida albicans* or other fungi;[31–33] or (D) a young patient or a disillusioned older one who does not wish to face possible future revision arthroplasties. Occasionally, fusion may be the best choice for a very heavy patient with a septic TKA failure. Although certain patients insist on TKA reimplantation following septic TKA, some do not want to risk recurrent infection and choose arthrodesis as definitive treatment.

Deficiency of the extensor mechanism is a compelling indication for arthrodesis when it occurs in the setting of an infected knee arthroplasty. The patient generally displays a profound extensor lag with poor results if reimplantation TKA is performed. Despite various reconstructive techniques, disruption of the extensor mechanism often yields a compromised result.[34] The patient will never be able to adequately extend the knee and will generally display a profound extensor lag if reimplantation TKA is attempted. Repair of the extensor mechanism is often impossible because of extensive tissue destruction that occurs secondary to the infection. An extensor mechanism allograft may be needed to reconstruct the extensor deficit but is relatively contraindicated in the setting of previous sepsis.

ARTHRODESIS TECHNIQUES

Arthrodesis of the knee may be accomplished by one of 4 techniques: (A) compression arthrodesis with external fixation; (B) compression arthrodesis with compression plating;[35,36] (C) intramedullary rod fixation; and (D) a combination of intramedullary rod fixation and compression plating.[37]

A suitable cancellous surface on both the femoral and tibial surfaces optimizes fusion. Bone shortening relaxes the hamstrings and increases flexibility at the hip joint, which is desirable if both knees have to be fused.[7] Charnley reported that patients considered limb shortening advantageous for dressing and foot care.[7] The desired alignment is 0 to 5 degrees of valgus, with the knee flexed 10 to 15 degrees. Less flexion can be accepted in the presence of marked bone loss. The patella can be left alone or used to augment the fusion mass.

When arthrodesis is indicated after failed total knee arthroplasty with bone loss, further host bone should not be resected; the surfaces must be thoroughly debrided and their irregular surfaces opposed to give the best possible contact. Intramedullary reamings as well as the patella can be used as graft to fill large defects.

Compression Arthrodesis

Compression arthrodesis using an external pin and frame technique was popularized by Key[38] and Charnley.[7,8,39,40] Multiple transfixation pins are now used. Half-pins (6.5 mm Schantz screws) at right angles to the transfixation pins augment stability. Other configurations, such as triangular frames with half-pin fixation, result in a high degree of anteroposterior and mediolateral stability.[9,41] Furthermore, success with Ilizarov external fixation systems has been achieved.

The advantages of external fixation are: (A) stable compression across the fusion site,[9,41] especially if half-pins are added anteriorly; (B) limb stabilization for management of extensive soft tissue infection; (C) technical ease of application and removal; and (D) *dynamization* and loading across the fusion site. The disadvantages include: (A) external pin tract problems; (B) poor patient compliance; (C) frequent need for premature removal and cast immobilization; and (D) nonrigid fixation in cases of severe bone loss.

Success has been achieved with external fixation compression arthrodesis.[7,8,38–41] Fusion rates of 50% occurred in series that included large numbers of failed hinged prostheses. In this situation, external fixation does not always provide the stability necessary for bone healing. Knutson and colleagues reported 91 attempted fusions for failed knee arthroplasty. Fusions after surface replacement arthroplasties were much more successful than those after hinged prostheses. They believed that both intramedullary rod and external fixation methods were successful and that repeated attempts at fusion were worthwhile.[42] External fixator devices must be in place for approximately 3 months; then cast immobilization is necessary until the arthrodesis is healed. One advantage of external fixation for treatment of septic knee replacements is that the device may be removed, leaving no retained hardware in the knee.

The use of compression plate fixation to achieve knee fusion has been frequently described.[35,36] Dual plate fixation has been recommended to achieve rigid biplanar fixation, and Nichols achieved solid fusion of 11 knees after failed TKA at an average of 5.6 months.[42] A more extensive dissection is required, and the technique is demanding, especially in severely osteoporotic patients with significant bone loss where screw purchase may be compromised.

Surgical Technique

External Fixation Compression Arthrodesis Existing midline incisions are used; transverse incisions that divide the quadriceps mechanism may be used in primary cases. Joint surfaces are prepared with a saw. Cutting jigs from a total knee arthroplasty tray are used to make accurate resections and obtain the correct alignment. Three parallel transfixation pins are passed through the distal femur, and 3 more through the upper tibia. If the knee still demonstrates anteroposterior instability after the frame is applied, additional half-pins, 3 above and 3 below the knee, are inserted under radiographic control. The pins are connected to the frame, and compression is applied. Fixation is usually secure enough to allow weightbearing. Currently, the triangular frame configuration is popular, using half-pins 6.5 mm in diameter at an angle 45 degrees to the anteroposterior and mediolateral planes. This configuration yields rigid stability in both planes and is more tolerable.

Intramedullary Rod Arthrodesis Intramedullary rod fixation has been reported to achieve union in a high percentage of patients[43–52] (Figure 27-1). Knutson obtained fusion in 9 out of 10 knees treated with this method.[49] Donley et al. obtained an 85% fusion rate in 20 knees using intramedullary rod fixation and arthrodesis for the treatment of giant cell tumor, nonunion of a distal femur or proximal tibia fracture, aseptic loosening of a total knee replacement, and septic total knee replacement.[43] In

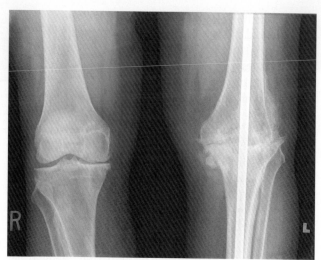

FIGURE 27-1. A 70-year-old man with successful arthrodesis following failed 2-stage reimplantation.

addition, Harris,[47] Mazet,[50] and Griend[46] have reported successful results using this technique. Wilde, however, successfully fused only 6 of 9 knees using an intramedullary rod technique.[52]

Advantages of the intramedullary rod technique include: (A) immediate weightbearing and easier rehabilitation; (B) the elimination of problems associated with external transfixation pins and frames; (C) high fusion rate; (D) the potential for dynamization and load sharing; and (E) increased stability in bone weakened by atrophy or osteopenia in which screws or pins may pull out. The disadvantages include: (A) the risk of proximal rod migration requiring removal; (B) difficulty achieving accurate alignment; (C) intramedullary dissemination of infection; (D) risk of fat embolism; and (E) potential incompatibility with ipsilateral total hip arthroplasty.

After failure of a hinged arthroplasty, the femur and tibia may resemble hollow cones with little or no remaining cancellous bone. In this setting, external fixation devices cannot provide the stability required for arthrodesis (Figure 27-2). Cortical bone is often irregular, partially devascularized, or impregnated with metallic debris. Kaufer et al.[48] recommended an initial period of prolonged immobilization. If this results in a stable, painless, fibrous ankylosis, then no further treatment is indicated.[53] After removal of the prosthetic components, a period of up to 1 year is allowed to pass before performing formal arthrodesis by intramedullary rod fixation.

Intramedullary arthrodesis has gained widespread favor for the salvage of severely infected knee replacements. Most authors recommend performing the procedure in 2 stages, although Puranen has reported single-stage arthrodesis in a few patients who were infected with organisms exquisitely sensitive to antibi-

otics.[51] However, the best results occurred with a staged arthrodesis after administration of 4 to 6 weeks of intravenous antibiotic therapy between prosthetic removal and arthrodesis.[51] Kaufer recommended a curved nonmodular Kuntscher rod that was cut down to an appropriate length during the procedure.[43,47] In severe infections in which a 2-stage reimplantation of a new total knee replacement is less likely to succeed, e.g., *Clostridium perfringens*[32] and *Candida albicans*,[54] successful arthrodesis has been achieved. New, safer, fungal-specific antimicrobial drugs may make salvage of the latter infection possible in the future. In our series, we reported the results of intramedullary arthrodesis of the knee after failed septic TKA.[55] Union occurred in 16 out of 17 patients (94%) at an average of 16 weeks.

Stiehl has reported 8 cases of knee arthrodesis using combined intramedullary rodding and plate fixation.[37] By adding a compression plate, intramedullary nail arthrodesis can be extended to situations in which bone loss requires a segmental allograft.

Nonmodular Intramedullary Rod Our technique of intramedullary arthrodesis of the knee has been previously described.[56] The original longitudinal incision is

FIGURE 27-2. Extensive bone loss precludes the use of extramedullary fixation. An intramedullary rod approximates remaining cortical bone, which is supplemented with autologous bone graft, and if necessary, morsellized allograft.

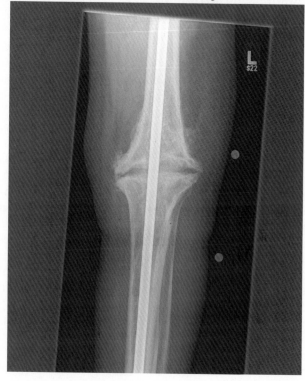

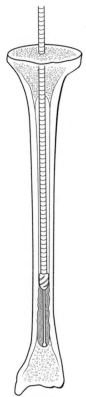

FIGURE 27-3. An intramedullary ball-tipped guidewire is introduced into the tibial shaft to the plafond of the ankle. The canal is sequentially reamed until the cortex is engaged at the tibial isthmus. This canal width determines the intramedullary rod diameter. The tibial length is measured using the guide rod as a reference.

the guidewire, and dissection is carried down through the gluteal musculature to the piriformis recess. The recess is reamed progressively to a size 1 mm larger than the tibial and femoral reamer size (Figure 27-6). After reaming, an arthrodesis nail of the appropriate length is inserted (Figure 27-7). Compression is applied to the arthrodesis site by applying a retrograde force to the tibia by striking the heel (Figure 27-8). The patella may be used to augment the fusion by using two 6.5 mm cancellous screws for fixation at the level of the resection.

In the treatment of traumatic femoral shaft fractures, an intramedullary nail is inserted with its curve following the anterolateral bow of the femur. However, in intramedullary knee arthrodesis, if the rod follows the anterolateral bow of the femur, it creates varus alignment with slight hyperextension. For this reason, the rod is inserted with the curve positioned anteromedially down the femoral shaft. The rod then comes through the tibia in valgus and slight flexion at the knee, which is a pre-

FIGURE 27-4. The ball-tipped guidewire is removed from the tibial canal and inserted into the femoral shaft until it contacts the piriformis recess. The femoral canal is reamed until it matches the size of the tibial reamer. The femoral length is measured using the guide rod at the piriformis fossa as a reference.

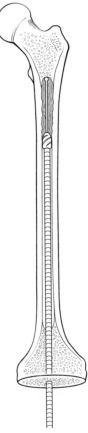

used whenever possible. The knee joint is exposed in a manner similar to that used in revision arthroplasty, and all scar tissue is resected. Cancellous bone is completely exposed on the distal femur and proximal tibia. An intramedullary ball-tip guidewire is introduced into the tibial shaft to the plafond of the ankle (Figure 27-3). The canal is sequentially reamed until the cortex is engaged at the tibial isthmus. This canal width determines the intramedullary rod diameter. The tibial length is measured using the guide rod as a reference.

The ball-tip guidewire is removed from the tibial canal and inserted into the femoral shaft until it contacts the piriformis recess (Figure 27-4). The femoral canal is reamed until it matches the size of the tibial reamer. The femoral length is measured using the guide rod at the piriformis fossa as a reference. Subtracting 1 cm from the combined length of the femur and tibial measurements determines the appropriate rod length. The guidewire is tapped proximally through the piriformis recess with a mallet (Figure 27-5). The guidewire is advanced until it can be easily palpated under the skin of the thigh, with the leg in an adducted position. An incision is made over

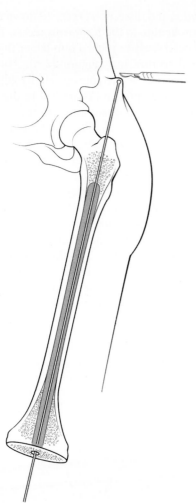

Wichita nail (Stryker, Allendale, NJ), which is comprised of independent femoral and tibial rods coupled at the knee joint (Figure 27-9A, B). Advantages of this technique include: (A) independent sizing of the femoral and tibial diaphysis; (B) the elimination of proximal or distal rod migration; (C) the elimination of a surgical incision about the hip; and (D) the ability to accommodate a future ipsilateral total hip arthroplasty.

The intramedullary canal is sequentially reamed until the cortex is engaged at the tibial and femoral isthmus. This canal width of the tibia and femur determines the size of the tibial and femoral portions of the nail. The bony surfaces of the tibia and femur are prepared to maximize bony contact. The tibial and femoral lengths are measured using fluoroscopy. The appropriately sized tibial and femoral components are selected. As the components are of a fixed length, any shortening of the components is accomplished with a Midas Rex diamond-tipped cutting wheel. After preparing the femoral and tibial metaphyses to accept the articulated

FIGURE 27-6. The recess is reamed progressively to a size 1 mm larger than the tibial and femoral reamer size.

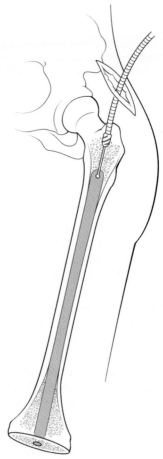

FIGURE 27-5. The guidewire is tapped proximally through the piriformis recess with a mallet. The guidewire is advanced until it can be easily palpated under the skin of the thigh, with the leg in an adducted position. An incision is made over the guidewire, and dissection is carried down through the gluteal musculature to the piriformis recess.

ferred position of arthrodesis. An axial load is placed on the proximal tibia against the distal end of the femur during rod insertion. Sometimes the rod forces the anterior tibial flare forward, making closure of the arthrotomy difficult. If this occurs, the surgeon may modify the anterior flare with a reciprocating saw. Resected bone and intramedullary reamings should be used as autograft, although some authors consider this unnecessary.[43] Interlocking screws or wiring of the proximal portion of the rod has been recommended, to prevent proximal migration.[43,47]

Modular Intramedullary Nail Alternatively, intramedullary rodding may be accomplished using the Neff femorotibial nail (Zimmer, Inc., Warsaw, IN) or the

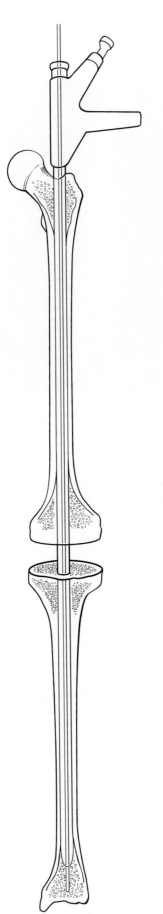

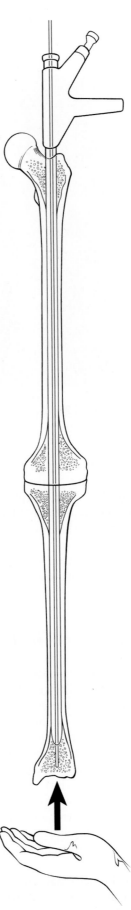

FIGURE 27-7. After reaming, an arthrodesis nail of the appropriate length is inserted.

FIGURE 27-8. Compression is applied to the arthrodesis site by applying a retrograde force to the tibia by striking the heel.

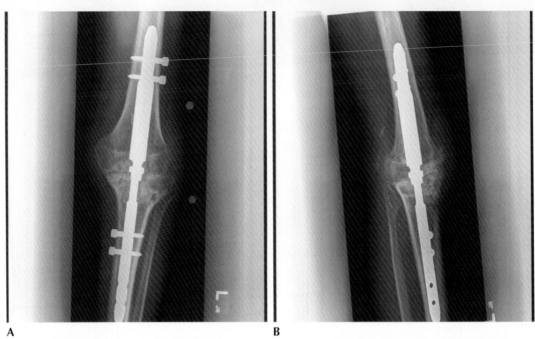

A   **B**

FIGURE 27-9. (A and B) Successful intramedullary arthrodesis using the modular Wichita nail.

portion of the nail, the actual components are inserted into the tibia and femur, respectively. The male and female portions of the nail are coupled. Several blows to the heel secure compression of the Morse taper, which is then reinforced with 2 set screws. Autologous bone from the intramedullary reamings is then packed about the fusion site. The patella may be used as an additional source of autologous graft and is secured using two 6.5 mm cancellous screws.

COMPLICATIONS OF ARTHRODESIS

In our report of 17 intramedullary knee arthrodeses for the treatment of failed septic TKA, complications occurred in 10 patients, including recurrent infection, nonunion with subsequent nail breakage, proximal migration of the nail, and perforation of the ankle joint.[55] Regardless of the technique, union may not occur. If the resulting pseudarthrosis is painful, the arthrodesis should be revised. Failed intramedullary fusion with pseudarthrosis may eventually cause breakage of the rod. Fatigue fracture of the rod occurs at or near the pseudarthrosis site. Arthrodesis may be revised using a larger intramedullary nail supplemented by autologous bone grafting.

A successful arthrodesis may remain actively infected, particularly if foreign material or necrotic tissue remains. With external fixation, pin tract infections may require premature removal of the apparatus and can seed the intramedullary canal if followed by intramedullary rod fixation.

Hip pain can be related to proximal migration of an intramedullary nail, especially if no interlocking screws are used. Femoral or tibial fractures can occur after successful arthrodesis secondary to increased forces generated from a large single bone moment arm. Back pain has been reported, and patient satisfaction is modest, even with the best arthrodesis. Shortening of the lower extremity is common with an average of 3 cm and needs to be discussed with the patient thoroughly preoperatively. A stiff limb, although painless and functional, can be socially unacceptable. Furthermore, a patient considering knee arthrodesis may benefit from a trial in a cylinder cast to understand the permanent disadvantages of a stiff limb.

Conversion of a solid knee arthrodesis to TKA has been reported.[11] This procedure is relatively contraindicated for the following reasons: (A) collateral ligament integrity is compromised; (B) long-standing fusion may result in permanent contracture and scarring of surrounding musculature, limiting knee flexion after conversion; (C) muscle atrophy may not be irreversible and leaves a residual extension lag; (D) the new arthroplasty is at greater risk of infection or mechanical problems than are routine knee replacements; and (E) if subsequent septic or aseptic failure occurs, there is probably a decreased chance of successful fusion.

RESECTION ARTHROPLASTY

Resection arthroplasty is accomplished by excising the opposing articular surfaces of the distal femur and proximal tibia (Figure 27-10). Complete removal of scar tissue, synovium, and all foreign material, including metallic hardware, knee replacement components, and acrylic cement is mandatory.[53,57] This option is generally reserved for medically fragile patients who cannot tolerate a 2-stage reimplantation protocol. It may also serve as an intermediate step for the patient who has reservations about arthrodesis. Fallahee et al. reported 28 knees that underwent resection arthroplasty for infected total knee arthroplasty.[53] Six patients with prior monarticular osteoarthritis found the resection arthroplasty unacceptable and underwent successful arthrodesis. In 3 patients, spontaneous bony fusion developed after the resection, with the knee in satisfactory alignment. Patients with more severe disability before the original knee arthroplasty were more likely to be satisfied with the functional results of the resection arthroplasty. Conversely, patients with less disability originally were more likely to find the resection arthroplasty unacceptable. Fifteen patients walked independently. Five of those patients were able to stand and walk without external limb support. The other 10 patients used either a knee-ankle-foot orthosis or a universal knee splint. All 15 patients, however, required either a cane or walker and remained either moderately or severely restricted in their overall walking capacity.

Definitive resection arthroplasty is useful for the severely disabled sedentary patient. The procedure is least suitable for patients with relatively minor disability before their original total joint replacement. In the latter group, arthrodesis or reimplantation of a total knee replacement is recommended, if possible, depending on the sensitivity of the organism and adequacy of the antibiotic treatment. The advantage of the resection arthroplasty is that some motion is preserved for sitting and transferring into and out of automobiles. The disadvantages are persistent pain and instability with walking.

A modified resection arthroplasty has been presented for problem cases with sepsis or excessive loss of bone stock, in which exchange arthroplasty or arthrodesis is inadvisable or impossible.[58] The space between the femur and tibia is filled with a bolus of antibiotic-impregnated polymethylmethacrylate after implant removal. The cement spacer improves initial stability and diminishes functional limb length discrepancy. Furthermore, the spacer maintains a potential space for easier reimplantation of a TKA after spacer removal in the future.[59-61]

SUMMARY

Arthrodesis as a salvage procedure remains a durable, time-proven technique for treatment of sepsis, tumor, failed arthroplasty, and the flail limb. It should be performed selectively, especially in light of modern arthroplasty and the increasingly favorable results of 2-stage reimplantation.[62] Arthrodesis of the knee can be performed via various techniques. Each technique has a role in these difficult salvage knee cases.

REFERENCES

1. Windsor RE, Bono JV. Infected total knee replacements. *J Am Acad Orthop Surg.* 1994;2(1):44–53.
2. Broderson MP, Fitzgerald RH Jr, Peterson LFA, Coventry MB, Bryan, RS. Arthrodesis of the knee following failed total knee arthroplasty. *J Bone Joint Surg Am.* 1979;61:181–185.
3. Green DP, Parkes JC II, Stinchfiled, FE. Arthrodesis of the knee. a follow-up study. *J Bone Joint Surg Am.* 1967;49:1065–1078.
4. Hagemann WF, Woods GW, Tullos HS. Arthrodesis in failed total knee replacement. *J Bone Joint Surg Am.* 1978;60:790–794.
5. Stulberg SD. Arthrodesis in failed total knee replacements. *Orthop Clin North Am.* 1982;13(1):213–224.
6. Enneking WF, Shirley PD. Resection-arthrodesis for malignant and potentially malignant lesions about the knee using an intramedullary rod and local bone gra fts. *J Bone Joint Surg Am.* 1977;59:223–236.
7. Charnley J, Baker SL. Compression arthrodesis of the knee. a clinical and historical study. *J Bone Joint Surg Br.* 1952;34:187–199.

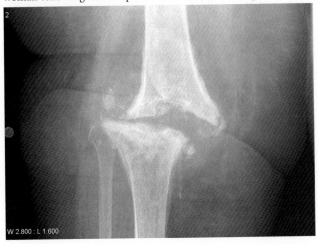

FIGURE 27-10. Resection arthroplasty in an obese elderly woman following failed septic TKA with recurrent sepsis.

8. Charnley J, Lowe HG. A study of the end results of compression arthrodesis of the knee. *J Bone Joint Surg Br.* 1958; 40:633–635.

9. Briggs B, Chao EYS. The mechanical performance of the standard Hoffmann-Vidal external fixation apparatus. *J Bone Joint Surg Am.* 1982;64:566–573.

10. Siller TN, Hadjiipavlou A. Arthrodesis of the knee. In: *The American Academy of Orthopaedic Surgeons Symposium on Reconstructive Surgery of Knee.* St. Louis: C.V. Mosby; 1978:161.

11. Dee R. The case for arthrodesis of the knee. *Orthop Clin North Am.* 1979;10:(1)249–261.

12. Holden DL, Jackson DW. Considerations in total knee arthroplasty following previous knee fusion. *Clin Orthop.* 1988;227:223–228.

13. Montgomery WH, Becker MW, Windsor RE, Insall JN. Primary total knee arthroplasty in stiff and ankylosed knees. *Orthop Trans.* 1991;15:54–55.

14. Krackow KA, Weiss A-PC. Recurvatum deformity complicating performance of TKA. *J Bone Joint Surg Am.* 1990; 72:268–271.

15. Drennan DB, Fahey JJ, Maylahn DJ. Important factors in achieving arthrodesis of the Charcot knee. *J Bone Joint Surg Am.* 1971;53:1180–1193.

16. Soudry M, Binazzi R, Johanson NA, Bullough PG, Insall JN. Total knee arthroplasty in Charcot and Charcot-like joints. *Clin Orthop.* 1986;208:199–204.

17. Edmonson AS, Crenshaw AH. *Campbell's Operative Orthopaedics.* St. Louis: C.V. Mosby; 1980:1108.

18. Higinbotham ML, Coley BL. The treatment of bone tumors by resection and replacement with massive grafts. In: Ebert RH, ed. *Instructional Course Lectures, The American Academy of Orthopaedic Surgeons.* 1950;26–33. Ann Arbor, MI: JW Edwards; 1950.

19. Lexer E. Joint transplantations and arthroplasty. *Surg Gynecol Obstet.* 1925;40:782–809.

20. Marcove RC, Lyden JP, Huvos AG, Bullough PB. Giant-cell tumors treated by cryosurgery. a report of twenty-five cases. *J Bone Joint Surg Am.* 1973;55:1633–1644.

21. Merle D'Aubigne R, Dejouany JP. Diaphyso-epiphyseal resection for bone tumor at the knee. with reports of nine cases. *J Bone Joint Surg Br.* 1958;40:385–395.

22. Ottolenghi CE. Massive osteoarticular bone grafts. transplant of the whole femur. *J Bone Joint Surg Br.* 1966; 48:646–659.

23. Ottolenghi CE. Massive osteo and osteo-articular bone grafts. technique and results of 62 cases. *Clin Orthop.* 1972; 87:156–164.

24. Parrish FF. Treatment of bone tumors by total excision and replacement with massive autologous and homologous grafts. *J Bone Joint Surg Am.* 1966;48:968–990.

25. Parrish FF. Homografts of bone. *Clin Orthop.* 1972; 87:36–42.

26. Tuli SM. Bridging of bone defects by massive bone grafts in tumorous conditions and in osteomyelitis. *Clin Orthop.* 1972;87:60–73.

27. Volkov M. Allotransplantation of joints. *J Bone Joint Surg Br.* 1970;52:49–53.

28. Wilson PD Jr. A clinical study of the biomechanical behavior of massive bone transplants used to reconstruct large bone defects. *Clin Orthop.* 1972;87:81–109.

29. Wilson PD, Lance EM. Surgical reconstruction of the skeleton following segmental resection for bone tumors. *J Bone Joint Surg Am.* 1965;47:1629–1656.

30. Lexer E. Substitution of whole or half joints from freshly amputated extremities by free plastic operation. *Surg Gynecol Obstet.* 1908;6:601–607.

31. Iskander MK, Khan, MA. *Candida albicans* infection of a prosthetic knee replacement [letter]. *J Rheumatol.* 1988; 15(10):1594–1595.

32. Koch AE. *Candida albicans* infection of a prosthetic knee replacement: a report and review of the literature. *J Rheumatol.* 1988;15(2):362–365.

33. Wilde AH, Sweeney RS, Borden LS. Hematogenously acquired infection of a total knee arthroplasty by *Clostridium perfringens. Clin Orthop.* 1988;229:228–231.

34. Cadambi A, Engh GA. Use of a semitendinosus tendon autogenous graft for rupture of the patellar ligament after total knee arthroplasty. *J Bone Joint Surg Am.* 1992;74: 974–979.

35. Lucas DB, Murray WR. Arthrodesis of the knee by double plasting. *J Bone Joint Surg Am.* 1964;43:795.

36. Nichols SJ, Landon GC, Tullos HS. Arthrodesis with dual plates after failed total knee arthroplasty. *J Bone Joint Surg Am.* 1991;73:1020.

37. Stiehl JB, Hanel DP. Knee arthrodesis using combined intramedullary rod and plate fixation. *Clin Orthop.* 1993: 294:238–246.

38. Key JA. Positive pressure in arthrodesis for tuberculosis of the knee joint. *South Med J.* 1932;25:909.

39. Charnley JC. Positive pressure in arthrodesis of the knee joint. *J Bone Joint Surg Br.* 1948;30:478–486.

40. Charnley J. Arthrodesis of the knee. *Clin Orthop.* 1960; 18:37–42.

41. Knutson K, Bodelind B, Lindgren L. Stability of external fixators used for knee arthrodesis after failed knee arthroplasty. *Clin Orthop.* 1984;186:90–95.

42. Knutson K, Hovelius L, Lindstrand A, Lindgren L. Arthrodesis after failed knee arthroplasty a nationwide multicenter investigation of 91 cases. *Clin Orthop.* 1984; 191:202–211.

43. Donley BG, Matthews LS, Kaufer H. Arthrodesis of the knee with an intramedullary nail. *J Bone Joint Surg Am.* 1991; 73:907–913.

44. Fern Ed, Stewart HD, Newton G. Curved Kuntscher nail arthrodesis after failure of knee replacement. *J Bone Joint Surg Br.* 1989;71:588–590.

45. Figgie HE III, Brody GA, Inglis AE, Sculco TP, Goldberg VM, Figgie MP. Knee arthrodesis following total knee arthroplasty in rheumatoid arthritis. *Clin Orthop.* 1987; 224:2237–243.

46. Griend RV. Arthrodesis of the knee with intramedullary fixation. *Clin Orthop.* 1983;181:146–150.

47. Harris CM, Froehlich J. Knee fusion with intramedullary rods for failed total knee arthroplasty. *Clin Orthop.* 1985; 197:209–216.

48. Kaufer H, Irvine G, Matthews LS. Intramedullary arthrodesis of the knee. *Orthop Trans.* 1983;7:547–548.

49. Knutson K, Lindstrand A, Lidgren L. Arthrodesis for failed knee arthroplasty. *J Bone Joint Surg Br.* 1985;67:47–52.

50. Mazet R, Urist MR. Arthrodesis of the knee with intramedullary nail fixation. *Clin Orthop.* 1960;18:43–52.

51. Puranen J, Kortelainen P, Jalovaara P. Arthrodesis of the knee with intramedullary nail fixation. *J Bone Joint Surg Am.* 1990;72:433–442.

52. Wilde AH, Stearns KL. Intramedullary fixation for arthrodesis of the knee after infected total knee arthroplasty. *Clin Orthop.* 1989;248:87–92.

53. Falahee MH, Matthews LS, Kaufer H. Resection arthroplasty as a salvage procedure for a knee with infection after total arthroplasty. *J Bone Joint Surg Am.* 1987;69:1013–1021.

54. Levine M, Rehm SJ, Wilde AH. Infection with *Candida albicans* of a total knee arthroplasty. case report and review of the literature. *Clin Orthop.* 1988;226:235–239.

55. Bono JV, Windsor RE, Sherman P, Laskin R, Sculco T, Adelman R, Fuchs M, Figgie M, Inglis A. Intramedullary arthrodesis following failed TKA. *Orthop Trans.* 1995; 19(2):336.

56. Windsor RE, Bono JV. Arthodesis and resection arthroplasty. In: Fu F, Harner C, Vince K, eds. *Knee Surgery.* Baltimore: Williams & Wilkins; 1994:1587–1595.

57. Lettin AW, Neil MJ, Citron ND, August A. Excision arthroplasty for infected constrained total knee replacements. *J Bone Joint Surg Br.* 1990;72:220–224.

58. Jones WA, Wroblewski BM. Salvage of failed total knee arthroplasty: "beefburger" procedure. *J Bone Joint Surg Br.* 1989;71:856–857.

59. Booth RE Jr, Lotke PA. The results of spacer block technique in revision of infected total knee arthroplasty. *Clin Orthop.* 1989;248:57–60.

60. Cohen JC, Hozack WJ, Cuckler JM, Booth RE. Two-stage reimplantation of septic total knee arthroplasty. *J Arthroplasty.* 1988;3:369–377.

61. Wilde AH, Ruth JT. Two-stage reimplantation in infected total knee arthroplasty. *Clin Orthop.* 1988;236:23–35.

62. Adelman R, Bono JV, Haas S, Windsor RE, Brause B. Two-stage reimplantation for total knee arthroplasty salvage: further follow-up and enlargement of cohort group. Scientific Presentation, 63rd Annual Meeting of The American Academy of Orthopaedic Surgeons, Atlanta, Georgia, February 21–27, 1996.

INDEX